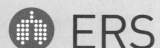

MW01275621

New Developments in Mechanical Ventilation

Published by European Respiratory
Society ©2012
March 2012
Print ISBN: 978-1-84984-021-7
Online ISBN: 978-1-84984-022-4
Print ISSN: 1025-448x
Online ISSN: 2075-6674
Printed by Latimer Trend & Co. Ltd,
Plymouth, UK

Managing Editor: Fiona Marks
European Respiratory Society
442 Glossop Road, Sheffield,
S10 2PX, UK
Tel: 44 114 2672860
E-mail: Monograph@ersj.org.uk

Edited by M. Ferrer and P. Pelosi

Editor in Chief
T. Welte

This book is one in a series of *European Respiratory Monographs*. Each individual issue provides a comprehensive overview of one specific clinical area of respiratory health, communicating information about the most advanced techniques and systems needed to investigate it. It provides factual and useful scientific detail, drawing on specific case studies and looking into the diagnosis and management of individual patients. Previously published titles in this series are listed at the back of this Monograph.

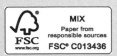

MIX
Paper from
responsible sources
FSC® C013436
FSC
www.fsc.org

Contents

Number 55   March 2012

Guest Editors   v

Preface   vi

Introduction   viii

1. Ventilator-induced lung injury   1
   T. Maron-Gutierrez, P. Pelosi and P.R.M. Rocco

2. Ventilator strategies in severe hypoxaemic respiratory failure   19
   A. Esan, D. Hess, C. Sessler, L. George, C. Oribabor, F. Khusid and S. Raoof

3. Recruitment manoeuvres in patients with acute lung injury   40
   T. Paterson and E. Fan

4. Surfactant therapy in acute lung injury/acute respiratory distress syndrome   54
   J. Kesecioglu and M.M.J. van Eijk

5. NIV in hypoxaemic acute respiratory failure   65
   J-C Lefebvre, S. Dimassi and L. Brochard

6. Biphasic PAP/airway pressure release ventilation in ALI   81
   A. Güldner, N.C. Carvalho P. Pelosi and M. Gama de Abreu

7. Proportional assist ventilation   97
   E. Akoumianaki, E. Kondili and D. Georgopoulos

8. Neurally adjusted ventilatory assist   116
   P. Navalesi, D. Colombo, G. Cammarota and R. Vaschetto

9. Helium as a therapeutic gas: an old idea needing some new thought   124
   J. Carr, B. Jung, G. Chanques and S. Jaber

10. Extracorporeal membrane oxygenation   133
    A. Zanella, V. Scaravilli, G. Grasselli, N. Patroniti, and A. Pesenti

11. Extracorporeal lung support to remove carbon dioxide   142
    P. Terragni, A. Birocco and V.M. Ranieri

12. Prevention of VAP: role of the artificial airway, body position and
    setting the ventilator   153
    G. Li Bassi, M. Ferrer, O.T. Ranzani, J-D. Marti, L. Berra, L. Fernandez
    and A. Torres

13. Predictors of weaning from mechanical ventilation   169
    F. Laghi and D. Morales

14. NIV in withdrawal from mechanical ventilation   191
    M. Ferrer, J. Sellares and A. Torres

15. Tracheostomy in mechanical ventilation   206
    P. Terragni, A. Trompeo, C. Faggiano, and V.M. Ranieri

16. Mechanical ventilation with advanced closed-loop systems   217
    F. Lellouche, A. Bojmehrani and K. Burns

17. Update on sedation and analgesia in mechanical ventilation   229
    T. Strøm and P. Toft

|C|O|P|E| COMMITTEE ON PUBLICATION ETHICS

This journal is a member of and subscribes to
the principles of the Committee on Publication
Ethics.

Guest Editors

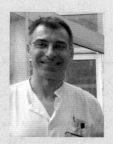

M. Ferrer

M. Ferrer is currently a consultant physician at the Respiratory Intensive and Intermediate Care Unit in the Pneumology Department within the Hospital Clinic of Barcelona (Barcelona, Spain). He gained his degree in medicine from the University of Barcelona in 1985. After this, he specialised in pneumology at the Hospital Clinic of Barcelona from 1987 to 1990, and subsequently obtained a doctorate in medicine in 1993. He attained the position of staff physician within the Pneumology Department in 1992 and is also Clinic Professor in the Department of Medicine at the University of Barcelona. M. Ferrer is a member of the research group Applied Research in Respiratory Diseases of the Institute of Biomedical Investigations August Pi i Sunyer (IDIBAPS), as well as a member of the Network of Biomedical Research in Respiratory Diseases (CIBERES) of the "Carlos III" Health Institute, Spanish Ministry of Science and Technology. He currently participates in several activities related to scientific societies, including the Spanish Society of Pneumology and Thoracic Surgery (SEPAR), and was a member of the committee that developed the Spanish guidelines for Hospital-Acquired Pneumonia published in 2011. As an active European Respiratory Society (ERS) member he is part of the Noninvasive Ventilatory Support Group within the ERS Respiratory Intensive Care Assembly and is part of the long-range planning committee for this Assembly. He is also involved in the Harmonised Education in Respiratory Medicine for European Specialists (HERMES) Critical Care Project and is part of the ERS and American Thoracic Society (ATS) Task Force on the indications of use for noninvasive ventilation in acute respiratory failure.

M. Ferrer's research interests include noninvasive ventilation, weaning from invasive mechanical ventilation, severe community-acquired pneumonia and nosocomial pneumonia in the intensive care unit. He has authored or co-authored some 170 articles, including original investigations, reviews, editorials and book chapters.

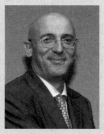

P. Pelosi

P. Pelosi grew up in Milan (Italy) and attended the University of Milan, graduating as *magna cum laude* in medicine and surgery. After graduation, he completed his studies first as a specialist in anaesthesia and intensive care and then as Research Fellow at the University of Milan. He served as Associate Professor in Anaesthesia and Intensive Care Medicine at the University of Insubria (Varese, Italy) from 1999 to 2010. He is currently Chief Professor in Anaesthesia and Intensive Care and Director of the Speciality School in Anaesthesiology at the University of Genoa (Genoa, Italy) and Head of the Intensive Care Unit at the IRCCS Azienda Ospedaliera San Martino Genoa – IST. His professional activities have always been directed both at the clinical and research fields.

P. Pelosi's main research interests are respiratory physiology during anaesthesia and respiratory failure. He has developed numerous collaborations with European and international countries for research in the field of mechanical ventilation. He is actively involved in the Fellow and Resident educational programme at the University of Genoa. He is the current Head of the Respiratory Intensive Care Assembly of the ERS. He is author or co-author of over 170 medical and scientific peer review papers, 60 book chapters, and has lectured in more than 800 national and international meetings on ventilation management during the perioperative period and on the pathophysiology and treatments of acute respiratory failure.

Eur Respir Mon 2012; 55: v.
Printed in UK – all rights reserved
Copyright ERS 2012
European Respiratory Monograph
ISSN: 1025-448x
DOI: 10.1183/1025448x.10000612

Preface

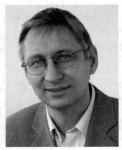

There is no other discipline in medicine that has developed as quickly as intensive care medicine has in recent decades. Substantial progress has mainly been made in the field of mechanical ventilation. Thirty years ago, it was thought that it was not possible to survive for more than one week on a ventilator due to ventilator-associated lung injury (VALI) on the one hand, and ventilator-associated infections on the other. Since then, we have learnt a lot about the pathophysiology of VALI, leading to the concept of ventilation-induced volutrauma (an injury from excess distension) and atelectrauma (local shear injury from tidal opening and closing). Stretch and shear forces induce inflammation and initiate a myriad of signalling cascades, which enhance lung damage and worsen the long-term prognosis of patients.

With the fast technical development of ventilator technology, protective mechanical ventilation that avoids lung distension and tidal opening became possible. In 2000, the NIH ARDS (National Institute of Health Acute Respiratory Distress Syndrome) Network was able to demonstrate for the first time the tremendous effect of such ventilatory modes on patient morbidity and mortality. Since then, mortality in ARDS patients has come down from close to 50% to about 25%, and it is still dropping.

While research focused on the initial ventilation phase for decades, the process of weaning patients from the ventilator eventually began to receive more and more attention. It was recognised that the weaning process is normally longer than the period of acute respiratory failure. A better understanding of the pathophysiology of weaning failure, which no longer focused only on the lung but also took the respiratory muscle pump and pulmonary haemodynamics into account, led to further development of new ventilator modes supporting the patient's own breathing efforts and allowing earlier determination of analgosedation. In a similar manner to protective ventilation in the acute phase of respiratory failure, the improvement and standardisation of the weaning process had an impressive impact on the long-term prognosis of ventilated patients.

Optimisation of both parts of ventilation, the period of acute lung injury and the weaning phase, is still not complete. New ventilatory modes, *i.e.* high-frequency oscillatory ventilation for the acute phase or neurally adjusted ventilatory assistance for the weaning period, have been demonstrated to reduce complications of mechanical ventilation and may therefore improve long-term outcome. Nevertheless, the next step in development has yet to begin. Extracorporeal lung assist (ECLA) systems that remove carbon dioxide and improve oxygenation have become far smaller and offer better handling than 20 years ago. Complications such as massive bleeds or cytokine burst due to activation of the inflammatory cells by the device itself have been

Eur Respir Mon 2012; 55: vi. Printed in UK – all rights reserved. Copyright ERS 2012. European Respiratory Monograph. ISSN: 1025-448x. DOI: 10.1183/1025448x.10000812.

reduced. ECLA systems can now be used for weeks and allow a further reduction in the pressure applied by the ventilator. The amount of inflammation seems to be reduced in comparision with ventilation alone. Close to the time of writing, implementation of awake extracorporeal membrane oxygenation in patients on the lung transplant waiting list, with no analgosedation and intubation for critical hypoxaemia, was reported, and a 30% improvement in survival was shown in comparison with a historical control group.

The future vision of this kind of development is the engineering of a biocompatible membrane for lung assist, which can be used in chronic cases for months and years. This may take time; however, 30 years ago nobody even considered this possibility.

This volume of the *European Respiratory Monograph* provides a summary of the current state-of-the-art in mechanical ventilation, beginning with the actual pathophysiological concepts and ending with developing technologies.

I want to congratulate the Guest Editors of this excellent *Monograph*, which will be of interest to basic scientists and clinicians, and may have an impact on clinical practice in intensive care medicine. I am convinced that this *Monograph* will be useful in daily practice.

T. Welte
Editor in Chief

Introduction

M. Ferrer[+,#,¶] and P. Pelosi[+]

[*]Respiratory Intensive Care Unit, Thorax Institute, Hospital Clínic, [#]Institut d'Investigacions Biomèdiques August Pi i Sunyer (IDIBAPS), [¶]Centro de Investigación Biomédica en Red de Enfermedades Respiratorias (CIBERES), Barcelona, Spain. [+]Dept of Surgical Sciences and Integrated Diagnostics, University of Genoa, Genoa, Italy.

Correspondence: M. Ferrer, Servei de Pneumologia, Hospital Clinic, Villarroel 170, 08036, Barcelona, Spain. Email miferrer@clinic.ub.es

S evere acute respiratory failure is one of the most frequent causes for patient admission to the intensive care unit (ICU). In the most severe conditions, invasive mechanical ventilation is required life support in these patients.

The polio epidemic that occurred in Denmark in 1952 demonstrated how careful airway management and the application of positive-pressure ventilation could dramatically reduce mortality in patients presenting with paralysis of the respiratory muscles. The focus on airway care and ventilator management encouraged the way forward for critical care facilities. Technological advances in the 1960s led to the development of sophisticated, physiological monitoring equipment. Later, further developments were introduced that included: improved understanding of mechanical ventilation pathophysiology in patients with severe-acute respiratory failure; the production of ventilators with improved technology, new ventilator modes that were aimed at improving patient outcomes; and since the early 1990s, the introduction of noninvasive ventilation (NIV) as a less invasive mode of ventilatory support in patients with intermediate severity of respiratory failure.

Mechanical ventilation is currently the life support technique most frequently used in critically ill patients who are admitted to the ICU, and an extensive body of literature has been published within this topic. The appropriate knowledge on mechanical indications and settings is mandatory in order to develop and implement protective ventilation strategies and avoid possible iatrogenic effects.

This *European Respiratory Monograph* is intended as an update on various aspects and novel developments that have occurred in recent years within the field of mechanical ventilation. Topics that have been included are conventional and innovative ventilator modalities, adjuvant therapies that include sedation and analgesia, modes of extracorporeal support, weaning from mechanical ventilation, ventilator strategies in different clinical conditions, complications of mechanical ventilation and prevention, and NIV.

As Guest Editors we invited international experts to write up-to-date reviews based on their expertise and long-time experiences within this field. We would like to take this opportunity to warmly thank all the contributors for their enthusiasm and hard work. We are also indebted to Professor Tobias Welte, Editor in Chief of the *European Respiratory Monograph*, as well as all those at the European Respiratory Society Publications Office for their excellent technical help with producing this fifty-fifth issue of the *European Respiratory Monograph*.

Eur Respir Mon 2012; 55: viii. Printed in UK – all rights reserved. Copyright ERS 2012. European Respiratory Monograph. ISSN: 1025-448x. DOI: 10.1183/1025448x.10000712

Chapter 1

Ventilator-induced lung injury

T. Maron-Gutierrez*, P. Pelosi# and P.R.M. Rocco*

Summary

Mechanical ventilation has become essential for the support of critically ill patients; however, it can cause ventilator-induced lung injury (VILI) or aggravate ventilator-associated lung injury (VALI), contributing to the high mortality rates observed in acute respiratory distress syndrome. This chapter discusses the mechanisms leading to VILI/VALI, the diagnostic procedures of early detection and how to prevent it.

The clinical relevance of low lung volume injury and the application of high positive end-expiratory pressure levels remain debatable. Furthermore, researchers were not successful in transferring the measurement of inflammatory mediators during VILI/VALI from bench to bedside. Therefore, the following issues still require elucidation: 1) the best ventilator strategy to be adopted; 2) which ventilator parameters should be managed; 3) how to monitor VILI/VALI (arterial blood gases, lung mechanics, proinflammatory mediators); 4) the role of imaging (computed tomography scan, lung ultrasound and positron emission tomography; and 5) how to prevent VILI/VALI (new ventilatory and pharmacological strategies).

Keywords: Assisted mechanical ventilation, computed tomography scan, lung ultrasound, positive end-expiratory pressure, tidal volume, transpulmonary pressure

*Laboratory of Pulmonary Investigation, Carlos Chagas Filho Institute of Biophysics, Federal University of Rio de Janeiro, Rio de Janeiro, Brazil.
#Dept of Surgical Sciences and Integrated Diagnostics, University of Genoa, Genoa, Italy.

Correspondence: P.R.M. Rocco, Laboratory of Pulmonary Investigation, Carlos Chagas Filho Biophysics Institute, Federal University of Rio de Janeiro, Centro de Ciências da Saúde, Avenida Carlos Chagas Filho, s/n, Bloco G-014, Ilha do Fundão, 21941-902, Rio de Janeiro, Brazil.
Email prmrocco@biof.ufrj.br

Eur Respir Mon 2012; 55: 1–18.
Printed in UK – all rights reserved
Copyright ERS 2012
European Respiratory Monograph
ISSN: 1025-448x
DOI: 10.1183/1025448x.10001311

Over the past 50 years, mechanical ventilation has become essential for the support of critically ill patients [1]. Nevertheless, mechanical ventilation can also cause ventilator-induced lung injury (VILI) or aggravate ventilator-associated lung injury (VALI), contributing to the high mortality rates observed in acute respiratory distress syndrome (ARDS) [2].

The histological changes observed in VILI are nonspecific [3–5]; similar to acute lung injury (ALI)/ ARDS [6]. However, there is a direct relationship between histological findings, mechanical ventilation duration and the intensity of the injury stimulus. Mechanical ventilation with high transpulmonary pressure (PL) can lead to alveolar injury characterised by the presence of hyaline membrane, alveolar haemorrhage and neutrophilic infiltration [7]. Endothelial and epithelial lesions can be visualised by electron microscopy a few minutes after the start of mechanical ventilation with high airway pressures [3, 4], including disruption of type II pneumocytes [8], endothelial cell/basement membrane

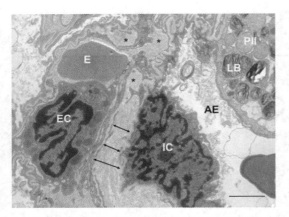

Figure 1. Electron microscopy of the alveolar–capillary membrane in acute lung injury rats ventilated with high tidal volume (12 mL·kg^{-1}) for 1 hour. Interstitial (indicated with arrows) and alveolar oedema (AE) and collagen fibres (indicated with asterisks) can be observed. PII: type II pneumocytes; LB: lamellar body; IC: interstitial cell; E: erythrocyte; EC: endothelial cell. Scale bar: 2 μm. Provided courtesy of V. Capelozzi (Dept of Pathology, School of Medicine, University São Paulo, São Paulo, Brazil).

detachment, endothelial disruption and alveolar oedema (fig. 1) [9]. With the progression of the injury, proliferation of fibroblasts and type II pneumocytes can be observed, similar to those seen in the late stage of ARDS [10].

In this chapter we will discuss: 1) the mechanisms leading to VILI and VALI (table 1 and fig. 2); 2) the diagnostic procedures of early detection of VILI and VALI; and finally 3) how to prevent VILI and VALI (table 1).

Pulmonary oedema and effects of surfactant inactivation

The lungs are intrinsically protected against the accumulation of fluid in the extravascular space and the development of oedema. Protection is conferred by three components: 1) capillary filtration pressure, 2) ability of the interstitial space to absorb and buffer extravascular fluids, and 3) ability of the pulmonary lymphatic system to transport fluid out of the lung.

WEBB and TIERNEY [7] conducted the first comprehensive study showing that mechanical ventilation may induce pulmonary oedema in intact animals. Oedema occurs with high peak inspiratory pressure (PIP) of 30 and 45 cmH$_2$O, even though it develops faster with 45 cmH$_2$O PIP. However, at PIP $\leqslant$30 cmH$_2$O [11], this deleterious effect acts synergistically with pre-existing injury [12].

Initially, it was believed that mechanical ventilation-induced pulmonary oedema resulted from an increase in vascular transmural pressure at both extra-alveolar and alveolar levels [7, 13, 14]. Nevertheless, microscopic analysis of pulmonary oedema fluid showed eosinophilic infiltration and large amounts of protein, suggesting a change in the permeability of the alveolar–capillary barrier. In this context, major alterations in lung epithelial and endothelial permeability have been reported in isolated lungs, confirmed by open-chest and intact animals subjected to high airway pressures [1]. Moreover, regional differences in pulmonary perfusion and atelectasis may result in increased filtration forces in specific alveolar–capillary units, leading to oedema formation. VILI also compromises the ability of the lung to reabsorb fluid [13]. Inhibition of active transport of Na$^+$ and reduced Na, K-ATPase activity in type II pneumocytes have been demonstrated in rats subjected to mechanical ventilation with hyperinflation [15].

Among its effects on fluid filtration, surfactant inactivation and elevated alveolar surface tension may increase alveolar epithelial permeability. In the pathophysiology of VILI, surfactant deficiency exacerbates ventilator-induced lesions; however, mechanical ventilation itself can affect the surfactant system, favouring the development of lung injury [16]. Surfactant is present in alveolar spaces as small (functionally inferior) or large (functionally superior) aggregates. Changes in the relative proportions of these structural forms were reported in animal models of ALI [17], in patients with ARDS [18] and during mechanical ventilation with high volumes [16]. Deeper changes in the surfactant system are observed in the injured lung subjected to mechanical ventilation with high tidal volume (VT) [19]. The conversion of surfactant aggregates induced by high VT is related to two mechanisms: 1) changes in surface area, and 2) increased activity of proteases in the air spaces [12]. Surfactant deficiency increases surface tension and can contribute to the genesis of VILI in several ways: 1) the alveoli and the airways become more prone to collapse, 2) the unequal expansion of lung units increases stress through the regional mechanism of interdependence, and 3) increased vascular filtration pressure can cause oedema formation.

Table 1. Factors inducing or preventing ventilator-associated/ventilator-induced lung injury

Induction	Prevention
High Vt	Low Vt (6 mL·kg^{-1} PBW)
High Pplat of the respiratory system (high stress)	Pplat of the respiratory system <28–30 cmH$_2$O
High Pplat of the lung, *i.e.* PL (high stress)	Pplat of the PL <26–24 cmH$_2$O
High Vt/end expiratory lung volume ratio (high strain)	Prone position, strain <2.0
	Upright position, according to haemodynamics
Dishomogeneous distribution of PL and alveolar ventilation	Prone position when Pa,O$_2$/Fi,O$_2$ <150 mmHg and PEEP >10 cmH$_2$O
	Assisted ventilation when Pa,O$_2$/Fi,O$_2$ >150 mmHg and PEEP ≤10 cmH$_2$O
PEEP (low or high)	PEEP set according to physiological response of each patient based on: best oxygenation, best respiratory system or lung compliance, best physiological dead space and lower inflection point of the pressure–volume curve of the respiratory system or lung
	PEEP set according to lung morphology based on: CT scan at two pressures, lung ultrasound and electric impedance tomography
High respiratory rate	Lowest respiratory rate to achieve: physiological pHa (7.25–7.30)
	Lowest auto-PEEP or no expiratory flow at end-expiration
High inspiratory flow	Lowest inspiratory flow according to respiratory rate, inspiratory to expiratory time and Vt
Fi,O$_2$	Lowest inspiratory oxygen fraction to achieve a peripheral oxygen saturation between 88–92%
	Prone position
	Deep sedation and paralysis within the first 48 hours
Patient ventilator asynchronies and fluid overload	Optimisation of fluids according to central venous and pulmonary pressures, intrathoracic blood volumes, cardiac output, oxygen delivery, central venous or mixed oxygen saturation
	Vasoactive drugs
Primary or secondary infection	Correct diagnosis and antimicrobial agents
Early and late fibrogenic remodelling process	Low dose of corticosteroids

Vt: tidal volume; PBW: predicted body weight; Pplat; plateau pressure; PL: transpulmonary pressure; Pa,O$_2$: arterial oxygen tension; Fi,O$_2$: inspiratory oxygen fraction; PEEP: positive end-expiratory pressure; CT: computed tomography; pHa: arterial hydrogen ion concentration.

Main determinants of VILI/VALI

Barotrauma and volutrauma

High-pressure mechanical ventilation induces rupture of air spaces and hence air leakage. This phenomenon produces many clinical manifestations, recognised as gross barotrauma, such as pneumomediastinum, subcutaneous emphysema, pneumothorax, pneumopericardium, pneumoperitoneum and interstitial emphysema [20]. Therefore, for many years VILI has been synonymous with gross barotrauma. Although the macroscopic consequences of these events are fairly evident, morphological and subtler physiological changes were described much later. It was not until 1974 that WEBB and TIERNEY [7] showed ultrastructural lesions associated with mechanical ventilation even in the absence of air leakage. Subsequent studies confirmed the diffuse alveolar damage induced by high PIP.

However, it is noteworthy that the absolute pressure in the airways is not harmful in itself, as confirmed by the observation that trumpet players commonly achieve airway pressures of 150 cmH$_2$O without developing lung injury [21]. Additionally, experimental evidence indicates that the degree of lung inflation seems to be more important in the genesis of lung injury than the level of pressure. The

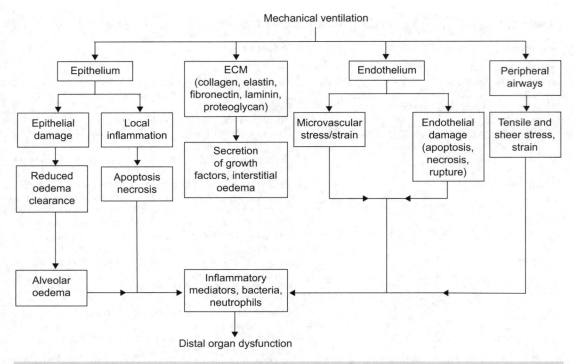

Figure 2. Potential mechanisms of ventilator-induced lung injury (VILI)/ventilator associated lung injury (VALI). Critical physical forces contributing to VILI/VALI have been defined as "stress" (force per unit of area) or "strain" (force along longitudinal axis), and their primary possible targets include: epithelial and endothelial cells, the extracellular matrix (ECM) and peripheral airways. These forces result in increased permeability, oedema, rupture of the alveolar–capillary barrier, and increased concentrations of proinflammatory mediators, bacteria and neutrophils, which may lead to distal organ dysfunction.

relative contribution of PIP and V_T to lung injury was evaluated primarily in healthy rats ventilated with restriction of thoracoabdominal motion. A high PIP (45 cmH$_2$O) without high V_T did not produce severe lung injury. However, animals ventilated without restriction of thoracoabdominal motion (in which a high V_T was achieved) developed severe lung injury, with either positive or negative pressures. These findings were further confirmed [22, 23], resulting in the coinage of the word volutrauma, damage caused by overdistension, sometimes called high volume or high end-inspiratory volume injury. These experimental data suggested that it is not airway pressure *per se*, but rather P_L that determines VILI and VALI. This was a major step forward in the understanding of the mechanisms of VILI and VALI, and translated into a shift from the concept of gross barotrauma to barotrauma and volutrauma. Patients with ARDS are more susceptible to alveolar overdistension, especially when submitted to high V_T with conventional MV (10–15 mL·kg^{-1}), since the number of alveolar units available to be ventilated is reduced due to fluid accumulation, consolidation and atelectasis [24]. Low V_T ventilation reduced the mortality rate in patients with ARDS [25]; even though a V_T of 6 mL·kg^{-1} is not necessarily safe, it implies a better prognosis than a V_T of 12 mL·kg^{-1}.

Atelectrauma and biotrauma

Mechanical ventilation with low volumes at end-expiration can also induce lung damage. This injury is related to the opening and closing cycles of distal airways, ducts and/or alveolar units, hence the term atelectrauma. The recruitment and repeated collapse of alveolar units can increase local shear stress with every respiratory cycle. The opening of airways is associated with two types of stress, tensile stress, an action perpendicular to the surface, and shear stress, parallel to the surface of action [9].

The classic concept of barotrauma implies that injury occurs only when stress/strain is high enough to rupture the lung; however, since the early 1990s, several studies have suggested that unphysiological stress/strain can promote the release of proinflammatory cytokines and neutrophilic recruitment, leading to lung inflammation even in the absence of structural damage [26]. The term biotrauma describes a process of injury in which biophysical forces can alter the normal physiology of lung cells, increasing the levels of inflammatory mediators and promoting changes in the process of repair/remodelling of lung tissue. Clinical and experimental studies have shown that injurious ventilation strategies can initiate or perpetuate a local and systemic inflammatory response, which, in turn, can contribute significantly to multiple organ dysfunction syndrome (MODS) (fig. 2) [26–28]. TREMBLAY et al. [28] reported increased levels of tumour necrosis factor (TNF)-α and interleukin (IL)-6 after 2 hours of mechanical ventilation with elevated V_T [28]. RICARD et al. [29] did not detect higher levels of TNF-α and macrophage inflammatory protein (MIP)-2 in bronchoalveolar lavage fluid of healthy lungs ventilated with high V_T (42 mL·kg^{-1}) for 2 hours; however, those authors noticed a significant increase in the level of IL-1β. Additionally, mechanical ventilation with high V_T and positive end-expiratory pressure (PEEP) of zero led to lung injury and release of inflammatory mediators [30]. Accordingly, several studies have shown that protective ventilation reduces the levels of IL-1, IL-6, IL-10 and TNF-α, underscoring the influence of mechanical ventilation on the release of pro- and anti-inflammatory mediators in the lung, as well as the role of mechanical ventilation in the genesis and perpetuation of local and systemic inflammatory response. In this context, the mechanisms involved in the peripheral organ dysfunction observed in VILI appear to be derived from direct mechanical pulmonary damage, which enhances the inflammatory response and subsequent inflammatory cascades in lung tissue, including translocation of mediators, endotoxins and bacteria from the lung to the systemic circulation [31].

Other potential mechanisms of VILI/VALI

Respiratory frequency

VILI/VALI can also be induced by cyclic mechanical stress determined by high frequency [32, 33]. High frequency ventilation can cause microfractures in lung parenchyma, which can increase in number and become wider with each cycle until the fracture line is large enough to cause tissue failure [32]. In normal volumes, the alveolar–capillary membrane supports a certain amount of stress because epithelial and endothelial cells adapt to a certain degree of deformation without suffering injury. However, in the presence of previous lung injury and injurious ventilatory strategies, the reduction in respiratory frequency provides additional protection against VILI [32, 33]. The question is if the increase in P_L that determines VILI/VALI depends on the respiratory rate or the distribution of P_L during the different respiratory cycles. SPIETH and co-workers [34, 35] have recently shown that variability of pressures and V_T, i.e. applying different P_L (higher and lower than usual), may be associated with less VILI and VALI compared with monotonous mechanical ventilation, both during controlled and assisted ventilation. This suggests that the generally accepted concept of VILI/VALI due to P_L should also be revisited. It seems that it is not P_L per se, but rather the modality of delivery that causes VILI/VALI.

Reversed inspiratory time and expiratory time ratio

Mechanical ventilation with reverse inspiratory:expiratory time ratio (I:E) has been used in patients with ARDS to reduce PEEP and/or PIP and improve arterial oxygenation [36]. This strategy also targeted a more homogeneous distribution of air, with less risk of alveolar overdistension. However, experimental studies have shown that increased inspiratory time can exacerbate lung injury, worsening ventilation–perfusion, reducing lung compliance and increasing pulmonary oedema [37].

Inspiratory flow

High inspiratory flows increase tensile stress, resulting in transmission of kinetic energy to underlying structures. It also increases shear stress, with parenchymal distortion and deformation of the epithelial surface [38]. During mechanical ventilation with high PIP, high pulmonary airflow triggers microvascular injury [39], whereas reduced inspiratory flow leads to protection and a lower degree of shunt, histological injury, pulmonary neutrophil infiltration and alveolar oedema [40].

Cellular response to mechanical forces

During mechanical ventilation, lungs (epithelium, endothelium, extracellular matrix and peripheral airways) are subjected to abnormal mechanical forces, which can trigger deleterious effects on their cellular components, altering structure, function and metabolism (fig. 2) [41]. In homogeneous lungs, P_L is transmitted equally to all lung regions. However, P_L is not evenly distributed in heterogeneous lungs, as observed in patients with ALI/ARDS, leading to excessive local stress [9].

Mechanotransduction is the conversion of a mechanical stimulus, such as cell deformation, into intracellular biochemical and molecular alterations. The means by which mechanical stimuli are converted into chemical signals is not fully understood. Mechanisms such as stretch-activated ion channels, extracellular pathways between the matrix, integrin and cytoskeleton, and changes in intercellular junctions appear to be involved in mechanotransduction [9, 42]. Intracellular signalling includes the generation of second messengers, activation of specific protein kinases, phosphorylation and activation of signalling molecules, amplification of signals by enzymatic cascades and modulation of gene expression [9]. Accordingly, several studies have shown that lung tissue deformation activates nuclear factor (NF)-κB signalling, regulating the production of IL-6, IL-8, IL-1β and TNF-α [43].

Different mechanical stimuli can also affect the gene expression of extracellular matrix components [44]. In this context, GARCIA et al. [44] demonstrated that healthy lung parenchyma strips subjected to sinusoidal oscillations with high amplitude (strain) and constant force (stress) increase type III procollagen mRNA expression.

Translocation of bacteria and/or bacterial products from the lung

Mechanical ventilation can also promote harmful translocation of bacteria and bacterial products from the lung into the bloodstream, contributing to the development of MODS [45]. Lung distention, associated with the cyclic opening and collapse of alveolar units, facilitates the translocation of bacteria that are intratracheally instilled into the bloodstream as a result of injury to the alveolar–capillary barrier [45]. This effect can be reduced by PEEP. Ventilation strategies, such as high V_T and zero PEEP can also promote the translocation of endotoxins from the lung into the systemic circulation (fig. 2) [46].

Apoptosis and necrosis

Apoptosis, or programmed cell death, is a common component of the development and health of multicellular organisms. It differs from necrosis, in which uncontrolled cell death leads to cell lysis and more pronounced inflammatory responses [9]. The balance between apoptosis and necrosis may be relevant not only for the repair of the alveolar–capillary membrane, but also for the reabsorption of fibrin exudates, resulting in recovery of normal architecture and lung function.

Lung apoptosis has been described in experimental models of ALI with protective mechanical ventilation, whereas necrosis, in addition to apoptosis in distal organs, kidneys, intestines and liver, predominated after injurious ventilatory strategies [47, 48]. Different approaches are needed to explain the apoptosis observed in distal organs. One of the suggested mechanisms is an increase in plasma levels of inflammatory mediators and proaptotic soluble factors, such as Fas ligand [25, 27, 47].

Protection against VILI/VALI

As discussed previously, VILI/VALI is the result of a succession of events, beginning with mechanical alteration of the lung parenchyma due to disproportionate stress and strain. The resulting structural tension can initiate an inflammatory cascade; however, the tension can reach the limits of stress, with structural destruction. VILI/VALI may be attenuated and even prevented by interfering with the sequence of inflammatory response [41, 49].

Mechanical approach to prevent VILI/VALI

As nonphysiological stress and strain appear to be the first trigger of VILI/VALI, the possibilities available for limiting and preventing this excessive stress and strain are reviewed (table 1).

Low tidal volume

Since the late 1990s, numerous studies have been performed in order to evaluate the clinical outcome with low and high V_T ventilation [25, 50–53]. Some of these studies were not able to show any differences between V_T of 7 and 10–10.5 mL·kg^{-1} ideal body weight [50, 52, 53]. The key variable in determining pulmonary overdistension is the P_L [41, 54]. Therefore, it is evident that measuring V_T can lead to controversy, since a given V_T can yield different airway pressure (P_{aw}) depending on the respiratory system elastance (E_{rs}) E_{rs} ($P_{aw} = E_{rs}/V_T$). In turn, a given P_{aw} produces different P_L according to the ratio of lung elastance (E_L) to E_{rs} ($P_L = P_{aw}E_L/E_{rs}$), indicating that the relationship between V_T and the resulting P_L may be greatly altered [41]. Certainly, in a relatively small population, randomisation may be unable to distribute equally between groups of different E_L and chest wall elastance present in the population under study. This bias should be attenuated in a large population. However, even in this case, the linkage between V_T and P_L is weak [55]. However, the discussion regarding the importance of V_T *versus* the importance of P_{aw} and P_L as VILI determinants is still debatable.

In this context, disproportionate stress at end-inflation can result in an overdistension injury (volutrauma), probably due to high P_L [1, 56]. The National Institutes of Health (NIH) ARDS network showed a reduction in mortality of 22% when patients were ventilated with V_T of 6 mL·kg^{-1} compared with V_T of 12 mL·kg^{-1}, while plateau pressures (P_{plat}) were maintained at less than 30 cmH$_2$O [25]. This trial distinctly defined a "lung protective" strategy to minimise the effects of volutrauma.

However, atelectrauma may be induced by repetitive opening and closing of alveolar units [57], presumably due to levels of PEEP that are insufficient to prevent derecruitment. A subsequent trial by the ARDS network investigators (ALVEOLI) endeavoured to address the mechanism of atelectrauma by evaluating the effects of higher compared with lower levels of PEEP [58]. Previous studies suggested that minimising derecruitment of alveoli at end-exhalation with higher levels of PEEP would mitigate lung injury. In this study, patients diagnosed with ALI/ARDS were randomised to either high or low PEEP set by two different sliding scales, based only on the patient's oxygenation. The resulting average level of PEEP in the two groups was approximately 14 cmH$_2$O and 8 cmH$_2$O, in the high and low PEEP groups, respectively [58]. The authors were unable to establish improvement in the intensive care unit (ICU) mortality [59]. In this context, GRASSO et al. [60] have postulated that the aforementioned ALVEOLI trial did not show beneficial effects because the study protocol failed to individualise PEEP to each patient's respiratory system features. Using measurements of gas exchange and respiratory mechanics, they demonstrated that applying higher PEEP resulted in an extensively variable response. More precisely, nine out of 19 patients had a favourable response to higher PEEP, measured by alveolar recruitment, *via* pressure–volume curves plotted during low-flow tidal inflation, increased oxygenation and a reduction in static E_L. Contrariwise, the remaining patients, termed "non-recruiters", failed to show improvement in any of these. The authors concluded that random application of high PEEP, not only failed to induce recruitment in many patients, but could also lead to over distension [60].

In the lung open ventilation (LOV) trial, MEADE et al. [61] randomised 983 ARDS patients to either "conventional" levels of PEEP or an "open lung" approach, whereby PEEP was increased but still based on a predetermined inspiratory oxygen fraction (F_{I,O_2}) scale. The methods in this study were similar to the ALVEOLI trial, with the exception that recruitment manoeuvres were permitted in the study group. Nevertheless, there was no statistical difference in the mortality rate. In the ExPress study, MERCAT et al. [62] randomised 767 ARDS patients to either a moderate PEEP strategy or a high PEEP strategy. This protocol allowed the titration of PEEP in the study group to a quantifiable variable of respiratory mechanics, rather than simply oxygenation. The primary end-point was mortality at 28 days and secondary end-points were hospital mortality at 60 days, ventilator-free days and organ failure-free days. The results showed no significant difference in either 28 day or hospital mortality. However, the study group had a higher median number of ventilator-free days and organ failure-free days. Although the ExPress study utilised physiological variables of respiratory system mechanics and demonstrated improvement in some important secondary end-points, the use of Pplat to titrate PEEP may still fail to account for other important variables of the respiratory system, for example, chest wall elastance [59, 63]. In the trials by AMATO et al. [51] and VILLAR et al. [64], PEEP was set at 2 cmH$_2$O above the lower inflection point on the pressure–volume curve. Nevertheless, these trials are difficult to interpret since the control group received VT that would now be considered potentially injurious. Additionally, the measurement of static and quasi-static pressure–volume loops, and the determination of Pflex (the airway pressure corresponding to the lower inflection point on the inspiratory pressure–volume curve measured with zero expiratory-end pressure (ZEEP)), to set PEEP has proven to be challenging [65].

Positive end-expiratory pressure

As discussed previously, while surpassing pulmonary elastic limits is known to induce lung injury, ventilation with low volumes can induce atelectrauma, therefore inducing lung injury. Since alveolar collapse usually occurs at end-expiration, an adequate distending pressure can be applied to avoid the derecruitment of the alveolar units [66]. Therefore, the usage of a proper PEEP is essential to maintain end-expiratory lung volume above the derecruitment level [1]. Nevertheless, PEEP induces an increase in mean PL, which can cause more stress in lung parenchyma. A reasonable explanation is that, when an area of the lung is collapsed, and cannot expand during inspiration, the adjacent regions have increased tension and strain. Therefore, if PEEP is able to maintain the collapsed areas opened after the end of expiration, the applied force in the next respiratory cycle can be shared more homogeneously [41]. However, setting the level of PEEP to provide protection against VILI may be guided by constructing a respiratory pressure–volume curve, still, the optimal level of PEEP has been difficult to determine. In a study by TALMOR et al. [67] PL was estimated with the use of oesophageal balloon catheters. The authors hypothesised that the use of pleural–pressure measurements, despite technical limitations to the accuracy of such measurements, would enable the finding of an optimal PEEP value to maintain oxygenation while preventing lung injury due to repeated alveolar collapse and/or overdistention.

Additionally, the importance of setting PEEP above the lower inflection of a ZEEP pressure–volume curve has been questioned [68]. Some studies showed that moderate levels of PEEP are able to protect against VILI, in which PEEP is effective in keeping open most of the lung, thus attenuating the stress/ strain misdistribution [3, 7]. In another experimental study, rats ventilated with peak pressure of 45 cmH$_2$O presented less haemorrhage and oedema when a PEEP of 10 cmH$_2$O was applied [7]. DREYFUSS et al. [3] reported that PEEP markedly reduced ventilator-associated pulmonary oedema, and additionally preserved the alveolar epithelium ultrastructure, reporting a protective effect of PEEP during permeability oedema.

CAIRONI et al. [69] studied how lung recruitability influences the effects of high PEEP in patients with ARDS and showed a beneficial impact of reducing intratidal alveolar opening and closing by increasing PEEP, which prevailed over the effects of increasing alveolar strain. Additionally, the authors showed that the higher the quantity of tidal opening and closing tissue, the higher the mortality. Nevertheless, some studies of randomised trials on low versus high PEEP in ALI patients did not present any significant difference in mortality [25, 61, 62]. From the database of these studies, BRIEL et al. [70] performed an individual meta-analysis demonstrating that treatment with higher versus lower levels of PEEP were not associated with improved hospital survival. Conversely, higher levels were associated with improved survival among the subgroup of patients with ARDS, as opposed to ALI non-ARDS.

High PEEP led to haemodynamic impairment impeding venous return and increasing right ventricular afterload. The recent PEEP trials used low VT and high PEEP [25, 61, 62]. This approach is different from that used in the past, when high V_T generated very high P_{plat} [71]. In this context, FOUGÈRES *et al.* [72] evaluated the haemodynamic effect of increasing PEEP when V_T and the P_{plat} are limited. Echocardiography and pulmonary artery catheterisation were performed in 21 patients with ARDS ventilated with low V_T. They hypothesised that the increase in central blood volume may recruit pulmonary microvessels previously collapsed by PEEP. Since capillaries are directly exposed to alveolar pressures, a better knowledge of the effects of PEEP on local perfusion may be clinically relevant [71]. While the use of recruitment manoeuvres (RMs) and high PEEP is not routinely recommended, they seem effective at improving oxygenation with minor adverse effects [73], in addition, RMs associated with higher PEEP have been shown to reduce hypoxaemia-related deaths [61].

Recruitment manoeuvres

As described earlier, a protective mechanical ventilation strategy characterised by low V_T has been associated with reduced mortality in patients with ALI/ARDS. Nevertheless, this "protective" strategy can result in alveolar collapse [74]. Therefore, RMs are required to open up collapsed lungs, while adequate PEEP levels may counteract alveolar derecruitment during low V_T ventilation, improving respiratory function and minimising VALI [74]. However, the optimal RM is still a controversial topic. RMs involve a dynamic process of intentional transient increase in P_L to open collapsed alveoli and increase end-expiratory lung volume, improving lung mechanics and gas exchange. Nonetheless, these beneficial effects did not improve patient outcomes such as mortality and length of ventilation [73]. The most common RM is conventional sustained inflation [75–78]. It is associated with respiratory and cardiovascular side-effects that may be minimised by newly proposed strategies: prolonged or incremental PEEP elevation [79]; pressure-controlled ventilation (PCV) with fixed PEEP and increased driving pressure; PCV applied with escalating PEEP and constant driving pressure; and long and slow increase in pressure [38]. Various factors can affect the efficiency of RMs, such as the nature and extent of lung injury, the ability to increase inspiratory P_L, patient positioning and cardiac preload. In an experimental model, SANTIAGO *et al.* [80] observed that in the presence of alveolar oedema, regional mechanical heterogeneities and hyperinflation, RMs promoted a modest, however consistent increase in inflammatory and fibrogenic response, which may have worsened lung function. In an elegant study, SILVA *et al.* [81] investigated the effects of the rate of airway pressure increase and duration of RMs on lung function and activation of inflammation, fibrogenesis and apoptosis in experimental ALI. The authors reported an improvement in lung function, with less biological impact, longer-duration RMs and slower airway pressure increase. The development of new recruitment strategies with fewer haemodynamic and biological effects on the lungs, as well as randomised clinical trials analysing the impact of RMs on morbidity and mortality in ALI/ARDS patients, are urgently required [74].

Transient increases in intrathoracic pressure during RMs may lead to haemodynamic instability [82]. Nevertheless, RMs have been recognised as effective for improving oxygenation, at least transiently [73], and even reducing the need for rescue therapies in severe hypoxaemia [61]. Fluid management has been used to minimise haemodynamic instability associated with RMs [79]; however, fluid management itself may have an impact on lung and distal organ injury [83, 84]. Although fluid restriction may cause distal organ damage [83], hypervolemia has been associated with increased lung injury [85, 86]. In an experimental study, Silva *et al.* [87] investigated the effects of RMs on lung and distal organs in the presence of hypovolemia, normovolemia and hypervolemia. The authors observed an increase in lung wet-to-dry ratio with impairment of oxygenation and static E_L, and alveolar and endothelial cell damage, together with increased levels of IL-6, vascular cell adhesion molecule (VCAM)-1, and intercellular adhesion molecule (ICAM)-1 in the hypervolemia group. Conversely, in hypervolemic animals, RM improved oxygenation, however, it also increased lung injury and led to higher inflammatory and fibrogenetic responses, suggesting that volemic status should be taken into account during RMs.

Prone positioning

The prone position has been proposed to improve gas exchange and respiratory mechanics in ALI/ARDS patients, although prospective, randomised clinical trials [24, 88–90] have failed to demonstrate an improvement in clinical outcome [49]. Nevertheless, it is well known that P_L is not uniformly distributed in either humans or experimental animals, with a gradient along the vertical axis, with nondependent lung regions experiencing greater P_L and tension of the fibres than dependent lung regions [49]. This phenomenon is even improved in a nonhomogeneous lung. In the prone position, in both humans [41, 91, 92] and experimental models [93], regional inflation is more uniformly distributed along the vertical axis, indicating a significant reduction in P_L gradient, and thus suggesting that the stress and strain are more homogeneously distributed within the lung parenchyma. Experimental studies on healthy [48, 94] and injured lung animals [95] ventilated with high V_T and PEEP have shown that prone position causes less extensive histological changes in dorsal regions when compared with supine position. Additionally, other studies with high V_T suggest that prone position is effective in delaying VILI [96, 97]. In an experimental model, VALENZA et al. [96] observed a more homogeneous distribution of lung strain during mechanical ventilation in the prone position, suggesting that the delayed occurrence of VILI could be explained by a better distribution of alveolar ventilation in the prone position compared with the supine position. In another study, MENTZELOPOULOS et al. [98] analysed parenchymal lung stress and strain in ARDS patients, estimated from the transpulmonary P_{plat} and the V_T to end-expiratory lung volume ratio. Both parameters were reduced in the prone position compared with the semirecumbant position, indicating that lung tissue damage by VILI can be reduced by the prone position. The beneficial effects of prone position leading to the reduction of VILI can be related to: 1) a more homogeneous distribution of P_L gradient [93, 99], yielding a redistribution of ventilation; 2) increased end-expiratory lung volume resulting in a reduction in stress and strain [41, 96]; and 3) changes in regional perfusion [100, 101]. In an experimental model of ALI, SANTANA et al. [102] demonstrated that prone position led to increased end-expiratory lung volume, less atelectasis, more homogeneous distribution of aeration and increased distribution of blood flow in both ventral and dorsal regions, resulting in an improvement in lung mechanics and oxygenation compared with the supine position, suggesting that prone position may lead to reduced VALI due to lower regional stress and strain. Nevertheless, there were no differences in kidney, brain and intestinal apoptosis comparing the supine and prone positions [48].

Assisted mechanical ventilation

Assisted mechanical ventilation has been suggested to minimise the development of VALI by increasing lung volume and reducing atelectasis, leading to improvement in E_L, with consequent reduction in P_L and in the amount of opening and closing of peripheral airways and atelectasis. Also, pleural pressures (P_{pl}) are redistributed. However, spontaneous breathing during assisted mechanical ventilation may exacerbate lung injury by increasing patient-ventilator asynchrony and rapid shallow breathing, and inducing further atelectasis and tidal recruitment–derecruitment [103]. Additionally, negative P_{pl} may increase intrathoracic blood volume, worsening pulmonary oedema and lung damage [104]. During controlled mechanical ventilation, P_{pl} depends on V_T and E_L. The resulting alveolar pressure (P_A) depends on V_T as well as lung and chest wall elastances. During assisted mechanical ventilation, P_A does not necessarily reflect P_{pl} since the degree of activation of respiratory muscles and the consequent reduction in P_{pl} must be taken into account. In other words, even with constant P_A, the increase in inspiratory effort and P_{pl} determines higher P_L.

Few experimental studies have evaluated the effects of assisted mechanical ventilation on VALI. SADDY et al. [105] compared the effects of different assisted-ventilation modes (pressure-assist control ventilation (PACV) with I:E of 1:2 and 1:1, and Bi-Vent, a variant of bilevel positive airway pressure (BiPAP) that allows spontaneous breaths assisted by pressure support in both the lower and the higher P_{aw} levels) with PCV on lung histology, arterial blood gases, inflammatory and fibrogenic mediators in experimental ALI in rats. Interestingly, the V_T delivered and the inspiratory effort was higher during assisted mechanical ventilation modes. However, the inspiratory effort estimated by mouth occlusion pressure at 100 ms ($P_{0.1}$) was lower with Bi-Vent and pressure support ventilation (PSV), and higher during assisted-pressure control modes. The main findings were that assisted ventilation modes had more beneficial effects on respiratory function and reduced lung injury compared with PSV. Among assisted ventilation modes, Bi-Vent and PSV demonstrated better functional results with less lung damage and expression of inflammatory mediators. This study raised interesting points for assisted mechanical ventilation: 1) V_T, within certain limits, and increased P_L might not be specific determinants of VALI; 2) higher inspiratory effort during assisted mechanical ventilation could increase injury, and the "safe" level of inspiratory effort should be determined in the near future; 3) $P_{0.1}$ could be useful to optimise assisted ventilation, by achieving optimal recruitment with minimal stress and strain; and 4) modalities of assisted ventilation that favour lower I:E may lead to less hyperinflation. Interestingly, Bi-Vent and PSV were associated with lower hyperinflation compared with PACV 1:1, which could be due to a better animal–ventilator interaction that reduced respiratory drive, with consequent decrease in the inspiratory P_L. GAMA DE ABREU et al. [106] have recently shown that in saline lung lavage, protective ventilation with PSV and noisy PSV was associated with reduced histological lung damage and reduction in IL-6 in the lung tissue compared with protective controlled mechanical ventilation.

Different factors could have promoted reduced lung injury during assisted ventilation by: 1) recruitment of dependent atelectatic lung regions, reducing opening and closing during tidal breath, thus limiting shear stress forces; 2) more homogeneous distribution of regional P_L; 3) variability of breathing pattern; 4) redistribution of perfusion towards non-atelectatic injured areas; and 5) improved lymphatic drainage. Taken together, these observations suggest that the type of assisted mechanical ventilation and the amount of inspiratory effort play a relevant role in VALI, especially in more severe ARDS patients.

Sedation and paralysis

Sedation has become a standard treatment strategy for critically ill patients undergoing mechanical ventilation [71]. Recent studies explored different strategies aimed at limiting or interrupting daily intravenous sedation to constrain the time under mechanical ventilation. STROM et al. [107] aimed to establish whether duration of mechanical ventilation could be reduced with a protocol of no sedation *versus* daily interruption of sedation in critically ill patients. The no sedation protocol was associated with an increase in days without ventilation and shorter ICU length of stay, without modifying self-extubation occurrence. Although studies have shown that reducing sedation of critically ill patients shortens time on the ventilator and in ICU, limiting sedation strategies may affect long-term cognitive psychological and functional outcome [71]. JACKSON et al. [108] aimed to determine the long-term effects of a wake up and breathe protocol that interrupts and reduces sedative exposure in the ICU, which resulted in similar cognitive, psychological and functional outcomes among patients tested 3 and 12 months post-ICU, implying that the immediate benefit associated with the awakening approach tested in this study was not offset by a potential long-term cognitive and psychological adverse outcome. GIRARD et al. [109] aimed to assess a protocol that paired spontaneous awakening trials and daily interruption of sedatives with spontaneous breathing trials, and observed that a wake up and breathe protocol that pairs daily spontaneous awakening trials with daily spontaneous breathing trials resulted in better outcomes for patients undergoing mechanical ventilation than the current standard approaches. Depressive disorders were present in 42% of patients transferred to a long-term facility for weaning, and were associated with a higher risk of weaning failure and death [110]. Functional dependence and history of psychiatric disorders before ICU admission were independently associated with the occurrence of such disorders, suggesting that specific attention should be paid to this subgroup of patients [71].

In mechanically ventilated patients with ARDS, neuromuscular blocking agents may improve oxygenation and decrease VALI; however, these agents may also cause muscle weakness [111]. In this line, PAPAZIAN et al. [112] evaluated clinical outcomes after 2 days of therapy with neuromuscular blocking agents in patients with ARDS. The authors found that early administration of a neuromuscular blocking agent improved the adjusted 90-day survival and increased the time off the ventilator without increasing muscle weakness, suggesting that low V_T ventilation associated with the administration of a neuromuscular blocking agent may improve outcomes. Nevertheless, more studies are needed to confirm and develop these findings before they can be used in the clinical setting.

New approaches to prevent VILI/VALI

Neurally adjusted ventilatory assist (NAVA), an alternative mode of ventilation that has been recently developed and tested in patients with respiratory failure [113], was as effective as the low V_T strategy in attenuating VILI/VALI and in attenuating systemic and remote organ dysfunction [114]. During NAVA, an array of electrodes attached to a nasogastric tube are used to measure diaphragmatic electrical activity, which triggers the ventilator-assisted mode; pressure at the airway opening is provided in proportion [54, 113]. The ventilator therefore acts as a muscle under patient neural command [71]. NAVA can improve synchrony between the patient and ventilator in a similar way to proportional assist ventilation (PAV) [115]; however, NAVA prevents over assistance because excessive assist downregulates respiratory centre activity and, thus, inspiratory pressure. Nevertheless, clinicians still need to adjust the NAVA level [71].

Mechanical ventilation is a life-saving intervention in acute respiratory failure without alternative; however, even protective ventilation strategies applying minimal mechanical stress may induce VILI/VALI. Therefore, adjuvant pharmacological strategies in addition to lung-protective ventilation to attenuate VILI/VALI are necessary. MÜLLER et al. [116] showed that adrenomedullin, an endogenous peptide that is important in maintaining endothelial barrier integrity, significantly reduced lung permeability, thus attenuating the accumulation of leukocytes in the lung, leading to improved oxygenation in mice ventilated with high V_T.

How to identify VILI/VALI

Pressure–volume curves

Pressure–volume curves of the respiratory system can be measured by static methods with constant or sinusoidal flow, and quasi-static methods for breath-to-breath determination [74]. Pressure–volume curves have been proposed to identify patients with a higher potential for recruitment [117–120] as: 1) the inspiratory pressure–volume curve may help identify patients with higher recruitment potential, identification of inflection point and curvilinear or S-shaped pressure–volume curve, and patients with a lower potential for recruitment, no inflection point and linear pressure–volume curve; and 2) the expiratory pressure–volume curve should also be performed in order to evaluate hysteresis [74]. In this context, DEMORY et al. [120] proposed using the hysteresis of the pressure–volume curve to assess the lung recruitability in ARDS patients, and to identify those patients requiring RM before setting PEEP. This technique has advantages such as: pressure–volume curves guide PEEP titration in protective ventilation strategies, consequently reducing mortality in patients with ARDS [51] and are automatically performed by the mechanical ventilator. Unfortunately, pressure–volume curves normally require interruption of mechanical ventilation that could generate data artefacts. Moreover, pressure–volume curves do not allow inference on regional elastic properties of the respiratory system [74].

Imaging

Computed tomography scan

Computed tomography (CT) techniques have been proposed [121] to identify patients with a high or low potential for recruitment [24, 74, 122]. The main advantages of using CT to assess lung recruitment are: the regional response to recruitment can be determined; the technique is objective; and the morpho-functional correlations obtained can be useful for a comprehensive patient evaluation [74, 122]. CT scans should be performed at different pressure levels to identify potential for recruitment. Initially, one single whole-lung CT scan should be performed at PEEP equal to 5–10 cmH$_2$O to evaluate the distribution of aeration and to compute lung weight. Subsequently, two to three lung CT slices, taken at the lung apex, hilum and basis, should be performed to assess lung recruitability. Nevertheless, there are important limitations, such as radiation exposure, the need to move patients outside the ICU, unavailability of CT at the bedside, lack of information on lung mechanical stress, CT densities may not correlate with overdistension and high cost [74, 122]. Additionally, CT scans should be performed as early as possible after the onset of ALI/ARDS and repeated after 1 week in the absence of clinical improvement. The use of a CT scan at the start of mechanical ventilation may be helpful to assess the nature and extent of the patient's response to mechanical ventilation when performed early in the course of ALI/ARDS. Lung recruitability at CT scan has been associated with the severity of lung injury as well as mortality, with no significant correlation with respiratory physiological variables, particularly changes in oxygenation [123]. In ALI/ARDS patients, CT reveals discrepancies between bedside chest radiograph and various clinical and physiological parameters [74, 122]. In order to minimise radiation, the lung is usually imaged at one single level, with different ventilator settings. The use of different pressure levels helps to distinguish between areas of alveolar collapse and consolidation, providing useful information about mechanical ventilation parameters [74, 122]. Alternative techniques, measurement of end-expiratory lung volume and lung ultrasound, should be taken into account whenever CT cannot be performed and to monitor the patient at the bedside.

Lung ultrasound

Lung ultrasound at the bedside is a noninvasive technique that is easily repeatable, providing accurate information regarding lung morphology, such as focal or diffuse aeration loss [74, 124]. Therefore, it is useful for optimising PEEP. Additionally, lung ultrasound can replace bedside chest radiography and lung CT for assessment of pleural effusion, pneumothorax, alveolar–interstitial syndrome, lung consolidation, pulmonary abscess and lung recruitment/derecruitment [124]. Consequently, it is one of the most promising bedside techniques for monitoring patients with ARDS, and therefore a useful tool to avoid VILI [124]; however, a precise interpretation of lung ultrasound data requires experience.

Positron emission tomography

Positron emission tomography (PET) has recently gained attention among investigators as a novel imaging tool for monitoring VILI, and to study lung pathophysiology *in vivo* noninvasively on a regional basis [125]. PET studies have demonstrated that: 1) the redistribution of pulmonary perfusion away from oedematous shunting regions is variable among individuals and correlated with arterial oxygen tension $(Pa,O_2)/FI,O_2$ ratio [126, 127]; 2) PEEP and RM can shift perfusion back toward shunting regions, attenuating the beneficial effect of alveolar recruitment on gas exchange [128, 129]; 3) prone positioning improves gas exchange by reducing shunt in dorsal lung regions [130, 131]; and 4) neutrophil metabolic activation is increased in the early stages of ALI/ARDS and VILI/VALI, and is amplified by endotoxin and reduced by PEEP [132, 133]. Therefore, PET has added important data to the field. PET is a versatile imaging tool for physiological investigation. By imaging the regional effects of interventions commonly performed in patients with ALI/ARDS, PET has improved the understanding of the positive or negative effects mechanisms produced by different mechanical ventilation interventions, as well as of the pathophysiology of ALI/ARDS and VILI/VALI [125].

Conclusions

Mechanical ventilation is essential for the support of critically ill patients, but can aggravate and even trigger lung damage. The clinical relevance of low lung volume injury and the application of high PEEP levels remain debatable. Furthermore, researchers were not successful in transferring the measurement of inflammatory mediators during VILI/VALI from bench to bedside. Therefore, many issues still require elucidation: 1) the best ventilator strategy to be adopted; 2) which ventilator parameters should be managed; 3) how to monitor VILI/VALI: arterial blood gases, lung mechanics, proinflammatory mediators; 4) the role of imaging; and 5) how to prevent VILI/VALI (new ventilatory and pharmacological strategies, as well as stem cell therapy).

Support statement

T. Maron-Gutierrez and P.R.M. Rocco are supported by the Centers of Excellence Program (PRONEX-FAPERJ; Rio de Janeiro, Brazil), Brazilian Council for Scientific and Technological

Development (CNPq), Carlos Chagas Filho, Rio de Janeiro State Research Supporting Foundation (FAPERJ), and Coordination for the Improvement of Higher Education Personnel (CAPES) (Brazil).

Statement of interest

None declared.

References

1. Dreyfuss D, Saumon G. Ventilator-induced lung injury: lessons from experimental studies. *Am J Respir Crit Care Med* 1998; 157: 294–323.
2. Han B, Lodyga M, Liu M. Ventilator-induced lung injury: role of protein-protein interaction in mechanosensation. *Proc Am Thorac Soc* 2005; 2: 181–187.
3. Dreyfuss D, Soler P, Basset G, *et al.* High inflation pressure pulmonary edema. Respective effects of high airway pressure, high tidal volume, and positive end-expiratory pressure. *Am Rev Respir Dis* 1988; 137: 1159–1164.
4. Dreyfuss D, Basset G, Soler P, *et al.* Intermittent positive-pressure hyperventilation with high inflation pressures produces pulmonary microvascular injury in rats. *Am Rev Respir Dis* 1985; 132: 880–884.
5. Dreyfuss D, Soler P, Saumon G. Spontaneous resolution of pulmonary edema caused by short periods of cyclic overinflation. *J Appl Physiol* 1992; 72: 2081–2089.
6. Bachofen M, Weibel ER. Structural alterations of lung parenchyma in the adult respiratory distress syndrome. *Clin Chest Med* 1982; 3: 35–56.
7. Webb HH, Tierney DF. Experimental pulmonary edema due to intermittent positive pressure ventilation with high inflation pressures. Protection by positive end-expiratory pressure. *Am Rev Respir Dis* 1974; 110: 556–565.
8. John E, McDevitt M, Wilborn W, *et al.* Ultrastructure of the lung after ventilation. *Br J Exp Pathol* 1982; 63: 401–407.
9. dos Santos CC, Slutsky AS. The contribution of biophysical lung injury to the development of biotrauma. *Annu Rev Physiol* 2006; 68: 585–618.
10. Tsuno K, Prato P, Kolobow T. Acute lung injury from mechanical ventilation at moderately high airway pressures. *J Appl Physiol* 1990; 69: 956–961.
11. Nolop KB, Maxwell DL, Royston D, *et al.* Effect of raised thoracic pressure and volume on 99mTc-DTPA clearance in humans. *J Appl Physiol* 1986; 60: 1493–1497.
12. Dreyfuss D, Soler P, Saumon G. Mechanical ventilation-induced pulmonary edema. Interaction with previous lung alterations. *Am J Respir Crit Care Med* 1995; 151: 1568–1575.
13. Albert RK, Lakshminarayan S, Kirk W, *et al.* Lung inflation can cause pulmonary edema in zone I of *in situ* dog lungs. *J Appl Physiol* 1980; 49: 815–819.
14. Pattle RE. Properties, function and origin of the alveolar lining layer. *Nature* 1955; 175: 1125–1126.
15. Lecuona E, Saldias F, Comellas A, *et al.* Ventilator-associated lung injury decreases lung ability to clear edema in rats. *Am J Respir Crit Care Med* 1999; 159: 603–609.
16. Ito Y, Veldhuizen RA, Yao LJ, *et al.* Ventilation strategies affect surfactant aggregate conversion in acute lung injury. *Am J Respir Crit Care Med* 1997; 155: 493–499.
17. Lewis JF, Veldhuizen R, Possmayer F, *et al.* Altered alveolar surfactant is an early marker of acute lung injury in septic adult sheep. *Am J Respir Crit Care Med* 1994; 150: 123–130.
18. Veldhuizen RA, McCaig LA, Akino T, *et al.* Pulmonary surfactant subfractions in patients with the acute respiratory distress syndrome. *Am J Respir Crit Care Med* 1995; 152: 1867–1871.
19. Malloy JL, Veldhuizen RA, Lewis JF. Effects of ventilation on the surfactant system in sepsis-induced lung injury. *J Appl Physiol* 2000; 88: 401–408.
20. Tobin MJ. Advances in mechanical ventilation. *N Engl J Med* 2001; 344: 1986–1996.
21. Bouhuys A. Physiology and musical instruments. *Nature* 1969; 221: 1199–1204.
22. Hernandez LA, Peevy KJ, Moise AA, *et al.* Chest wall restriction limits high airway pressure-induced lung injury in young rabbits. *J Appl Physiol* 1989; 66: 2364–2368.
23. Carlton DP, Cummings JJ, Scheerer RG, *et al.* Lung overexpansion increases pulmonary microvascular protein permeability in young lambs. *J Appl Physiol* 1990; 69: 577–583.
24. Gattinoni L, Caironi P, Pelosi P, *et al.* What has computed tomography taught us about the acute respiratory distress syndrome? *Am J Respir Crit Care Med* 2001; 164: 1701–1711.
25. Ventilation with lower tidal volumes as compared with traditional tidal volumes for acute lung injury and the acute respiratory distress syndrome. The Acute Respiratory Distress Syndrome Network. *N Engl J Med* 2000; 342: 1301–1308.
26. Tremblay LN, Slutsky AS. Ventilator-induced injury: from barotrauma to biotrauma. *Proc Assoc Am Physicians* 1998; 110: 482–488.

27. Ranieri VM, Suter PM, Tortorella C, *et al.* Effect of mechanical ventilation on inflammatory mediators in patients with acute respiratory distress syndrome: a randomized controlled trial. *JAMA* 1999; 282: 54–61.

28. Tremblay L, Valenza F, Ribeiro SP, *et al.* Injurious ventilatory strategies increase cytokines and c-fos m-RNA expression in an isolated rat lung model. *J Clin Invest* 1997; 99: 944–952.

29. Ricard JD, Dreyfuss D, Saumon G. Production of inflammatory cytokines in ventilator-induced lung injury: a reappraisal. *Am J Respir Crit Care Med* 2001; 163: 1176–1180.

30. Bregeon F, Delpierre S, Chetaille B, *et al.* Mechanical ventilation affects lung function and cytokine production in an experimental model of endotoxemia. *Anesthesiology* 2005; 102: 331–339.

31. Tremblay LN, Slutsky AS. Ventilator-induced lung injury: from the bench to the bedside. *Intensive Care Med* 2006; 32: 24–33.

32. Conrad SA, Zhang S, Arnold TC, *et al.* Protective effects of low respiratory frequency in experimental ventilator-associated lung injury. *Crit Care Med* 2005; 33: 835–840.

33. Hotchkiss JR Jr, Blanch L, Murias G, *et al.* Effects of decreased respiratory frequency on ventilator-induced lung injury. *Am J Respir Crit Care Med* 2000; 161: 463–468.

34. Spieth PM, Carvalho AR, Pelosi P, *et al.* Variable tidal volumes improve lung protective ventilation strategies in experimental lung injury. *Am J Respir Crit Care Med* 2009; 179: 684–693.

35. Spieth PM, Carvalho AR, Guldner A, *et al.* Pressure support improves oxygenation and lung protection compared to pressure-controlled ventilation and is further improved by random variation of pressure support. *Crit Care Med* 2011; 39: 746–755.

36. Wang SH, Wei TS. The outcome of early pressure-controlled inverse ratio ventilation on patients with severe acute respiratory distress syndrome in surgical intensive care unit. *Am J Surg* 2002; 183: 151–155.

37. Casetti AV, Bartlett RH, Hirschl RB. Increasing inspiratory time exacerbates ventilator-induced lung injury during high-pressure/high-volume mechanical ventilation. *Crit Care Med* 2002; 30: 2295–2299.

38. Rzezinski AF, Oliveira GP, Santiago VR, *et al.* Prolonged recruitment manoeuvre improves lung function with less ultrastructural damage in experimental mild acute lung injury. *Respir Physiol Neurobiol* 2009; 169: 271–281.

39. Peevy KJ, Hernandez LA, Moise AA, *et al.* Barotrauma and microvascular injury in lungs of nonadult rabbits: effect of ventilation pattern. *Crit Care Med* 1990; 18: 634–637.

40. Rich PB, Reickert CA, Sawada S, *et al.* Effect of rate and inspiratory flow on ventilator-induced lung injury. *J Trauma* 2000; 49: 903–911.

41. Gattinoni L, Carlesso E, Cadringher P, *et al.* Physical and biological triggers of ventilator-induced lung injury and its prevention. *Eur Respir J* 2003; 22: Suppl. 47, 15s–25s.

42. Plataki M, Hubmayr RD. The physical basis of ventilator-induced lung injury. *Expert Rev Respir Med* 2010; 4: 373–385.

43. Schwartz MD, Moore EE, Moore FA, *et al.* Nuclear factor-kappa B is activated in alveolar macrophages from patients with acute respiratory distress syndrome. *Crit Care Med* 1996; 24: 1285–1292.

44. Garcia CS, Rocco PR, Facchinetti LD, *et al.* What increases type III procollagen mRNA levels in lung tissue: stress induced by changes in force or amplitude? *Respir Physiol Neurobiol* 2004; 144: 59–70.

45. Verbrugge SJ, Sorm V, van't Veen A, *et al.* Lung overinflation without positive end-expiratory pressure promotes bacteremia after experimental *Klebsiella pneumoniae* inoculation. *Intensive Care Med* 1998; 24: 172–177.

46. Murphy DB, Cregg N, Tremblay L, *et al.* Adverse ventilatory strategy causes pulmonary-to-systemic translocation of endotoxin. *Am J Respir Crit Care Med* 2000; 162: 27–33.

47. Imai Y, Parodo J, Kajikawa O, *et al.* Injurious mechanical ventilation and end-organ epithelial cell apoptosis and organ dysfunction in an experimental model of acute respiratory distress syndrome. *JAMA* 2003; 289: 2104–2112.

48. Nakos G, Batistatou A, Galiatsou E, *et al.* Lung and "end organ" injury due to mechanical ventilation in animals: comparison between the prone and supine positions. *Crit Care* 2006; 10: R38.

49. Gattinoni L, Protti A, Caironi P, *et al.* Ventilator-induced lung injury: the anatomical and physiological framework. *Crit Care Med* 2010; 38: Suppl. 10, S539–S548.

50. Stewart TE, Meade MO, Cook DJ, *et al.* Evaluation of a ventilation strategy to prevent barotrauma in patients at high risk for acute respiratory distress syndrome. Pressure- and Volume-Limited Ventilation Strategy Group. *N Engl J Med* 1998; 338: 355–361.

51. Amato MB, Barbas CS, Medeiros DM, *et al.* Effect of a protective-ventilation strategy on mortality in the acute respiratory distress syndrome. *N Engl J Med* 1998; 338: 347–354.

52. Brochard L, Roudot-Thoraval F, Roupie E, *et al.* Tidal volume reduction for prevention of ventilator-induced lung injury in acute respiratory distress syndrome. The Multicenter Trail Group on Tidal Volume reduction in ARDS. *Am J Respir Crit Care Med* 1998; 158: 1831–1838.

53. Brower RG, Shanholtz CB, Fessler HE, *et al.* Prospective, randomized, controlled clinical trial comparing traditional *versus* reduced tidal volume ventilation in acute respiratory distress syndrome patients. *Crit Care Med* 1999; 27: 1492–1498.

54. Del Sorbo L, Slutsky AS. Ventilatory support for acute respiratory failure: new and ongoing pathophysiological, diagnostic and therapeutic developments. *Curr Opin Crit Care* 2010; 16: 1–7.

55. Tobin MJ. Culmination of an era in research on the acute respiratory distress syndrome. *N Engl J Med* 2000; 342: 1360–1361.

56. Dos Santos CC, Slutsky AS. Invited review: mechanisms of ventilator-induced lung injury: a perspective. *J Appl Physiol* 2000; 89: 1645–1655.

57. Slutsky AS. Lung injury caused by mechanical ventilation. *Chest* 1999; 116: Suppl. 1, 9S–15S.

58. Brower RG, Lanken PN, MacIntyre N, *et al*. Higher *versus* lower positive end-expiratory pressures in patients with the acute respiratory distress syndrome. *N Engl J Med* 2004; 351: 327–336.

59. Sarge T, Talmor D. Transpulmonary pressure: its role in preventing ventilator-induced lung injury. *Minerva Anestesiol* 2008; 74: 335–339.

60. Grasso S, Fanelli V, Cafarelli A, *et al*. Effects of high *versus* low positive end-expiratory pressures in acute respiratory distress syndrome. *Am J Respir Crit Care Med* 2005; 171: 1002–1008.

61. Meade MO, Cook DJ, Guyatt GH, *et al*. Ventilation strategy using low tidal volumes, recruitment maneuvers, and high positive end-expiratory pressure for acute lung injury and acute respiratory distress syndrome: a randomized controlled trial. *JAMA* 2008; 299: 637–645.

62. Mercat A, Richard JC, Vielle B, *et al*. Positive end-expiratory pressure setting in adults with acute lung injury and acute respiratory distress syndrome: a randomized controlled trial. *JAMA* 2008; 299: 646–655.

63. Sarge T, Talmor D. Targeting transpulmonary pressure to prevent ventilator induced lung injury. *Minerva Anestesiol* 2009; 75: 293–299.

64. Villar J, Kacmarek RM, Perez-Mendez L, *et al*. A high positive end-expiratory pressure, low tidal volume ventilatory strategy improves outcome in persistent acute respiratory distress syndrome: a randomized, controlled trial. *Crit Care Med* 2006; 34: 1311–1318.

65. Harris RS, Hess DR, Venegas JG. An objective analysis of the pressure-volume curve in the acute respiratory distress syndrome. *Am J Respir Crit Care Med* 2000; 161: 432–439.

66. Muscedere JG, Mullen JB, Gan K, *et al*. Tidal ventilation at low airway pressures can augment lung injury. *Am J Respir Crit Care Med* 1994; 149: 1327–1334.

67. Talmor D, Sarge T, Malhotra A, *et al*. Mechanical ventilation guided by esophageal pressure in acute lung injury. *N Engl J Med* 2008; 359: 2095–2104.

68. Adams AB, Cakar N, Marini JJ. Static and dynamic pressure-volume curves reflect different aspects of respiratory system mechanics in experimental acute respiratory distress syndrome. *Respir Care* 2001; 46: 686–693.

69. Caironi P, Cressoni M, Chiumello D, *et al*. Lung opening and closing during ventilation of acute respiratory distress syndrome. *Am J Respir Crit Care Med* 2010; 181: 578–586.

70. Briel M, Meade M, Mercat A, *et al*. Higher *vs* lower positive end-expiratory pressure in patients with acute lung injury and acute respiratory distress syndrome: systematic review and meta-analysis. *JAMA* 2010; 303: 865–873.

71. Richard JC, Lefebvre JC, Tassaux D, *et al*. Update in mechanical ventilation 2010. *Am J Respir Crit Care Med* 2011; 184: 32–36.

72. Fougères E, Teboul JL, Richard C, *et al*. Hemodynamic impact of a positive end-expiratory pressure setting in acute respiratory distress syndrome: importance of the volume status. *Crit Care Med* 2010; 38: 802–807.

73. Hodgson C, Keating JL, Holland AE, *et al*. Recruitment manoeuvres for adults with acute lung injury receiving mechanical ventilation. *Cochrane Database Syst Rev* 2009; 2: CD006667.

74. Rocco PR, Pelosi P, de Abreu MG. Pros and cons of recruitment maneuvers in acute lung injury and acute respiratory distress syndrome. *Expert Rev Respir Med* 2010; 4: 479–489.

75. Lapinsky SE, Aubin M, Mehta S, *et al*. Safety and efficacy of a sustained inflation for alveolar recruitment in adults with respiratory failure. *Intensive Care Med* 1999; 25: 1297–1301.

76. Rimensberger PC, Cox PN, Frndova H, *et al*. The open lung during small tidal volume ventilation: concepts of recruitment and "optimal" positive end-expiratory pressure. *Crit Care Med* 1999; 27: 1946–1952.

77. Kloot TE, Blanch L, Melynne Youngblood A, *et al*. Recruitment maneuvers in three experimental models of acute lung injury. Effect on lung volume and gas exchange. *Am J Respir Crit Care Med* 2000; 161: 1485–1494.

78. Grasso S, Stripoli T, Sacchi M, *et al*. Inhomogeneity of lung parenchyma during the open lung strategy: a computed tomography scan study. *Am J Respir Crit Care Med* 2009; 180: 415–423.

79. Borges JB, Okamoto VN, Matos GF, *et al*. Reversibility of lung collapse and hypoxemia in early acute respiratory distress syndrome. *Am J Respir Crit Care Med* 2006; 174: 268–278.

80. Santiago VR, Rzezinski AF, Nardelli LM, *et al*. Recruitment maneuver in experimental acute lung injury: the role of alveolar collapse and edema. *Crit Care Med* 2010; 38: 2207–2214.

81. Silva PL, Moraes L, Santos RS, *et al*. Impact of pressure profile and duration of recruitment maneuvers on morphofunctional and biochemical variables in experimental lung injury. *Crit Care Med* 2011; 39: 1074–1081.

82. Fan E, Wilcox ME, Brower RG, *et al*. Recruitment maneuvers for acute lung injury: a systematic review. *Am J Respir Crit Care Med* 2008; 178: 1156–1163.

83. Rivers EP. Fluid-management strategies in acute lung injury – liberal, conservative, or both? *N Engl J Med* 2006; 354: 2598–2600.

84. Schuster DP. Fluid management in ARDS: "keep them dry" or does it matter? *Intensive Care Med* 1995; 21: 101–103.

85. Jia X, Malhotra A, Saeed M, *et al*. Risk factors for ARDS in patients receiving mechanical ventilation for >48 h. *Chest* 2008; 133: 853–861.

86. Rosenberg AL, Dechert RE, Park PK, *et al*. Review of a large clinical series: association of cumulative fluid balance on outcome in acute lung injury: a retrospective review of the ARDSnet tidal volume study cohort. *J Intensive Care Med* 2009; 24: 35–46.

87. Silva PL, Cruz FF, Fujisaki LC, *et al.* Hypervolemia induces and potentiates lung damage after recruitment maneuver in a model of sepsis-induced acute lung injury. *Crit Care* 2010; 14: R114.

88. Guerin C, Gaillard S, Lemasson S, *et al.* Effects of systematic prone positioning in hypoxemic acute respiratory failure: a randomized controlled trial. *JAMA* 2004; 292: 2379–2387.

89. Mancebo J, Fernandez R, Blanch L, *et al.* A multicenter trial of prolonged prone ventilation in severe acute respiratory distress syndrome. *Am J Respir Crit Care Med* 2006; 173: 1233–1239.

90. Fernandez R, Trenchs X, Klamburg J, *et al.* Prone positioning in acute respiratory distress syndrome: a multicenter randomized clinical trial. *Intensive Care Med* 2008; 34: 1487–1491.

91. Gattinoni L, Bombino M, Pelosi P, *et al.* Lung structure and function in different stages of severe adult respiratory distress syndrome. *JAMA* 1994; 271: 1772–1779.

92. Pelosi P, D'Andrea L, Vitale G, *et al.* Vertical gradient of regional lung inflation in adult respiratory distress syndrome. *Am J Respir Crit Care Med* 1994; 149: 8–13.

93. Mutoh T, Guest RJ, Lamm WJ, *et al.* Prone position alters the effect of volume overload on regional pleural pressures and improves hypoxemia in pigs *in vivo. Am Rev Respir Dis* 1992; 146: 300–306.

94. Broccard A, Shapiro RS, Schmitz LL, *et al.* Prone positioning attenuates and redistributes ventilator-induced lung injury in dogs. *Crit Care Med* 2000; 28: 295–303.

95. Broccard AF, Shapiro RS, Schmitz LL, *et al.* Influence of prone position on the extent and distribution of lung injury in a high tidal volume oleic acid model of acute respiratory distress syndrome. *Crit Care Med* 1997; 25: 16–27.

96. Valenza F, Guglielmi M, Maffioletti M, *et al.* Prone position delays the progression of ventilator-induced lung injury in rats: does lung strain distribution play a role? *Crit Care Med* 2005; 33: 361–367.

97. Nishimura M, Honda O, Tomiyama N, *et al.* Body position does not influence the location of ventilator-induced lung injury. *Intensive Care Med* 2000; 26: 1664–1669.

98. Mentzelopoulos SD, Roussos C, Zakynthinos SG. Prone position reduces lung stress and strain in severe acute respiratory distress syndrome. *Eur Respir J* 2005; 25: 534–544.

99. Albert RK, Leasa D, Sanderson M, *et al.* The prone position improves arterial oxygenation and reduces shunt in oleic-acid-induced acute lung injury. *Am Rev Respir Dis* 1987; 135: 628–633.

100. Lamm WJ, Graham MM, Albert RK. Mechanism by which the prone position improves oxygenation in acute lung injury. *Am J Respir Crit Care Med* 1994; 150: 184–193.

101. Richter T, Bellani G, Scott Harris R, *et al.* Effect of prone position on regional shunt, aeration, and perfusion in experimental acute lung injury. *Am J Respir Crit Care Med* 2005; 172: 480–487.

102. Santana MC, Garcia CS, Xisto DG, *et al.* Prone position prevents regional alveolar hyperinflation and mechanical stress and strain in mild experimental acute lung injury. *Respir Physiol Neurobiol* 2009; 167: 181–188.

103. Thille AW, Rodriguez P, Cabello B, *et al.* Patient-ventilator asynchrony during assisted mechanical ventilation. *Intensive Care Med* 2006; 32: 1515–1522.

104. Kallet RH, Alonso JA, Luce JM, *et al.* Exacerbation of acute pulmonary edema during assisted mechanical ventilation using a low-tidal volume, lung-protective ventilator strategy. *Chest* 1999; 116: 1826–1832.

105. Saddy F, Oliveira GP, Garcia CS, *et al.* Assisted ventilation modes reduce the expression of lung inflammatory and fibrogenic mediators in a model of mild acute lung injury. *Intensive Care Med* 2009; 36: 1417–1426.

106. Gama de Abreu M, Spieth PM, Carvalho AR, *et al.* Pressure support ventilation improves oxygenation with less lung injury and is further improved by random variation of pressure support. *Am J Respir Crit Care Med* 2010; 181: A4073.

107. Strom T, Martinussen T, Toft P. A protocol of no sedation for critically ill patients receiving mechanical ventilation: a randomised trial. *Lancet* 2010; 375: 475–480.

108. Jackson JC, Girard TD, Gordon SM, *et al.* Long-term cognitive and psychological outcomes in the awakening and breathing controlled trial. *Am J Respir Crit Care Med* 2010; 182: 183–191.

109. Girard TD, Kress JP, Fuchs BD, *et al.* Efficacy and safety of a paired sedation and ventilator weaning protocol for mechanically ventilated patients in intensive care (Awakening and Breathing Controlled trial): a randomised controlled trial. *Lancet* 2008; 371: 126–134.

110. Jubran A, Lawm G, Kelly J, *et al.* Depressive disorders during weaning from prolonged mechanical ventilation. *Intensive Care Med* 2010; 36: 828–835.

111. Slutsky AS. Neuromuscular blocking agents in ARDS. *N Engl J Med* 2010; 363: 1176–1180.

112. Papazian L, Forel JM, Gacouin A, *et al.* Neuromuscular blockers in early acute respiratory distress syndrome. *N Engl J Med* 2010; 363: 1107–1116.

113. Sinderby C, Navalesi P, Beck J, *et al.* Neural control of mechanical ventilation in respiratory failure. *Nat Med* 1999; 5: 1433–1436.

114. Brander L, Sinderby C, Lecomte F, *et al.* Neurally adjusted ventilatory assist decreases ventilator-induced lung injury and non-pulmonary organ dysfunction in rabbits with acute lung injury. *Intensive Care Med* 2009; 35: 1979–1989.

115. Younes M, Brochard L, Grasso S, *et al.* A method for monitoring and improving patient: ventilator interaction. *Intensive Care Med* 2007; 33: 1337–1346.

116. Müller HC, Witzenrath M, Tschernig T, *et al.* Adrenomedullin attenuates ventilator-induced lung injury in mice. *Thorax* 2010; 65: 1077–1084.

117. Gattinoni L, Pesenti A, Avalli L, *et al.* Pressure-volume curve of total respiratory system in acute respiratory failure. Computed tomographic scan study. *Am Rev Respir Dis* 1987; 136: 730–736.

118. Rouby J-J, Lu Q, Vieira S. Pressure/volume curves and lung computed tomography in acute respiratory distress syndrome. *Eur Respir J* 2003; 22: Suppl. 42, 27s–36s.

119. Koefoed-Nielsen J, Nielsen ND, Kjaergaard AJ, *et al.* Alveolar recruitment can be predicted from airway pressure-lung volume loops: an experimental study in a porcine acute lung injury model. *Crit Care* 2008; 12: R7.

120. Demory D, Arnal JM, Wysocki M, *et al.* Recruitability of the lung estimated by the pressure volume curve hysteresis in ARDS patients. *Intensive Care Med* 2008; 34: 2019–2025.

121. Brochard L. Watching what PEEP really does. *Am J Respir Crit Care Med* 2001; 163: 1291–1292.

122. Pelosi P, Rocco PR, de Abreu MG. Use of computed tomography scanning to guide lung recruitment and adjust positive-end expiratory pressure. *Curr Opin Crit Care* 2011; 17: 268–274.

123. Gattinoni L, Caironi P, Cressoni M, *et al.* Lung recruitment in patients with the acute respiratory distress syndrome. *N Engl J Med* 2006; 354: 1775–1786.

124. Arbelot C, Ferrari F, Bouhemad B, *et al.* Lung ultrasound in acute respiratory distress syndrome and acute lung injury. *Curr Opin Crit Care* 2008; 14: 70–74.

125. Musch G. Positron emission tomography: a tool for better understanding of ventilator-induced and acute lung injury. *Curr Opin Crit Care* 2011; 17: 7–12.

126. Schuster DP, Anderson C, Kozlowski J, *et al.* Regional pulmonary perfusion in patients with acute pulmonary edema. *J Nucl Med* 2002; 43: 863–870.

127. Musch G, Bellani G, Vidal Melo MF, *et al.* Relation between shunt, aeration, and perfusion in experimental acute lung injury. *Am J Respir Crit Care Med* 2008; 177: 292–300.

128. Richard JC, Le Bars D, Costes N, *et al.* Alveolar recruitment assessed by positron emission tomography during experimental acute lung injury. *Intensive Care Med* 2006; 32: 1889–1894.

129. Richard JC, Pouzot C, Gros A, *et al.* Electrical impedance tomography compared to positron emission tomography for the measurement of regional lung ventilation: an experimental study. *Crit Care* 2009; 13: R82.

130. Richard JC, Janier M, Lavenne F, *et al.* Effect of position, nitric oxide, and almitrine on lung perfusion in a porcine model of acute lung injury. *J Appl Physiol* 2002; 93: 2181–2191.

131. Musch G, Layfield JD, Harris RS, *et al.* Topographical distribution of pulmonary perfusion and ventilation, assessed by PET in supine and prone humans. *J Appl Physiol* 2002; 93: 1841–1851.

132. Costa EL, Musch G, Winkler T, *et al.* Mild endotoxemia during mechanical ventilation produces spatially heterogeneous pulmonary neutrophilic inflammation in sheep. *Anesthesiology* 2010; 112: 658–669.

133. Chen DL, Schuster DP. Positron emission tomography with [18F]fluorodeoxyglucose to evaluate neutrophil kinetics during acute lung injury. *Am J Physiol Lung Cell Mol Physiol* 2004; 286: L834–L840.

Chapter 2

Ventilator strategies in severe hypoxaemic respiratory failure

A. Esan*, D. Hess#, C. Sessler¶, L. George*, C. Oribabor+,
F. Khusid§ and S. Raoof*

Summary

Mechanical ventilation of patients with acute lung injury/acute respiratory distress syndrome (ARDS) should commence with low tidal volume (VT), low stretch and adequate positive end-expiratory pressure (PEEP), as proposed by the first ARDSnet trial. The majority of patients with ARDS will achieve their goals of oxygenation and plateau pressure, utilising the lung protective strategy. In the remaining minority of patients, these end-points may not be achieved. Such patients have a significantly high mortality and should be considered for rescue strategies relatively early on. If the patients respond positively to lung recruitment trials, using rescue strategies may open atelectatic alveoli and allow oxygenation or plateau pressure targets to be achieved. None of these rescue strategies have been shown to reduce mortality, although short-term objectives of improvement in oxygenation or reduction in plateau pressures may be achieved. Therefore, the selection of these strategies should be based on availability and level of comfort of the operators.

Keywords: Acute respiratory distress syndrome, alternative ventilator modes, hypoxaemic respiratory failure, mechanical ventilation, rescue strategies, ventilator strategies

*Depts of Pulmonary and Critical Care,
+Cardiothoracic Surgery,
§Respiratory Therapy, New York Methodist Hospital, Brooklyn, NY,
#Respiratory Care Services, Massachusetts General Hospital, Boston, MA, and
¶Medical College of Virginia Hospitals, Richmond, VA, USA.

Correspondence: A. Esan, Dept of Pulmonary and Critical Care, New York Methodist Hospital, 506 Sixth Street, Brooklyn, NY 11215, USA. Email bayoesan@yahoo.com

Eur Respir Mon 2012; 55: 19–39.
Printed in UK – all rights reserved
Copyright ERS 2012
European Respiratory Monograph
ISSN: 1025-448x
DOI: 10.1183/1025448x.10000412

Acute lung injury (ALI) and its more severe counterpart, acute respiratory distress syndrome (ARDS), are both syndromes of acute hypoxaemic respiratory failure that are associated with a wide variety of aetiologies. In 1994, the American-European Consensus Conference on ARDS standardised the definition of ALI and ARDS on the basis of certain clinical criteria, namely: 1) acute onset of severe respiratory distress; 2) bilateral infiltrates on a frontal chest radiograph; 3) the absence of left atrial hypertension or clinical signs of left heart failure, or a pulmonary capillary wedge pressure $\leqslant 18$ mmHg; and 4) severe hypoxaemia based on the ratio of arterial oxygen tension to the inspiratory oxygen concentration (Pa,O$_2$/FI,O$_2$ $\leqslant 300$ mmHg and 200 mmHg in ALI and ARDS, respectively) [1]. This widely used definition is limited by its inability to account for the diverse pulmonary and non-pulmonary aetiologies, or the level of positive end-expiratory pressure (PEEP) required in those patients requiring mechanical ventilation. This is further buttressed by a recent study showing that a moderate amount of PEEP was sufficient to reclassify patients from ARDS to ALI, resulting in a reduction in the expected mortality [2]. In an attempt to circumvent the problems associated with this existing definition, a new definition has been proposed [3]. The "Berlin definition" classifies ARDS into mild, moderate and severe based upon the following variables: timing, hypoxaemia, origin of oedema, radiological abnormalities and additional physiological derangements. This clinical definition aims to quantify the degree of hypoxaemia based upon the level of PEEP used. However, it has its own limitations and needs to be validated in clinical trials.

The vast majority of ALI/ARDS patients require mechanical ventilation for adequate gas exchange, as well as for alleviating the increased work of breathing. However, in addition to providing life-sustaining support, mechanical ventilation in ALI/ARDS patients can further worsen lung injury as a result of the heterogeneous manner in which the lungs are affected [4]. Ventilator-induced lung injury (VILI) is the collective term used to describe the various injuries that can occur, namely: barotrauma resulting from the the use of high inspiratory pressures; volutrauma due to over-distension from employing a large tidal volume (V_T); atelectrauma following cyclic collapsing and re-opening of unstable alveolar units; and biotrauma ensuing from the release of inflammatory mediators into the systemic circulation [5–11]. Consequently, not only is the goal to provide life-sustaining support with mechanical ventilation in ALI/ARDS patients, but to do so in a manner that minimises VILI, and thereby improve outcomes.

This chapter discusses different ventilator strategies that have been utilised to achieve these goals in the management of ALI/ARDS patients, as well as the evidence from clinical trials regarding the efficacy of these different ventilator strategies. The decision to employ a specific strategy should be based on an appraisal of the benefits, strength of evidence, possible risks, familiarity of use and availability of alternative modes of mechanical ventilation. A PubMed search was performed using each strategy as a key phrase. The article search was limited to those published in English and that studied primarily human subjects. The search was also expanded to comprise further articles, as suitable, from the reference lists of those identified from our initial search. The articles specifically excluded non-ventilatory strategies to maximise oxygenation (conservative fluid strategies, extra-corporeal membrane oxygenation, prone position, etc.), as well as noninvasive positive pressure ventilation.

Volume-targeted ventilation

The initial ventilator strategy that should be promptly utilised is low V_T and pressure ventilation, currently regarded as the standard of care in the management of patients with ALI/ARDS. This strategy attenuates the development of VILI, thus it is considered lung protective ventilation (LPV), and is the only method of mechanical ventilation that has been demonstrated to improve survival in randomised controlled trials (RCTs) of ARDS patients [12–14]. In the largest of these trials, conducted by the ARDS Network (ARDSnet), and generally considered a pivotal study, a 9% absolute reduction in mortality, and a greater number of both ventilator-free days and non-pulmonary organ failure-free days occurred in ALI/ARDS patients mechanically ventilated in the volume assist-control mode with a target V_T of $\leqslant 6$ mL·kg^{-1} predicted body weight (PBW) and a plateau pressure (P_{plat}) of $\leqslant 30$ cmH$_2$O [14]. This was performed using an empirically but prospectively determined F_{I,O_2}–PEEP table to obtain arterial saturations of 88–95% or a P_{a,O_2} of 55–88 mmHg, often resulting in initial decreases of the $P_{a,O_2}/F_{I,O_2}$ ratio, moderate increases in arterial carbon dioxide tension (P_{a,CO_2}), and the use of high respiratory rates with or without sodium bicarbonate to maintain pH goals, while minimising the development of intrinsic auto-PEEP [14].

In contrast, three earlier RCTs of LPV (table 1) did not demonstrate an improvement in outcome [15–17]. Like the ARDSnet study, these three studies had similar PEEP in both arms associated with low versus high V_T, unlike other studies with LPV that included both low V_T and high PEEP [13, 18]. This inconsistency with the earlier RCTs has been attributed to differences in sample size which may not have been sufficiently powered to detect survival differences, lower differences in the tidal volumes and P_{plat} utilised between groups, utilisation of lower pH thresholds, different methods for treating

Table 1. Randomised controlled trials of lung protective ventilation

First author [ref.]	Patients n	Intervention *versus* control group		Mortality rates %	p-value
		Tidal volume mL·kg^{-1}	Pressure cmH$_2$O		
AMATO [13]	53	$\leqslant$6 *versus* 12 ABW	<20 *versus* unlimited driving pressure[#]	38 *versus* 71[¶]	0.001
BROWER [15]	52	5–8 *versus* 10–12 PBW	$\leqslant$30 *versus* $\leqslant$45–55 Pplat	50 *versus* 46	0.61
STEWART [16]	120	$\leqslant$8 *versus* 10–15 IBW	$\leqslant$30 *versus* $\leqslant$50 P,peak	50 *versus* 47	0.72
BROCHARD [17]	116	6–10 *versus* 10–15 DBW	25–30 *versus* $\leqslant$60 Pplat *versus* P,peak	47 *versus* 38[+]	0.38
ARDSNET [14]	861	$\leqslant$6 *versus* 12 PBW	$\leqslant$30 *versus* $\leqslant$50 Pplat	31 *versus* 40	0.007
VILLAR [12]	103	5–8 *versus* 9–11 PBW	Unspecified Pplat	34 *versus* 56	0.04

Data for mortality rate are presented as the in-hospital mortality rates of intervention *versus* control groups, unless otherwise stated. ABW: actual body weight; PBW: predicted body weight; Pplat: plateau pressure; IBW: ideal body weight; P,peak: peak inspiratory pressure; DBW: dry body weight. [#]: Pplat–positive end-expiratory pressure; [¶]: 28-day mortality; [+]: 60-day mortality.

respiratory acidosis, as well as premature termination of the respective trials following interim analysis [19–21]. Similarly, different systemic reviews and meta-analyses of the heterogeneous LPV trials have had varying results [22–25]. In one of the early meta-analyses [23], it was reported that the two trials demonstrating a survival benefit with LPV did not represent standard of care in the control groups [13, 14], and that as long as Pplat was kept between 28–32 cmH$_2$O, there was no basis for the use of low VT. This meta-analysis has been critiqued as having significant methodological errors [24, 26]. In addition, a secondary analysis of the ARDSnet study [14] implied a higher, albeit nonsignificant mortality risk, even when a Pplat <31 cmH$_2$O was used in the control group compared with the LPV group (fig. 1) [27]. Moreover, a subsequent physiological study has shown that regional overdistention can occur at a Pplat of 28–30 cmH$_2$O even with a VT of 6 mL·kg^{-1} PBW [28]. The investigators indicate that although the existence of a "safe" Pplat limit remains unconfirmed, values <28 cmH$_2$O appear to be linked to more protective ventilatory parameters [28]. It is important to be mindful that although alveolar overdistension is usually estimated by Pplat measurement, it is the transalveolar pressure that accurately reflects the degree of alveolar distension. This is particularly important in patients with reductions in chest wall compliance such as in obesity, increased abdominal girth, abdominal compartment syndrome or pleural effusions when pleural pressures would be elevated. Such patients may consequently have elevated Pplat (>30 cmH$_2$O), but the transalveolar pressure would still be within acceptable levels. Therefore, measurement of the oesophageal pressure as a surrogate for the pleural pressure can provide an accurate assessment of the transalveolar pressure; this has been demonstrated in recent studies in ARDS patients and is suggested to have potential clinical benefit [29, 30]. However, the routine use of LPV is reported in several other meta-analyses to be beneficial to ALI/ARDS patients since it has been shown to improve hospital mortality [20, 22, 24, 25, 31].

Widespread adoption of LPV in the management of ALI/ARDS was initially reported to be slow in spite of its beneficial effects [32–35]. Even though

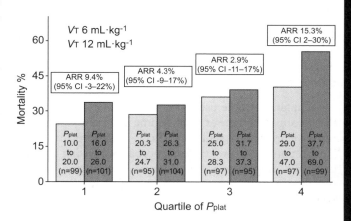

Figure 1. Mortality difference by quartile of day 1 plateau pressure (Pplat) in the ARDSnet trial. The range of Pplat in cmH$_2$O and the number of patients is detailed in each bar. ARR: absolute risk reduction; VT: tidal volume. Reproduced from [27] with permission from the publisher.

a ventilator strategy based on the ARDSnet study [14] serves as a rational starting point, certain barriers, such as failure to recognise patients with ALI/ARDS, unwillingness to relinquish ventilator control or follow a ventilatory strategy protocol, use of actual body weight instead of PBW in calculating tidal volumes, apprehension regarding patient–ventilator asynchrony, increased need for sedation or the development of auto-PEEP, tachypnoea, hypercapnia or acidosis, had limited extensive implementation [33–35]. Nonetheless, these barriers are unfounded [14, 36–41], and recent studies indicate that clinical practices are changing in response to current clinical evidence [42, 43]. In a recent study aiming to improve adherence to LPV, an electronic medical record-based VILI alert system was used to alert bedside providers *via* text paging notifications about potentially detrimental ventilator settings, ultimately reducing patient exposure to the latter [44]. LPV remains the primary ventilatory strategy recommended in the management of ALI/ARDS patients [12–14].

Pressure-targeted ventilation

Although volume-controlled ventilation (VCV), as was utilised in the ARDSnet study, is generally recommended in the management of ALI/ARDS patients [14], the use of pressure-controlled ventilation (PCV) has been proposed as an alternative in maintaining the goals of LPV, *i.e.* VT of 4– 8 mL·kg^{-1} PBW and end-inspiratory Pplat of <30–35 cmH$_2$O [45, 46]. The reasons for this originate from studies that have demonstrated reduced work of breathing by the patient, improved patient-ventilator synchrony and comfort, lower peak inspiratory pressures, higher mean airway pressures and, thus, improved oxygenation due to the variable-flow, pressure-controlled breaths of PCV as opposed to the fixed-flow, flow/volume-targeted breaths of VCV [47–51]. In addition, it has been argued that PCV is inherently safer than VCV because of its ability to restrain detrimental transalveolar forces that are produced and promoted by the fixed-flow and monotonous VT delivery of VCV [52]. In contrast, other studies have indicated that the aforementioned advantages with PCV can be achieved with VCV utilising a decelerating flow waveform as opposed to a square flow waveform [47, 53]. In acute respiratory failure patients, CHIUMELLO *et al.* [54] reported no difference in the work of breathing between PCV and VCV when VT and peak inspiratory flow were appropriately matched. Similarly, KALLET *et al.* [55] demonstrated no difference in the work of breathing when providing LPV to ALI/ ARDS patients using PCV in comparison to VCV with a high inspiratory flow rate. Furthermore, VT was not adequately controlled as a result of an active inspiratory effort in 40% of the patients during PCV [55]. SCHMIDT *et al.* [56] reiterated that VT and, hence, alveolar distension may be increased during active inspiratory efforts by the patient. While this may not translate to increased inspiratory pressures, it may culminate in volutrauma. Thus, one may conclude that paying particular attention to ventilator parameters such as VT, peak inspiratory flow, Pplat and waveform pattern minimises the differences seen between PCV and VCV. In a recent multicentre RCT, MEADE *et al.* [57] compared a low VT ventilation strategy using VCV with an experimental strategy (open lung approach) using PCV in which both arms targeted a VT of 6 mL·kg^{-1} ideal body weight. There were no difference in outcome; however, a direct comparison is confounded by the fact that different PEEP strategies were utilised in both arms [58].

An adaptation to the use of PCV in ALI/ARDS patients has involved employing an inspiratory time that is longer than the expiratory time in order to increase the mean airway pressure ($\bar{P}$aw), and thereby improve arterial oxygenation. This is called pressure-controlled inverted ratio ventilation (PC-IRV). Early reports of this ventilatory approach following failure of VCV indicated reductions in peak airway pressures, improvement in arterial oxygenation at lower minute ventilation and lower PEEP requirements without any worsening of haemodynamic parameters [59–63]. Although less common, volume-controlled (VC)-IRV has also being utilised in ARDS patients [64, 65]. However, later studies did not demonstrate any significant benefit of PC-IRV over VCV in terms of arterial oxygenation, haemodynamic compromise or risk of barotraumas resulting from the elevated $\bar{P}$aw and intrinsic PEEP, and that often led to the increased use of sedative and paralytic agents [66–70]. Based on current evidence, IRV is of unproven benefit in the ventilatory management of ARDS patients [71, 72]. Airway pressure release ventilation (APRV), another ventilatory mode that uses long inspiratory times will be discussed in a subsequent section.

Positive end-expiratory pressure

The use of PEEP in addition to LPV is a vital element in the ventilatory management of ALI/ARDS patients. Low V_T ventilation can lead to alveolar de-recruitment, particularly if an inadequate level of PEEP is utilised [73, 74]. The resultant cyclic collapsing and re-opening of alveoli during tidal ventilation are known to contribute to the development of VILI [5, 6, 9, 75]; thus, avoiding this situation by the addition of the necessary amount of PEEP to keep the lung open is essential in limiting its development [6, 76, 77]. Furthermore, the addition of PEEP results in enhanced oxygenation and the subsequent reduction in F_{I,O_2} requirements, believed to result from different mechanisms, namely, recruitment of alveoli, increased functional residual capacity, extravascular lung water redistribution and improvement in ventilation–perfusion matching [21, 78]. In addition, rescue therapies for severe hypoxaemia, such as inhaled nitric oxide, prone positioning, high frequency oscillation and extracorporeal membrane oxygenation, were used less frequently in some studies [57, 79]. Conversely, high levels of PEEP may result in a reduction in venous return and impairment in the right ventricle, ultimately leading to decreased cardiac output [80, 81]. However, the manner in which PEEP is selected has varied and the level required optimising its benefits while maintaining LPV has been the subject of multiple studies.

Several methods have been used to select the level of PEEP required in the ventilatory management of ALI/ARDS patients (table 2). The use of a table of F_{I,O_2}–PEEP combinations has commonly been used to select the level of PEEP required based on oxygenation targets ($Pa_{,O_2}$ 55–80 mmHg) [14, 57, 83]. Increases in these combinations are performed to maintain the oxygenation target, while also ensuring airway pressure limits are not exceeded i.e. $P_{plat} \leqslant 30$ cmH$_2$O. In contrast, regardless of its effect on oxygenation, MERCAT et al. [79] individually titrated PEEP to a level that did not exceed a P_{plat} of 28–30 cmH$_2$O. A decremental approach has been used by some authors, in which PEEP is set to $\geqslant 20$ cmH$_2$O, subsequently, stepwise decreases are made to identify the level that results in the best $Pa_{,O_2}$ and compliance [84, 85]. The pressure–volume (PV) curve has been used to assess the lower and upper inflection points (LIP and UIP, respectively) on the inspiratory limb of the curve to guide the level of PEEP and inflation pressure required [12, 13, 18]. The level of PEEP is usually set slightly higher than the LIP (e.g. 2–3 cmH$_2$O higher) [12, 13, 18]. GRASSO et al. [86] employed the stress index (SI) to determine the level of PEEP by using the pressure–time curve during constant-flow inhalation, i.e. tidal volume delivery. An SI >1 (upward sloping concave curve) represents overdistension, i.e. excessive PEEP, an SI <1 (downward sloping concave curve) represents ongoing recruitment, i.e. inadequate PEEP, and an SI equal to 1 (linear slope) represents no ongoing recruitment or overdistension i.e. adequate PEEP (fig. 2) [86, 87]. Finally, the use of an oesophageal balloon (fig. 3) to measure the

Table 2. Methods for selecting positive end-expiratory pressure (PEEP)

Method	Description
Incremental PEEP using empirical table	Combinations of F_{I,O_2} and PEEP are utilised to attain the desired oxygenation level or highest compliance
Incremental PEEP using P_{plat}	PEEP is individually titrated to a level such that P_{plat} is <30 cmH$_2$O
Decremental PEEP	A high level of PEEP is set (e.g. 20 cmH$_2$O); subsequently PEEP is decreased in a stepwise manner until de-recruitment takes place, typically with a decrease in $Pa_{,O_2}$ and compliance
Stress index measurement	Pressure–time curve is monitored during constant-flow inhalation for indications of tidal recruitment and over distension
Oesophageal pressure measurement	Intrapleural pressure is estimated by using an oesophageal balloon to measure oesophageal pressure; subsequently, the optimal PEEP level required is determined
Pressure–volume curve guidance	PEEP is set slightly higher than the lower inflection point

P_{plat}: plateau pressure; F_{I,O_2}: inspiratory oxygen fraction; $Pa_{,O_2}$: arterial oxygen tension. Reproduced from [82], with permission from the publisher.

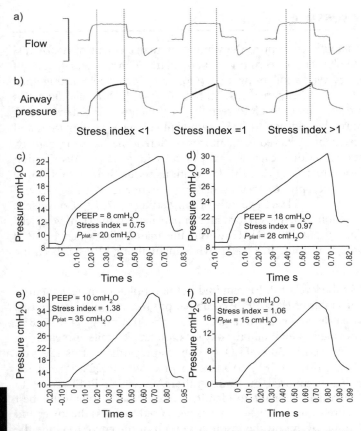

a)

Flow

b)

Airway pressure

Stress index <1   Stress index =1   Stress index >1

c)

Pressure cmH$_2$O

PEEP = 8 cmH$_2$O
Stress index = 0.75
P_{plat} = 20 cmH$_2$O

Time s

d)

Pressure cmH$_2$O

PEEP = 18 cmH$_2$O
Stress index = 0.97
P_{plat} = 28 cmH$_2$O

Time s

e)

Pressure cmH$_2$O

PEEP = 10 cmH$_2$O
Stress index = 1.38
P_{plat} = 35 cmH$_2$O

Time s

f)

Pressure cmH$_2$O

PEEP = 0 cmH$_2$O
Stress index = 1.06
P_{plat} = 15 cmH$_2$O

Time s

Figure 2. Stress index concept: a) flow and b) airway pressure *versus* time are demonstrated for three stress index concepts. The shape of the airway pressure waveform segment (bold lines) during constant-flow inflation of volume-cycled mechanical ventilation (·····) is used to determine the stress index. With a stress index <1, the airway pressure curve presents a downward concavity suggesting continuous decrease in elastance. With a stress index >1, the airway pressure curve presents an upward concavity suggesting continuous increase in elastance. With a stress index of 1, the airway pressure curve is straight, suggesting the absence of tidal variations in elastance. c–f) Stress index measurements in a patient with acute respiratory distress syndrome (ARDS). c, d) Early in the course of ARDS due to H1N1 infection. The stress index improves as positive end-expiratory pressure (PEEP) is increased. e, f) Late in the course of ARDS. The stress index improves as PEEP is decreased. a, c) Reproduced from [86] and c–f) reproduced from [87] with permission from the publisher.

oesophageal pressure and thereby estimate the intrapleural pressure has also been used to determine the optimal PEEP required [29, 30, 87]. Each of the aforementioned approaches has limitations, and there is currently no best method to selecting PEEP. Furthermore, most of the individualised approaches described can be technically challenging, consequently gas exchange targets using F_I,O_2–PEEP tables are more often clinically utilised to set PEEP.

Multiple randomised controlled studies (table 3) have been conducted to determine the optimal level of PEEP required in managing ALI/ARDS patients by comparing a lower/modest (conservative) *versus* a higher (aggressive) PEEP strategy, resulting in conflicting results [12, 13, 18, 30, 57, 79, 83]. Similarly, several meta-analyses of these studies (table 4) have been carried out to distinguish the outcomes in these patients when utilising a lower *versus* higher PEEP strategy, also resulting in varying results [20, 88–91]. Comparisons are challenging as the earlier studies [12, 13, 18] utilised ventilator strategies of high PEEP with low V_T against low PEEP with high V_T in ARDS patients, while the later studies [30, 57, 79, 83] compared high *versus* low PEEP with low V_T strategies in ALI/ARDS patients. In addition, different criteria were used for PEEP selection in the various aforementioned studies. Overall, there was a trend towards a mortality benefit in the high PEEP groups compared with the low PEEP groups in the different meta-analyses [20, 88–91]. In the only patient-level meta-analysis conducted using individual data from the three larger studies [91], as opposed to aggregated data used in other study-level meta-analyses [20, 88, 89], BRIEL *et al.* [91] concluded that although there was no overall difference in hospital mortality between the high and low PEEP groups, there was a significant reduction in mortality in the intensive care unit patients assigned to the high PEEP group. Furthermore, the subgroup of patients with ARDS at baseline had a reduced hospital mortality and were more likely to achieve liberation from ventilatory support earlier. Conversely, patients without ARDS at baseline who were assigned to the high PEEP group had a higher mortality risk. The authors conclude that higher levels of PEEP may be associated with reduction in hospital mortality in ARDS patients but may be detrimental to patients with less severe lung injury, *i.e.* ALI.

Although both the best strategy to determine PEEP and the most favourable level of PEEP required in the management of ALI/ARDS patients are unclear, it is vital to maintain the goals of LPV. High PEEP levels have been reported to result in lung overinflation in the caudal and non-dependent regions in ALI patients with a focal morphological pattern [92]. Similarly, as stated earlier, lung overinflation has been described in one-third of ARDS patients undergoing LPV with small, nondependent, normally aerated lung regions and large, dependent, nonaerated lung regions, resulting in the suggestion by the investigators of a more protective ventilator setting, *i.e.* Pplat <28 cmH$_2$O [28]. However, when determining the level of PEEP required, in order to avoid the development of VILI, it is important to consider both the potential for recruitment as well as the risk of alveolar overinflation, in addition to maintaining the goals of LPV [28, 92, 93].

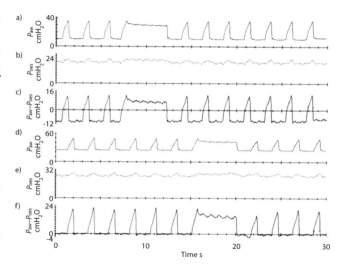

Figure 3. Positive end-expiratory pressure (PEEP) titration using oesophageal monitoring in a patient with morbid obesity. a) Oesophageal pressure (Poes), used as a surrogate for pleural pressure, is greater than the PEEP setting. b) The PEEP setting is increased so that the collapsing effect of the intrapleural pressure is offset. Although the plateau pressure is 40 cmH$_2$O, the alveolar distending pressure is only 14 cmH$_2$O. Paw: airway pressure. Reproduced from [87] with permission from the publisher.

Recruitment manoeuvres

A recruitment manoeuvre (RM) is a process whereby the reopening of collapsed alveoli occurs by means of a deliberate transient increase in the transpulmonary pressure, with the aim of improving gas exchange and respiratory mechanics [94–97]. As stated previously, in patients with ALI/ARDS, the use of LPV can result in alveolar collapse due to low VT [73, 74], and just like with PEEP, RMs have been utilised to open up collapsed lung [94]. However, there is currently no clear evidence demonstrating a beneficial clinical outcome with the use of RM in ALI/ARDS patients.

Various methods have been used to describe RMs [94, 96]. In a recent systematic review of 1,185 ALI/ARDS patients [94], the most frequently used methods were sustained inflation (45%), high PCV (23%), incremental PEEP (20%) and high VT/sigh (10%). The efficacy of sustained inflation, although the most commonly used RM, has been reported to be ineffective [98, 99], fleeting [100], coupled with haemodynamic impairment [101], associated with an increased risk of baro- and volutrauma [102], reduced net alveolar fluid clearance [103] and deterioration in oxygenation [104]. In a recent study [105], in contrast to the usual practice of applying a continuous pressure of 40 cmH$_2$O to the airways for up to 60 seconds, ARNAL *et al.* [105] demonstrated that most of the recruitment with sustained inflation occurs in the first 10 seconds in early-onset ARDS patients, subsequently followed by haemodynamic compromise after 10 seconds. In the corresponding article, it is suggested that sustained inflation should be abandoned for more effective RMs or, if utilised, should be closely monitored and applied for only a limited duration [106]. Some of these more effective techniques have recently been described and include [98]: 1) incremental increase in PEEP with limitation of the maximal inspiratory pressure [107]; 2) protracted lower pressure RM with elevation in PEEP of up to 15 cmH$_2$O and end-inspiratory pauses for 7 seconds twice a minute during a 15-minute period [108]; 3) PCV applied with increasing PEEP and constant driving pressure [99]; 4) intermittent sighs to reach a specific Pplat with either VCV or PCV [109]; and 5) a long slow increase in inspiratory pressure up to 40 cmH$_2$O [110]. The superiority of one method over the other remains undecided, and similarly the most favourable pressure, duration and regularity of RMs required is yet to be determined.

Table 3. Randomised controlled trials of high *versus* low positive end-expiratory pressure (PEEP) strategy

	First author [ref.]	Patients n	Intervention — High PEEP group	Intervention — Low PEEP group	Mortality %
High PEEP + low VT *versus* low PEEP + high VT	AMATO [13]	53	PEEP: 16.3 ± 0.7 cmH$_2$O VT: 6 mL·kg^{-1} Pplat: 31.8 ± 1.4 cmH$_2$O	PEEP: 6.9 ± 0.8 cmH$_2$O VT: 12 mL·kg^{-1} Pplat: 34.4 ± 1.9 cmH$_2$O	38 *versus* 71[#] (p<0.001) 45 *versus* 71[¶] (p=0.37)
	RANERI [18]	37	PEEP: 14.8 ± 2.7 cmH$_2$O VT: 7.6 ± 1.1 mL·kg^{-1} Pplat: 24.6 ± 2.4 cmH$_2$O	PEEP: 6.5 ± 1.7 cmH$_2$O VT: 11.1 ± 1.9 mL·kg^{-1} Pplat: 31.0 ± 4.5 cmH$_2$O	38 *versus* 58[#] (p=0.19)
	VILLAR [12]	95	PEEP: 14.1 ± 2.8 cmH$_2$O VT: 7.3 ± 0.9 mL·kg^{-1} Pplat: 30.6 ± 6.0 cmH$_2$O	PEEP: 9.0 ± 2.7 cmH$_2$O VT: 10.2 ± 1.2 mL·kg^{-1} Pplat: 32.6 ± 6.2 cmH$_2$O	32 *versus* 53.3[+] (p=0.040) 34 *versus* 55.5[¶] (p=0.041)
High PEEP + low VT *versus* low PEEP + low VT	BROWER [82]	549	PEEP: 14.7 ± 3.5 cmH$_2$O VT: 6.0 ± 0.9 mL·kg^{-1} Pplat: 27 ± 6 cmH$_2$O	PEEP: 8.9 ± 3.5 cmH$_2$O VT: 6.1 ± 0.8 mL·kg^{-1} Pplat: 24 ± 7 cmH$_2$O	25.1 *versus* 27.5[¶] (p=0.48)
	MERCAT [79]	767	PEEP: 14.6 ± 3.2 cmH$_2$O VT: 6.1 ± 0.3 mL·kg^{-1} Pplat: 27.5 ± 2.4 cmH$_2$O	PEEP: 7.1 ± 1.8 cm H$_2$O VT: 6.1 ± 0.4 mL·kg^{-1} Pplat: 21.1 ± 4.7 cmH$_2$O	27.8 *versus* 31.2[#] (p=0.31) 35.9 *versus* 39.5[¶] (p=0.31)
	MEADE [57]	983	PEEP: 15.6 ± 3.9 cmH$_2$O VT: 6.8 ± 1.4 mL·kg^{-1} Pplat: 30.2 ± 6.3 cmH$_2$O	PEEP: 10.1 ± 3.0 cmH$_2$O VT: 6.8 ± 1.3 mL·kg^{-1} Pplat: 24.9 ± 5.1 cmH$_2$O	36.4 *versus* 40.4[¶] (p=0.19) 28.4 *versus* 32.3[#] (p=0.20)
	TALMOR [30]	61	PEEP: 17 ± 6 cmH$_2$O VT: 7.1 ± 1.3 mL·kg^{-1} Pplat: 28 ± 7 cmH$_2$O	PEEP: 10 ± 4 cmH$_2$O VT: 6.8 ± 1 mL·kg^{-1} Pplat: 25 ± 6 cmH$_2$O	17 *versus* 39[#] (p=0.055)

Data for intervention were obtained on day 1, except for the study by TALMOR [30] when the data were obtained on day 3. VT: tidal volume; Pplat: plateau pressure. [#]: 28-day mortality; [¶]: hospital mortality; [+]: ICU mortality.

In the aforementioned review [94], an improvement in oxygenation was also reported following the RMs (Pa,O$_2$ 106 *versus* 193 mmHg (p=0.001) and Pa,O$_2$/FI,O$_2$ ratio 139 *versus* 251 mmHg (p<0.001)), although a rapid decline in the oxygenation benefits was reported to occur, sometimes within 15 to 20 minutes of the RM. Conversely, studies that have utilised a decremental PEEP strategy following an RM have sustained oxygenation benefits for up to 4–6 hours [83, 111], thus suggesting that the utilisation of higher PEEP levels after an RM may influence the sustainability of the effect. The timing of an RM also appears to play a role such that the longer the duration of ALI/ARDS, the less likely a beneficial effect will be derived [73, 112, 113]. GRASSO *et al.* [112] studied ARDS patients being ventilated with the ARDSnet strategy and demonstrated a response to a RM in those patients who received RM early, *i.e.* mean ± SD 1 ± 0.3 days, as opposed to no response in those who received it late, *i.e.* 7 ± 1 days. In the study by GATTINONI *et al.* [113], limited benefit was derived from an RM; however, the average duration of mechanical ventilation prior to recruitment was 5±6 days. Again, no significant improvement in oxygenation occurred in the study by VILLAGRA *et al.* [99] in both the early (ventilation <3 days) ARDS group as opposed to the late (ventilation >7 days) ARDS group, although oxygenation improvement in the latter group was less responsive to RMs than in the former group. However, baseline PEEP levels in the early and late ARDS groups were 14±1.3 and 15±1.9 cmH$_2$O, respectively [99]. Consequently, it was suggested that no benefit may be obtained from RMs if the lung has been optimally recruited from the level of PEEP applied [99]. Further modalities that are being employed to determine the potential for response to an RM include, pressure–volume curves by evaluating hysteresis [114], lung ultrasound [115, 116], electrical impedance tomography [117, 118] and computed tomography scan of the chest (not available at bedside) to determine lung morphology, *i.e.* focal, patchy or diffuse lung densities [113, 119].

Table 4. Meta-analyses of high *versus* low positive end-expiratory pressure (PEEP) strategy

Meta-analysis	RCT	Patients n	Summary of results

OBA [90]	A, C, D–F	2447	Small but significantly decreased hospital mortality with high PEEP[#]
			   RR 0.89; 95% CI 0.80–0.99; p=0.03[¶]
			Trend toward decreased 28-day mortality with high PEEP[#]
			   RR 0.88, 95% CI 0.76–1.01; p=0.06[+]
			No significant difference in incidence of barotraumas
			   OR 1.19, 95% CI 0.89–1.58; p=0.25
			No difference in ICU-free, ventilator-free and organ failure-free days
			Benefits of high PEEP are higher in patients with higher ICU severity scores

PHEONIX [89]	A–F	2484	Significantly decreased early and hospital mortality with high PEEP[#]
			   RR 0.87, 95% CI 0.78–0.96; p=0.007 (A – F)[§]
			   RR 0.87, 95% CI 0.77–0.97; p=0.0199 (A, C – F)[¶]
			In the three larger studies: trend towards decreased mortality in high PEEP[#]
			   RR 0.90, 95% CI 0.81–1.01; p=0.077 (D – F)[¶]
			No significant difference in incidence of barotraumas in all five trials,
			   but trend towards increased risk in three large trials with high PEEP[#]
			   RR 0.95, 95% CI 0.62–1.45; p=0.81 (A, C, D – F)
			   RR 1.17, 95% CI 0.90 1.52; p=0.25 (D – F)

PUTENSEN [20]	A, C, D–F	2447	No significant difference in hospital mortality or barotrauma
			   in studies D–F (lower Vt) with high PEEP[#]
			   OR 0.86, 95% CI 0.72–1.02; p=0.08[¶]
			   OR 1.19, 95% CI 0.89–1.58; p=0.25
			High PEEP reduced need of rescue therapy for life-threatening hypoxaemia and
			   reduced mortality in those patients receiving rescue therapy in studies E and F
			   OR 0.51, 95% CI 0.36–0.71; p<0.001
			   OR 0.51, 95% CI 0.36–0.71; p<0.001
			Decreased mortality and barotraumas with high PEEP in studies A and C[#]
			   OR 0.38, 95% CI 0.20–0.75; p=0.005[¶]
			   OR 0.20, 95% CI 0.06–0.63; p=0.006

BRIEL [91]	D–F	2299	No difference in hospital mortality between high *versus* low PEEP
			   (32.9% *versus* 35.2%)
			   RR 0.94, 95% CI 0.86–1.04; p=0.25[¶]
			Decreased ICU mortality with high PEEP (28.5% *versus* 32.8%)
			   RR 0.87, 95% CI 0.78–0.97; p=0.01[ƒ]
			High PEEP resulted in decreased hospital mortality in patients with ARDS
			   at baseline 34.1% *versus* 39.1%) but non-significant increase in patients
			   without ARDS at baseline (27.2% *versus* 19.4%)
			   RR 0.90, 95% CI 0.81–1.00; p=0.049[¶]
			   RR 1.37, 95% CI 0.98–1.92; p=0.07[¶]
			Increased ventilator-free days in ARDS patients with high PEEP (64.3%
			   versus 57.8% at 28 days), but decreased in non-ARDS patients (70.1%
			   versus 80.9%)
			   HR 1.16, 95% CI 1.03–1.30; p=0.01
			   HR 0.79, 95% CI 0.62–0.99; p=0.04
			Reduced use of rescue therapy or death following rescue therapy
			   with high PEEP
			   RR 0.64, 95% CI 0.54–0.75; p<0.001
			   RR 0.65, 95% CI 0.52–0.80; p<0.001
			No difference in incidence of barotraumas or vasopressor use
			   RR 1.19, 95% CI 0.89 .60; p=0.24
			   RR 0.93, 95% CI 0.75 .14; p=0.49

DASENBROOK [88]	D–G	2360	Non-significant 28-day mortality trend favouring high PEEP (27%
			   versus 30%), but no difference in hospital mortality[#]
			   RR 0.90, 95% CI 0.79–1.02 (D –G)[+]
			   RR 0.94, 95% CI 0.84–1.05; p=0.25 (D – F)[¶]
			Non-significant increase in barotraumas in high PEEP (9% *versus* 8%)[#]
			   RR 1.17, 95% CI 0.90–1.52

RCT: randomised controlled trials; ICU: intensive care unit; Vt: tidal volume; ARDS: acute respiratory distress syndrome. A: AMATO *et al.* [13]; B: RANIERI *et al.* [18]; C: VILLAR *et al.* [12]; D: BROWER *et al.* [83]; E: MERCAT *et al.* [79]; F: MEADE *et al.* [57]; G: TALMOR *et al.* [30]. [#]: pooled analysis; [¶]: hospital mortality; [+]: 28-day mortality; [§]: early mortality *i.e.* hospital plus 28-day mortality; [ƒ]: ICU mortality.

Patients occasionally require sedation and/or neuromuscular blockade during the utilisation of RMs. The most concerning complications that have been described are haemodynamic compromise and barotrauma. In their systemic review of RM, FAN *et al.* [94] reported the most common complications as being hypotension (10%) and desaturation (8%), with the more severe complications of barotraumas (1%) and arrhythmias (1%) being relatively rare. Consequently, the presence of clinical situations, such as haemodynamic compromise and barotrauma in ALI/ARDS patients, should preclude the use of RMs [120].

Current evidence suggests that the indiscriminate use of RMs in unselected ALI/ARDS patients may be non-beneficial. No prospective study has demonstrated a favourable clinical outcome. Considering its minimal risk for harm as well as the possibility for improvement in oxygenation, RMs may be considered on an individual basis in ALI/ARDS patients with life-threatening hypoxaemia with non-aerated lung zones, to aid in determining the appropriate level of PEEP required and also to recruit lungs that have undergone interventions associated with de-recruitment such as endotracheal suctioning or ventilator disconnections [94, 96, 121, 122].

Airway pressure release ventilation

APRV is a pressure-limited, time-cycled ventilatory approach that utilises a high continuous airway pressure level (Phigh) with a periodic pressure release to a lower airway pressure level (Plow), while simultaneously permitting patients to take spontaneous breaths at any point of the ventilator cycle (fig. 4) [123, 124]. Different time ratios for Phigh to Plow have been utilised with APRV, ranging from 1:1 to 9:1 in different studies [125, 126]. Optimising the time spent at Phigh, *i.e.* Thigh, potentially ensures adequate alveolar recruitment occurs, which in addition to the F_{I,O_2}, can determine and improve the level of oxygenation. The periodicity and usually short duration of the pressure release to Plow, together with the patient's ability to breathe spontaneously, determine the level of alveolar ventilation that takes place. Consequently, the VT generated is a function of the lung compliance, airway resistance, periodicity and duration of the pressure release phase [127]. The patient's spontaneous breathing can occur throughout the ventilator cycle as a result of an active exhalation valve; however, it tends to occur more frequently during Phigh which usually represents 80–95% of the ventilator cycle, as opposed to Plow which tends to last for 0.2–0.8 seconds in adults [128]. This short duration during Plow, *i.e.* Tlow, can result in an incomplete expiration resulting in the development of auto-PEEP from trapped gas volume [125].This is occasionally permitted to occur, particularly if the approach to APRV being used sets Plow at 0 cmH$_2$O, so as to prevent de-recruitment [128]. Notably, in the absence of spontaneous breathing, APRV is functionally identical to PC-IRV. In contrast, because spontaneous breathing is preserved, the need for heavy sedation and paralysis is unlikely [129, 130]. A further benefit of the maintenance of spontaneous breathing in APRV, particularly in ALI/ARDS patients, is the resultant diaphragmatic contractions that take place. In conventional mechanical ventilation, such as in VCV and PCV, diaphragmatic contraction is absent in fully ventilated patients. In addition, the dependent (dorsal) regions of the lung are inadequately ventilated in the supine patient. However, spontaneous breathing during APRV leads to recruitment of these dependent, juxtadiaphragmatic lung regions, thereby improving ventilation–perfusion matching, reducing intrapulmonary shunt, enhancing oxygenation and potentially reducing the likelihood of VILI [130–133]. However, care must be taken as spontaneous breaths during Phigh can potentially produce negative pleural pressures that add to the VT being generated by the ventilator, resulting in over-distension and subsequent volutrauma (fig. 4). Similarly, de-recruitment and subsequent atelectrauma can develop if Tlow is not sufficiently short in duration [128].

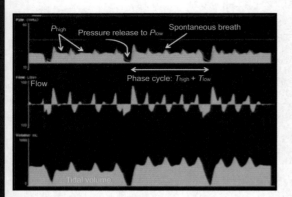

Figure 4. Airway pressure release ventilation in a spontaneously breathing patient. Airway pressure, flow and tidal volume are displayed during airway pressure release ventilation. Spontaneous breaths are seen occurring at Phigh, followed by a pressure release to Plow. The corresponding effect of spontaneous breaths during Phigh are seen on the tidal volumes generated (Thigh and Tlow), underscoring the possible risk of overinflation.

There are a small number of clinical studies evaluating the use the APRV in ALI/ARDS patients. In comparison to other forms of mechanical ventilation (*e.g.* synchronised intermittent mechanical ventilation (SIMV), PCV, VC-IRV, PC-IRV), some crossover studies have reported lower peak airway pressure requirements, less need for sedation or paralysis and improved oxygenation [129, 134–137]. A few moderately sized RCTs have also been performed with APRV [130, 138–140]. PUTENSEN *et al.* [130] randomised 30 multiple trauma patients who had or were at risk for developing ALI/ARDS to APRV *versus* PCV. The use of APRV resulted in increased lung compliance and oxygenation, as well as a reduction in the duration of ventilator support (15 *versus* 21 days), intensive care unit stay (23 *versus* 30 days) and less sedation and vasopressor requirements. However, these results are questionable because patients in the PCV group were initially paralysed for 72 hours. VARPULA *et al.* [139] initially randomised 45 ALI patients within 72 hours of mechanical ventilation to APRV *versus* pressure-controlled SIMV with pressure support (SIMV-PC/PS) in order to evaluate the effect of prone positioning on these ventilator strategies. The procedure for prone positioning was identical in both groups, and 33 out of the 45 patients who underwent prone positioning were analysed. Oxygenation was significantly improved in the APRV group following randomisation ($P_{a,O_2}/F_{I,O_2}$ 162 *versus* 123 mmHg; p=0.02) and this was further enhanced following two 6-hour sessions of prone positioning ($P_{a,O_2}/F_{I,O_2}$ 216 *versus* 180 mmHg; p=0.02). Sedation and analgesia requirements, incidence of adverse events and 28-day mortality were similar in both groups. In a subsequent RCT performed by the same investigators [140], 58 ALI patients were randomised to APRV *versus* SIMV-PC/PS. As in the previous study [139], it preceded the publication of the ARDSnet study [14], so liberal V_T (8–10 mL·kg^{-1}) was utilised in the ventilation protocol. However, this study was terminated early for futility after enrolling just 58 of the targeted 80 patients. There were no significant differences in ventilator-free days, sedation and analgesia requirements, as well as 28-day and 1-year mortality. In a recent randomised trial of 63 trauma patients (40% of them had ALI/ARDS) [138], APRV was compared to low V_T ventilation using volume-control SIMV with pressure support (SIMV-VC/PS). The results demonstrated a similar safety profile in both groups; however, there was a nonsignificant trend towards an increase in ventilator days (10.49 ± 7.23 *versus* 8.00 ± 4.01 days), intensive care unit length of stay (16.47 ± 12.83 *versus* 14.18 ± 13.26 days) and ventilator-associated pneumonia in the APRV group. Notably, low V_T ventilation was performed using SIMV-VC/PS instead of VCV which was in the ARDSnet study [14].

APRV is an alternative mode of mechanical ventilation that has potential benefits of lung recruitment, oxygenation and sedation requirements, and is being increasingly used as a primary ventilator strategy, as well as a rescue modality in ALI/ARDS patients. However, properly designed and powered RCTs are required to determine any potential outcome benefits with the use of APRV and thereby elucidate its precise role in the ventilatory management of ALI/ARDS patients. A concern with APRV is that at P_{high}, in an actively breathing patient, alveolar overdistension may occur. The mechanism is one of reduced pleural pressures during patient's inspiratory effort. This is especially true if the spontaneous breaths are supported by pressure support ventilation or automatic tube compensation.

High-frequency ventilation

High-frequency ventilation (HFV) can be broadly defined as a mechanical ventilatory strategy that utilises respiratory rates >100 breaths per minute in conjunction with the generation of small V_T, usually smaller than traditional estimations of both anatomical and physiological dead space, and ranging from ~1–5 mL·kg^{-1} [141, 142]. Different forms of HFV exist and include high-frequency oscillatory ventilation (HFOV), high-frequency percussive ventilation (HFPV), high-frequency positive pressure ventilation and high-frequency jet ventilation. The two forms of HFV that will be discussed in more detail are HFOV and HFPV. HFOV is more commonly described in ARDS compared to HFPV. Both modes, in theory, meet the goals of LPV from the generation of small V_T and constant lung recruitment [143]. Unlike in conventional ventilation where gas transport takes place by bulk delivery of gas, additional theoretical mechanisms believed to enhance gas exchange in these forms of HFV have been described in the literature and include: asymmetric velocity profiles, longitudinal (Taylor) dispersion, pendelluft, cardiogenic mixing and molecular diffusion [141, 144–146]. However, none of the forms of HFV have demonstrated clinical outcome benefit. Nonetheless,

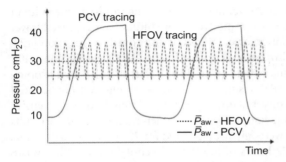

Figure 5. Schematic representation of perceived waveforms of high-frequency oscillatory ventilation (HFOV) and conventional pressure-controlled ventilation (PCV) in the distal airways. Large oscillatory pressure swings above and below a constant mean airway pressure ($\bar{P}$aw) are present at the proximal airways during HFOV, but are significantly reduced by the time the distal airways/alveoli are reached. The $\bar{P}$aw in HFOV tend to be higher than that in conventional ventilation contributing thereby to recruitment and increased oxygenation. Reproduced from [149] with permission from the publisher.

they both have been used as rescue modalities in ALI/ARDS patients with refractory/severe hypoxaemia.

High-frequency oscillatory ventilation

HFOV is characterised by the generation of small tidal volumes as a result of the oscillation of a bias gas flow resulting in pressure swings within the airway at frequencies ranging from 3 to 15 Hz (usually 3–6 Hz in adults) [147]. The oscillations are produced by an oscillatory diaphragm/piston pump, and result in an active inspiratory and expiratory phase. The rapid oscillations of gas are delivered at pressures above and below a constant $\bar{P}$aw which, in addition to F_I,O_2, determine the level of oxygenation. The $\bar{P}$aw at the outset is usually set approximately 5 cmH$_2$O above that obtained with conventional ventilation; however, the oscillatory pressure swings, which may be significant in the proximal airways, are substantially attenuated by the time the distal airways/alveoli are reached (fig. 5), resulting in the small VT [147, 148]. Ventilation, however, is directly related to the pressure amplitude of oscillation, *i.e.* degree of displacement by the oscillatory diaphragm/piston pump, but inversely related to the set frequency [149]. The combined effects of a high $\bar{P}$aw and small VT potentially result in improved recruitment of alveoli associated with a reduced risk of overdistension, thereby improving gas exchange and maintaining the goal of lung protection.

The majority of evidence associated with the use of HFOV in adults has been small observational (retrospective and prospective) studies in patients with refractory hypoxaemia or severe ARDS usually failing conventional ventilation [150–160]. These studies demonstrated that HFOV improved oxygenation without haemodynamic compromise, was safe and effective in patients failing conventional ventilation, was more likely to be beneficial if used early in the course of ARDS, and that failure to improve oxygenation was associated with high mortality. However, in several of these observational studies a high percentage of patients received sedation and paralysis [151, 153, 155–161]. To further improve gas exchange, HFOV has also been used in conjunction with RMs [152], prone positioning [162] and inhaled nitric oxide [161]. Other studies have been performed that have compared HFOV (occasionally in combination with other therapy) to conventional ventilation as the primary ventilatory strategy in ALI/ARDS, rather than as rescue therapy in refractory hypoxaemia. In the largest of the RCTs, DERDAK *et al.* [163] randomised 148 adult ARDS patients to HFOV *versus* conventional ventilation (PCV at 6–10 mL·kg^{-1} actual body weight), to compare safety and effectiveness. The applied $\bar{P}$aw was significantly higher in the HFOV group, and an early augmentation in the $P_a,O_2/F_I,O_2$ ratio was also seen. However, this did not continue beyond 24 hours. Furthermore, when comparing both the HFOV and conventional ventilation groups, there was no significant difference in terms of 30-day mortality (37 *versus* 52%; p=0.102), haemodynamic parameters, oxygenation and ventilation failure, barotraumas or mucus plugging. This study, in addition to being designed prior to the publication of the ARDSnet study [14], did not utilise 6 mL·kg^{-1} or lower VT in the control group and was not powered to evaluate mortality. BOLLEN *et al.* [164] similarly compared safety and effectiveness between HFOV and conventional ventilation (PCV) in 61 adult ARDS patients. There was no significant difference between both groups in terms of cumulative survival without oxygenation dependency or being on ventilatory support at 30 days (primary end-point), in addition there was no difference in mortality, therapy failure or cross-over rates of treatment arms. This study was, however, stopped early due to low patient recruitment which also contributed to an uneven randomisation of patients. Nonetheless, *post hoc* analysis suggested that HFOV may be more beneficial in patients with a higher baseline oxygenation index ($\bar{P}_{aw} \times F_{I,O_2}/P_{a,O_2}$). In a Cochrane database systemic review of RCTs comparing treatment with HFOV *versus* conventional ventilation in children and adults with ALI/ARDS, only two RCTs met the inclusion criteria [165]. The authors surmised that there was insufficient data to conclude whether HFOV reduced mortality or long-term morbidity in ALI/ARDS patients. In a subsequent systemic review of 419 patients [143], HFOV was compared to conventional ventilation as a primary ventilatory strategy for ALI/ARDS patients in contrast to rescue treatment for refractory hypoxaemia. A majority of the patients from the reviewed trials were adults (80%). In contrast to the earlier systemic review [165], HFOV was reported to significantly reduce mortality at hospital discharge or 30 days (risk ratio 0.77, 95% CI 0.61–0.98; p=0.03), but this was stated to be based on relatively few patients and outcome events, with analysis demonstrating wide confidence intervals. There was also a decreased risk of treatment failure with HFOV, but no difference in duration of mechanical ventilation or ventilator-free days. HFOV was also reported to increase the $P_{a,O_2}/F_{I,O_2}$ ratio by 16–24% within the first 72 hours and increased $\bar{P}_{aw}$ by 23–33% in comparison to conventional ventilation. No differences in adverse events such as barotrauma, hypotension and endotracheal obstruction were reported. The authors conclude that HFOV may decrease mortality in ARDS patients compared with conventional ventilation and is unlikely to cause harm. However, completion of ongoing multicentre randomised trials (OSCILLATE trial: ISRCTN 87124254; and OSCAR trial: ISRCT N10416500) comparing HFOV to current conventional LPV should provide more definitive data with regards to mortality and safety [143].

High-frequency percussive ventilation

HFPV is a pressure-limited, flow-regulated and time-cycled ventilator mode that delivers a sequence of high-frequency (200–900 cycles per minute), small volumes in a consecutive stepwise stacking pattern, leading to the formation of low-frequency (up to 40–60 cycles per minute), convective, pressure-limited breathing cycles (fig. 6) [87, 166–168]. Gas exchange is a function of the percussion frequency, such that at high percussion frequencies (300–600 cycles per minute) oxygenation is augmented, while at low percussion frequencies, carbon dioxide clearance is augmented [87, 167, 169, 170]. The volumetric diffusive respirator is the only ventilator that provides HFPV and an interplay of its control variables, either individually or in combination, play a role in determining the $\bar{P}_{aw}$ and degree of gas exchange [87, 167, 169, 171–173].

There are a limited number of small studies on the use of HFPV in ALI/ARDS patients. GALLAGHER *et al.* [174]

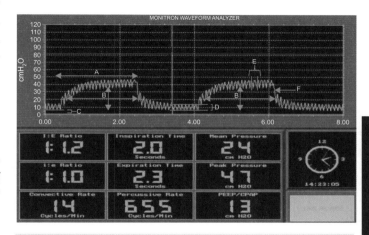

Figure 6. High-frequency percussive ventilation. An interplay of the percussive frequency, peak inspiratory pressure, inspiratory and expiratory times (of both percussive and convective breaths) and the oscillatory and demand continuous positive airway pressure (CPAP) levels either alone or in combination, are involved in determining mean arterial wedge pressure as well as the degree of gas exchange. The percussions are of lower amplitude at oscillatory CPAP (baseline oscillations) during exhalation, and are of higher amplitude during inspiration as a result of the selected pulsatile flow rate (see pressure-time display). During inspiration, the lung volumes progressively increase in a cumulative, stepwise manner by continually diminishing sub-tidal deliveries that result in stacking of breaths. Once an oscillatory pressure peak is reached and sustained, periodic programmed interruptions occur at specific times for predetermined intervals, allowing the return of airway pressures to baseline oscillatory pressure levels *i.e.* oscillatory CPAP, thereby passively emptying the lungs. A: pulsatile flow during inspiration at a percussive rate of 655 cycles·min^{-1}; B: convective pressure-limited breath with low-frequency cycle (14 cycles·min^{-1}); C: demand CPAP (provides static baseline pressure); D: oscillatory CPAP (provides high-frequency baseline pressure as a mean of the peak and nadir of the oscillations during exhalation); E: single percussive breath; F: periodic programmed interruptions signifying the end of inspiration and subsequent onset of exhalation. Reproduced from [87] with permission from the publisher.

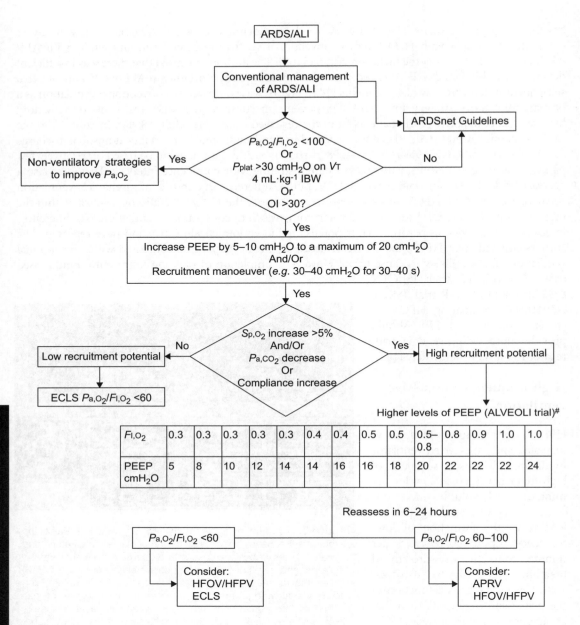

Figure 7. Ventilatory strategy algorithm for the management of acute respiratory distress syndrome (ARDS)/ acute lung injury (ALI) patients. The algorithm shows ventilator strategies that can be utilised in ARDS/ALI patients. The ARDSnet serves as the standard and the starting point. The other strategies can be employed following optimisation with the ARDSnet strategy. In patients with recruitable lungs, different methods can be used to determine the level of positive end-expiratory pressure (PEEP) required, such as higher levels of PEEP per the inspiratory oxygen fraction (F_{I,O_2})/PEEP table (PEEP may be set so as to reach a plateau pressure (P_{plat}) of 28–30 cmH$_2$O) use of oesophageal pressure monitoring or the stress index. V_T: tidal volume; IBW: ideal body weight; OI: oxygenation index; S_{p,O_2}: arterial oxygen saturation measured by pulse oximetry; P_{a,CO_2}: arterial carbon dioxide tension; ALVEOLI: Assessment of Low Tidal Volume and Elevated End-Expiratory Pressure to Obviate Lung Injury; ECLS: extracorporeal life support; HFOV: high-frequency oscillatory ventilation; APRV: airway pressure release ventilation; HFPV: high-frequency percussive ventilation. #: failure of the aforementioned can result in the use of the alternative ventilatory strategies in centres familiar with their use. Reproduced from [87] with permission from the publisher.

reported on seven ARDS patients who were switched from conventional ventilation to HFPV at the same level of airway pressure and F_{I,O_2}. There was a significant increase in P_{a,O_2}, a slight decrease in P_{a,CO_2} and no change in cardiac output. In an RCT comparing HFPV with conventional ventilation in 100 adult patients with acute respiratory failure, there was no difference between the two patient groups in the time it took to reach the therapeutic end-points of $P_{a,O_2}/F_{I,O_2}$ >225 mmHg or shunt <20%. However, in the subgroup of patients with ARDS, HFPV provided equivalent oxygenation and ventilation at significantly lower airway pressures. Nonetheless, there was no difference in mortality, intensive care unit days, hospital days or incidence of barotrauma. In two retrospective studies of ARDS patients failing conventional ventilation, HFPV was found to significantly improve oxygenation [172, 175]. In the former study [172], oxygenation is reported to have improved in association with a decreased peak inspiratory pressure but decreased $\bar{P}_{aw}$. However, in the latter study [175], improved oxygenation was not associated with an increase in $\bar{P}_{aw}$. The investigators suggest that other mechanisms of HFV may have contributed to the improvement in oxygenation. In a recent RCT, CHUNG et al. [168] compared HFPV with a low V_T ventilation-based strategy in 62 burns patients with respiratory failure. At baseline, 12 (39%) out of 31 of the patients in the HFPV group and 14 (45%) out of 31 of the patients in the low V_T group had ALI/ARDS. The investigators reported no significant difference between both groups in the primary outcome, i.e. mean ventilator-free days (12 ± 9 versus 11 ± 9 days). There was also no significant difference in secondary outcomes such as 28-day mortality, days free from non-pulmonary organ failure, ventilator-associated pneumonia and barotraumas. However, there was a significant difference in the need for a rescue modality as 29% (nine patients) of the low V_T group did not meet oxygenation and ventilation goals and were subsequently transitioned to a rescue mode as opposed to 6% (two patients) in the HFPV group. This was found to occur more commonly in the patients with inhalational injury. The investigators also reported the $P_{a,O_2}/F_{I,O_2}$ ratio was significantly higher in the HFPV group over the first week after randomisation in spite of equivalent $\bar{P}_{aw}$ and PEEP settings and lower peak inspiratory pressures in the HFPV group. There was also no significant difference in cytokine release between both groups over the first 7 days. The authors concluded by saying HFPV resulted in similar clinical outcomes when compared to a low V_T-based strategy.

No definitive conclusions can be made about the role of HFPV in the ventilatory management of ALI/ARDS patients. Oxygenation and ventilation improve at lower airway pressures in comparison to conventional ventilation; however, no mortality benefit has been demonstrated to date. Like the other alternative/rescue strategies that have been described, large RCTs are needed to accurately elucidate their role in the ventilatory management of ALI/ARDS patients.

Conclusions

A proposed algorithm to manage patients with severe hypoxaemic respiratory failure is depicted in figure 7. It is important to emphasise that patients with ARDS who are intubated and mechanically ventilated, should first be placed on low V_T lung protective strategy. In general, the patients are given V_T of 4–6 mL·kg^{-1} ideal body weight with adequate levels of PEEP. A vigilant eye is kept on the P_{plat}, with an endeavour to keep them <30 cmH$_2$O or as low as possible, ensuring adequate oxygenation. If within a reasonable period of time, usually a few hours, the end points of oxygenation or P_{plat} are not achieved, or if the patient demonstrates declining oxygenation or requires a PEEP of approximately >15 cmH$_2$O, the patient has a higher mortality and should be considered for rescue strategies. The first step may be to assess if the patient demonstrates alveolar recruitment in response to higher levels of PEEP. If so, a higher level of PEEP may be selected utilising different techniques outlined. However, if raising the level of PEEP does not improve oxygenation, or results in high P_{plat}, other rescue strategies may be utilised, including airway pressure release ventilation, HFOV and HFPV. In specialised centres where extra-corporeal membrane oxygenation may be available, such a mode may also be considered. It is important to point out that these modes have not been shown to reduce mortality. Selection of these modes should be based on availability and comfort of use of the operator. If these rescue modes are used, periodic assessment of end-points for their use should be checked.

Statement of interest

A. Esan has received consultancy fees from United Therapeutics Corporation. D. Hess is a consultant for Philips Respironics, ResMed, Breathe Technologies and Pari. He has also received honoraria from Covidien. S. Raoof received $1,000 from the ACCP for a postgraduate course that he had presented at the 2011 Chest meeting. He is in the process of donating the money to the Chest Foundation.

References

1. Bernard GR, Artigas A, Brigham KL, *et al.* The American-European Consensus Conference on ARDS. Definitions, mechanisms, relevant outcomes, and clinical trial coordination. *Am J Respir Crit Care Med* 1994; 149: 818–824.
2. Villar J, Perez-Mendez L, Lopez J, *et al.* An early PEEP/FIO2 trial identifies different degrees of lung injury in patients with acute respiratory distress syndrome. *Am J Respir Crit Care Med* 2007; 176: 795–804.
3. Ranieri M. Acute Respiratory Distress Syndrome (ARDS): The "Berlin Definition". European Society of Intensive Care Medicine, 24th Annual Congress. October 1–5, 2011. Available from: www.esicm.org/07-congresses/0A-annual-congress/webTv_ranieri.asp.
4. Gattinoni L, Caironi P, Pelosi P, *et al.* What has computed tomography taught us about the acute respiratory distress syndrome? *Am J Respir Crit Care Med* 2001; 164: 1701–1711.
5. Slutsky AS. Lung injury caused by mechanical ventilation. *Chest* 1999; 116: Suppl. 1, 9S–15S.
6. Muscedere JG, Mullen JB, Gan K, *et al.* Tidal ventilation at low airway pressures can augment lung injury. *Am J Respir Crit Care Med* 1994; 149: 1327–1334.
7. Dreyfuss D, Soler P, Basset G, *et al.* High inflation pressure pulmonary edema. Respective effects of high airway pressure, high tidal volume, and positive end-expiratory pressure. *Am Rev Respir Dis* 1988; 137: 1159–1164.
8. Tremblay LN, Slutsky AS. Ventilator-induced lung injury: from the bench to the bedside. *Intensive Care Med* 2006; 32: 24–33.
9. International consensus conferences in intensive care medicine: Ventilator-associated Lung Injury in ARDS. This official conference report was cosponsored by the American Thoracic Society, The European Society of Intensive Care Medicine, and The Societe de Reanimation de Langue Francaise, and was approved by the ATS Board of Directors, July 1999. *Am J Respir Crit Care Med* 1999; 160: 2118–2124.
10. Plotz FB, Slutsky AS, van Vught AJ, *et al.* Ventilator-induced lung injury and multiple system organ failure: a critical review of facts and hypotheses. *Intensive Care Med* 2004; 30: 1865–1872.
11. Ricard JD, Dreyfuss D, Saumon G. Production of inflammatory cytokines in ventilator-induced lung injury: a reappraisal. *Am J Respir Crit Care Med* 2001; 163: 1176–1180.
12. Villar J, Kacmarek RM, Perez-Mendez L, *et al.* A high positive end-expiratory pressure, low tidal volume ventilatory strategy improves outcome in persistent acute respiratory distress syndrome: a randomized, controlled trial. *Crit Care Med* 2006; 34: 1311–1318.
13. Amato MB, Barbas CS, Medeiros DM, *et al.* Effect of a protective-ventilation strategy on mortality in the acute respiratory distress syndrome. *N Engl J Med* 1998; 338: 347–354.
14. Ventilation with lower tidal volumes as compared with traditional tidal volumes for acute lung injury and the acute respiratory distress syndrome. The Acute Respiratory Distress Syndrome Network. *N Engl J Med* 2000; 342: 1301–1308.
15. Brower RG, Shanholtz CB, Fessler HE, *et al.* Prospective, randomized, controlled clinical trial comparing traditional *versus* reduced tidal volume ventilation in acute respiratory distress syndrome patients. *Crit Care Med* 1999; 27: 1492–1498.
16. Stewart TE, Meade MO, Cook DJ, *et al.* Evaluation of a ventilation strategy to prevent barotrauma in patients at high risk for acute respiratory distress syndrome. Pressure- and Volume-Limited Ventilation Strategy Group. *N Engl J Med* 1998; 338: 355–361.
17. Brochard L, Roudot-Thoraval F, Roupie E, *et al.* Tidal volume reduction for prevention of ventilator-induced lung injury in acute respiratory distress syndrome. The Multicenter Trail Group on Tidal Volume reduction in ARDS. *Am J Respir Crit Care Med* 1998; 158: 1831–1838.
18. Ranieri VM, Suter PM, Tortorella C, *et al.* Effect of mechanical ventilation on inflammatory mediators in patients with acute respiratory distress syndrome: a randomized controlled trial. *JAMA* 1999; 282: 54–61.
19. Wheeler AP, Bernard GR. Acute lung injury and the acute respiratory distress syndrome: a clinical review. *Lancet* 2007; 369: 1553–1564.
20. Putensen C, Theuerkauf N, Zinserling J, *et al.* Meta-analysis: ventilation strategies and outcomes of the acute respiratory distress syndrome and acute lung injury. *Ann Intern Med* 2009; 151: 566–576.
21. Yilmaz M, Gajic O. Optimal ventilator settings in acute lung injury and acute respiratory distress syndrome. *Eur J Anaesthesiol* 2008; 25: 89–96.
22. Moran JL, Bersten AD, Solomon PJ. Meta-analysis of controlled trials of ventilator therapy in acute lung injury and acute respiratory distress syndrome: an alternative perspective. *Intensive Care Med* 2005; 31: 227–235.

23. Eichacker PQ, Gerstenberger EP, Banks SM, *et al.* Meta-analysis of acute lung injury and acute respiratory distress syndrome trials testing low tidal volumes. *Am J Respir Crit Care Med* 2002; 166: 1510–1514.
24. Petrucci N, Iacovelli W. Ventilation with smaller tidal volumes: a quantitative systematic review of randomized controlled trials. *Anesth Analg* 2004; 99: 193–200.
25. Petrucci N, Iacovelli W. Lung protective ventilation strategy for the acute respiratory distress syndrome. *Cochrane Database Syst Rev* 2007; 3: CD003844.
26. Brower RG, Matthay M, Schoenfeld D. Meta-analysis of acute lung injury and acute respiratory distress syndrome trials. *Am J Respir Crit Care Med* 2002; 166: 1515–1517.
27. Hager DN, Krishnan JA, Hayden DL, *et al.* Tidal volume reduction in patients with acute lung injury when plateau pressures are not high. *Am J Respir Crit Care Med* 2005; 172: 1241–1245.
28. Terragni PP, Rosboch G, Tealdi A, *et al.* Tidal hyperinflation during low tidal volume ventilation in acute respiratory distress syndrome. *Am J Respir Crit Care Med* 2007; 175: 160–166.
29. Talmor D, Sarge T, O'Donnell CR, *et al.* Esophageal and transpulmonary pressures in acute respiratory failure. *Crit Care Med* 2006; 34: 1389–1394.
30. Talmor D, Sarge T, Malhotra A, *et al.* Mechanical ventilation guided by esophageal pressure in acute lung injury. *N Engl J Med* 2008; 359: 2095–2104.
31. Burns KE, Adhikari NK, Slutsky AS, *et al.* Pressure and volume limited ventilation for the ventilatory management of patients with acute lung injury: a systematic review and meta-analysis. *PLoS One,* 6: e14623.
32. Weinert CR, Gross CR, Marinelli WA. Impact of randomized trial results on acute lung injury ventilator therapy in teaching hospitals. *Am J Respir Crit Care Med* 2003; 167: 1304–1309.
33. Young MP, Manning HL, Wilson DL, *et al.* Ventilation of patients with acute lung injury and acute respiratory distress syndrome: has new evidence changed clinical practice? *Crit Care Med* 2004; 32: 1260–1265.
34. Rubenfeld GD, Cooper C, Carter G, *et al.* Barriers to providing lung-protective ventilation to patients with acute lung injury. *Crit Care Med* 2004; 32: 1289–1293.
35. Kalhan R, Mikkelsen M, Dedhiya P, *et al.* Underuse of lung protective ventilation: analysis of potential factors to explain physician behavior. *Crit Care Med* 2006; 34: 300–306.
36. Laffey JG, O'Croinin D, McLoughlin P, *et al.* Permissive hypercapnia-role in protective lung ventilatory strategies. *Intensive Care Med* 2004; 30: 347–356.
37. Hickling KG, Walsh J, Henderson S, *et al.* Low mortality rate in adult respiratory distress syndrome using low-volume, pressure-limited ventilation with permissive hypercapnia: a prospective study. *Crit Care Med* 1994; 22: 1568–1578.
38. Kahn JM, Andersson L, Karir V, *et al.* Low tidal volume ventilation does not increase sedation use in patients with acute lung injury. *Crit Care Med* 2005; 33: 766–771.
39. Bidani A, Tzouanakis AE, Cardenas VJ Jr, *et al.* Permissive hypercapnia in acute respiratory failure. *JAMA* 1994; 272: 957–962.
40. Cheng IW, Eisner MD, Thompson BT, *et al.* Acute effects of tidal volume strategy on hemodynamics, fluid balance, and sedation in acute lung injury. *Crit Care Med* 2005; 33: 63–70.
41. Hough CL, Kallet RH, Ranieri VM, *et al.* Intrinsic positive end-expiratory pressure in Acute Respiratory Distress Syndrome (ARDS) Network subjects. *Crit Care Med* 2005; 33: 527–532.
42. Esteban A, Ferguson ND, Meade MO, *et al.* Evolution of mechanical ventilation in response to clinical research. *Am J Respir Crit Care Med* 2008; 177: 170–177.
43. Checkley W, Brower R, Korpak A, *et al.* Effects of a clinical trial on mechanical ventilation practices in patients with acute lung injury. *Am J Respir Crit Care Med* 2008; 177: 1215–1222.
44. Herasevich V, Tsapenko M, Kojicic M, *et al.* Limiting ventilator-induced lung injury through individual electronic medical record surveillance. *Crit Care Med* 2011; 39: 34–39.
45. MacIntyre NR, Sessler CN. Are there benefits or harm from pressure targeting during lung-protective ventilation? *Respir Care,* 55: 175–180.
46. Haas CF. Mechanical ventilation with lung protective strategies: what works? *Crit Care Clin* 2011; 27: 469–486.
47. Davis K Jr, Branson RD, Campbell RS, *et al.* Comparison of volume control and pressure control ventilation: is flow waveform the difference? *J Trauma* 1996; 41: 808–814.
48. MacIntyre NR, McConnell R, Cheng KC, *et al.* Patient-ventilator flow dyssynchrony: flow-limited *versus* pressure-limited breaths. *Crit Care Med* 1997; 25: 1671–1677.
49. Cinnella G, Conti G, Lofaso F, *et al.* Effects of assisted ventilation on the work of breathing: volume-controlled *versus* pressure-controlled ventilation. *Am J Respir Crit Care Med* 1996; 153: 1025–1033.
50. Rappaport SH, Shpiner R, Yoshihara G, *et al.* Randomized, prospective trial of pressure-limited *versus* volume-controlled ventilation in severe respiratory failure. *Crit Care Med* 1994; 22: 22–32.
51. Yang LY, Huang YC, Macintyre NR. Patient-ventilator synchrony during pressure-targeted *versus* flow-targeted small tidal volume assisted ventilation. *J Crit Care* 2007; 22: 252–257.
52. Marini JJ. Point: is pressure assist-control preferred over volume assist-control mode for lung protective ventilation in patients with ARDS? Yes. *Chest* 2011; 140: 286–290.
53. Munoz J, Guerrero JE, Escalante JL, *et al.* Pressure-controlled ventilation *versus* controlled mechanical ventilation with decelerating inspiratory flow. *Crit Care Med* 1993; 21: 1143–1148.
54. Chiumello D, Pelosi P, Calvi E, *et al.* Different modes of assisted ventilation in patients with acute respiratory failure. *Eur Respir J* 2002; 20: 925–933.

55. Kallet RH, Campbell AR, Dicker RA, *et al.* Work of breathing during lung-protective ventilation in patients with acute lung injury and acute respiratory distress syndrome: a comparison between volume and pressure-regulated breathing modes. *Respir Care* 2005; 50: 1623–1631.

56. Schmidt UH, Hess DR. Does spontaneous breathing produce harm in patients with the acute respiratory distress syndrome? *Respir Care* 2010; 55: 784–786.

57. Meade MO, Cook DJ, Guyatt GH, *et al.* Ventilation strategy using low tidal volumes, recruitment maneuvers, and high positive end-expiratory pressure for acute lung injury and acute respiratory distress syndrome: a randomized controlled trial. *JAMA* 2008; 299: 637–645.

58. MacIntyre N. Counterpoint: is pressure assist-control preferred over volume assist-control mode for lung protective ventilation in patients with ARDS? No. *Chest* 2011; 140: 290–292.

59. Papadakos PJ, Halloran W, Hessney JI, *et al.* The use of pressure-controlled inverse ratio ventilation in the surgical intensive care unit. *J Trauma* 1991; 31: 1211–1214.

60. Abraham E, Yoshihara G. Cardiorespiratory effects of pressure controlled inverse ratio ventilation in severe respiratory failure. *Chest* 1989; 96: 1356–1359.

61. Gurevitch MJ, Van Dyke J, Young ES, *et al.* Improved oxygenation and lower peak airway pressure in severe adult respiratory distress syndrome. Treatment with inverse ratio ventilation. *Chest* 1986; 89: 211–213.

62. Tharratt RS, Allen RP, Albertson TE. Pressure controlled inverse ratio ventilation in severe adult respiratory failure. *Chest* 1988; 94: 755–762.

63. Lain DC, Di Benedetto R, Morris SL, *et al.* Pressure control inverse ratio ventilation as a method to reduce peak inspiratory pressure and provide adequate ventilation and oxygenation. *Chest* 1989; 95: 1081–1088.

64. Valta P, Takala J. Volume-controlled inverse ratio ventilation: effect on dynamic hyperinflation and auto-PEEP. *Acta Anaesthesiol Scand* 1993; 37: 323–328.

65. Cole AG, Weller SF, Sykes MK. Inverse ratio ventilation compared with PEEP in adult respiratory failure. *Intensive Care Med* 1984; 10: 227–232.

66. Zavala E, Ferrer M, Polese G, *et al.* Effect of inverse I:E ratio ventilation on pulmonary gas exchange in acute respiratory distress syndrome. *Anesthesiology* 1998; 88: 35–42.

67. Mancebo J, Vallverdu I, Bak E, *et al.* Volume-controlled ventilation and pressure-controlled inverse ratio ventilation: a comparison of their effects in ARDS patients. *Monaldi Arch Chest Dis* 1994; 49: 201–207.

68. Mercat A, Graini L, Teboul JL, *et al.* Cardiorespiratory effects of pressure-controlled ventilation with and without inverse ratio in the adult respiratory distress syndrome. *Chest* 1993; 104: 871–875.

69. Lessard MR, Guerot E, Lorino H, *et al.* Effects of pressure-controlled with different I:E ratios *versus* volume-controlled ventilation on respiratory mechanics, gas exchange, and hemodynamics in patients with adult respiratory distress syndrome. *Anesthesiology* 1994; 80: 983–991.

70. Mercat A, Titiriga M, Anguel N, *et al.* Inverse ratio ventilation (I/E=2/1) in acute respiratory distress syndrome: a six-hour controlled study. *Am J Respir Crit Care Med* 1997; 155: 1637–1642.

71. Duncan SR, Rizk NW, Raffin TA. Inverse ratio ventilation. PEEP in disguise? *Chest* 1987; 92: 390–392.

72. Shanholtz C, Brower R. Should inverse ratio ventilation be used in adult respiratory distress syndrome? *Am J Respir Crit Care Med* 1994; 149: 1354–1358.

73. Crotti S, Mascheroni D, Caironi P, *et al.* Recruitment and derecruitment during acute respiratory failure: a clinical study. *Am J Respir Crit Care Med* 2001; 164: 131–140.

74. Richard JC, Maggiore SM, Jonson B, *et al.* Influence of tidal volume on alveolar recruitment. Respective role of PEEP and a recruitment maneuver. *Am J Respir Crit Care Med* 2001; 163: 1609–1613.

75. Caironi P, Cressoni M, Chiumello D, *et al.* Lung opening and closing during ventilation of acute respiratory distress syndrome. *Am J Respir Crit Care Med* 2010; 181: 578–586.

76. Hemmila MR, Napolitano LM. Severe respiratory failure: advanced treatment options. *Crit Care Med* 2006; 34: Suppl. 9, S278–S290.

77. Ferguson ND, Frutos-Vivar F, Esteban A, *et al.* Airway pressures, tidal volumes, and mortality in patients with acute respiratory distress syndrome. *Crit Care Med* 2005; 33: 21–30.

78. Guerin C. The preventive role of higher PEEP in treating severely hypoxemic ARDS. *Minerva Anestesiol* 2011; 77: 835–845.

79. Mercat A, Richard JC, Vielle B, *et al.* Positive end-expiratory pressure setting in adults with acute lung injury and acute respiratory distress syndrome: a randomized controlled trial. *JAMA* 2008; 299: 646–655.

80. Schmitt JM, Vieillard-Baron A, Augarde R, *et al.* Positive end-expiratory pressure titration in acute respiratory distress syndrome patients: impact on right ventricular outflow impedance evaluated by pulmonary artery Doppler flow velocity measurements. *Crit Care Med* 2001; 29: 1154–1158.

81. Jardin F, Vieillard-Baron A. Right ventricular function and positive pressure ventilation in clinical practice: from hemodynamic subsets to respirator settings. *Intensive Care Med* 2003; 29: 1426–1434.

82. Esan A, Hess DR, Raoof S, *et al.* Severe hypoxemic respiratory failure: part 1– ventilatory strategies. *Chest* 2010; 137: 1203–1216.

83. Brower RG, Lanken PN, MacIntyre N, *et al.* Higher *versus* lower positive end-expiratory pressures in patients with the acute respiratory distress syndrome. *N Engl J Med* 2004; 351: 327–336.

84. Girgis K, Hamed H, Khater Y, *et al.* A decremental PEEP trial identifies the PEEP level that maintains oxygenation after lung recruitment. *Respir Care* 2006; 51: 1132–1139.

85. Badet M, Bayle F, Richard JC, *et al.* Comparison of optimal positive end-expiratory pressure and recruitment maneuvers during lung-protective mechanical ventilation in patients with acute lung injury/acute respiratory distress syndrome. *Respir Care* 2009; 54: 847–854.

86. Grasso S, Stripoli T, De Michele M, *et al.* ARDSnet ventilatory protocol and alveolar hyperinflation: role of positive end-expiratory pressure. *Am J Respir Crit Care Med* 2007; 176: 761–767.

87. Hess DR. Approaches to conventional mechanical ventilation of the patient with acute respiratory distress syndrome. *Respir Care* 2011; 56: 1555–1572.

88. Dasenbrook EC, Needham DM, Brower RG, *et al.* Higher PEEP in patients with acute lung injury: a systematic review and meta-analysis. *Respir Care* 2011; 56: 568–575.

89. Phoenix SI, Paravastu S, Columb M, *et al.* Does a higher positive end expiratory pressure decrease mortality in acute respiratory distress syndrome? A systematic review and meta-analysis. *Anesthesiology* 2009; 110: 1098–1105.

90. Oba Y, Thameem DM, Zaza T. High levels of PEEP may improve survival in acute respiratory distress syndrome: a meta-analysis. *Respir Med* 2009; 103: 1174–1181.

91. Briel M, Meade M, Mercat A, *et al.* Higher *vs* lower positive end-expiratory pressure in patients with acute lung injury and acute respiratory distress syndrome: systematic review and meta-analysis. *JAMA* 2010; 303: 865–873.

92. Nieszkowska A, Lu Q, Vieira S, *et al.* Incidence and regional distribution of lung overinflation during mechanical ventilation with positive end-expiratory pressure. *Crit Care Med* 2004; 32: 1496–1503.

93. Grasso S, Fanelli V, Cafarelli A, *et al.* Effects of high *versus* low positive end-expiratory pressures in acute respiratory distress syndrome. *Am J Respir Crit Care Med* 2005; 171: 1002–1008.

94. Fan E, Wilcox ME, Brower RG, *et al.* Recruitment maneuvers for acute lung injury: a systematic review. *Am J Respir Crit Care Med* 2008; 178: 1156–1163.

95. Hess DR, Bigatello LM. Lung recruitment: the role of recruitment maneuvers. *Respir Care* 2002; 47: 308–317.

96. Lapinsky SE, Mehta S. Bench-to-bedside review: recruitment and recruiting maneuvers. *Crit Care* 2005; 9: 60–65.

97. Rocco PR, Pelosi P, de Abreu MG. Pros and cons of recruitment maneuvers in acute lung injury and acute respiratory distress syndrome. *Expert Rev Respir Med* 2010; 4: 479–489.

98. Pelosi P, Gama de Abreu M, Rocco PR. New and conventional strategies for lung recruitment in acute respiratory distress syndrome. *Crit Care* 2010; 14: 210.

99. Villagra A, Ochagavia A, Vatua S, *et al.* Recruitment maneuvers during lung protective ventilation in acute respiratory distress syndrome. *Am J Respir Crit Care Med* 2002; 165: 165–170.

100. Brower RG, Morris A, MacIntyre N, *et al.* Effects of recruitment maneuvers in patients with acute lung injury and acute respiratory distress syndrome ventilated with high positive end-expiratory pressure. *Crit Care Med* 2003; 31: 2592–2597.

101. Odenstedt H, Aneman A, Karason S, *et al.* Acute hemodynamic changes during lung recruitment in lavage and endotoxin-induced ALI. *Intensive Care Med* 2005; 31: 112–120.

102. Meade MO, Cook DJ, Griffith LE, *et al.* A study of the physiologic responses to a lung recruitment maneuver in acute lung injury and acute respiratory distress syndrome. *Respir Care* 2008; 53: 1441–1449.

103. Constantin JM, Cayot-Constantin S, Roszyk L, *et al.* Response to recruitment maneuver influences net alveolar fluid clearance in acute respiratory distress syndrome. *Anesthesiology* 2007; 106: 944–951.

104. Musch G, Harris RS, Vidal Melo MF, *et al.* Mechanism by which a sustained inflation can worsen oxygenation in acute lung injury. *Anesthesiology* 2004; 100: 323–330.

105. Arnal JM, Paquet J, Wysocki M, *et al.* Optimal duration of a sustained inflation recruitment maneuver in ARDS patients. *Intensive Care Med* 2011; 37: 1588–1594.

106. Marini JJ. Recruitment by sustained inflation: time for a change. *Intensive Care Med* 2011; 37: 1572–1574.

107. Rzezinski AF, Oliveira GP, Santiago VR, *et al.* Prolonged recruitment manoeuvre improves lung function with less ultrastructural damage in experimental mild acute lung injury. *Respir Physiol Neurobiol* 2009; 169: 271–281.

108. Odenstedt H, Lindgren S, Olegard C, *et al.* Slow moderate pressure recruitment maneuver minimizes negative circulatory and lung mechanic side effects: evaluation of recruitment maneuvers using electric impedance tomography. *Intensive Care Med* 2005; 31: 1706–1714.

109. Steimback PW, Oliveira GP, Rzezinski AF, *et al.* Effects of frequency and inspiratory plateau pressure during recruitment manoeuvres on lung and distal organs in acute lung injury. *Intensive Care Med* 2009; 35: 1120–1128.

110. Riva DR, Oliveira MB, Rzezinski AF, *et al.* Recruitment maneuver in pulmonary and extrapulmonary experimental acute lung injury. *Crit Care Med* 2008; 36: 1900–1908.

111. Tugrul S, Akinci O, Ozcan PE, *et al.* Effects of sustained inflation and postinflation positive end-expiratory pressure in acute respiratory distress syndrome: focusing on pulmonary and extrapulmonary forms. *Crit Care Med* 2003; 31: 738–744.

112. Grasso S, Mascia L, Del Turco M, *et al.* Effects of recruiting maneuvers in patients with acute respiratory distress syndrome ventilated with protective ventilatory strategy. *Anesthesiology* 2002; 96: 795–802.

113. Gattinoni L, Caironi P, Cressoni M, *et al.* Lung recruitment in patients with the acute respiratory distress syndrome. *N Engl J Med* 2006; 354: 1775–1786.

114. Demory D, Arnal JM, Wysocki M, *et al.* Recruitability of the lung estimated by the pressure volume curve hysteresis in ARDS patients. *Intensive Care Med* 2008; 34: 2019–2025.

115. Arbelot C, Ferrari F, Bouhemad B, *et al.* Lung ultrasound in acute respiratory distress syndrome and acute lung injury. *Curr Opin Crit Care* 2008; 14: 70–74.

116. Bouhemad B, Brisson H, Le-Guen M, *et al.* Bedside ultrasound assessment of positive end-expiratory pressure-induced lung recruitment. *Am J Respir Crit Care Med* 2011; 183: 341–347.

117. Costa EL, Borges JB, Melo A, *et al.* Bedside estimation of recruitable alveolar collapse and hyperdistension by electrical impedance tomography. *Intensive Care Med* 2009; 35: 1132–1137.

118. Victorino JA, Borges JB, Okamoto VN, *et al.* Imbalances in regional lung ventilation: a validation study on electrical impedance tomography. *Am J Respir Crit Care Med* 2004; 169: 791–800.

119. Constantin JM, Grasso S, Chanques G, *et al.* Lung morphology predicts response to recruitment maneuver in patients with acute respiratory distress syndrome. *Crit Care Med* 2010; 38: 1108–1117.

120. Kacmarek RM, Kallet RH. Respiratory controversies in the critical care setting. Should recruitment maneuvers be used in the management of ALI and ARDS? *Respir Care* 2007; 52: 622–631.

121. Maggiore SM, Lellouche F, Pigeot J, *et al.* Prevention of endotracheal suctioning-induced alveolar derecruitment in acute lung injury. *Am J Respir Crit Care Med* 2003; 167: 1215–1224.

122. Marini JJ, Gattinoni L. Ventilatory management of acute respiratory distress syndrome: a consensus of two. *Crit Care Med* 2004; 32: 250–255.

123. Downs JB, Stock MC. Airway pressure release ventilation: a new concept in ventilatory support. *Crit Care Med* 1987; 15: 459–461.

124. Stock MC, Downs JB, Frolicher DA. Airway pressure release ventilation. *Crit Care Med* 1987; 15: 462–466.

125. Neumann P, Golisch W, Strohmeyer A, *et al.* Influence of different release times on spontaneous breathing pattern during airway pressure release ventilation. *Intensive Care Med* 2002; 28: 1742–1749.

126. Rose L, Hawkins M. Airway pressure release ventilation and biphasic positive airway pressure: a systematic review of definitional criteria. *Intensive Care Med* 2008; 34: 1766–1773.

127. Siau C, Stewart TE. Current role of high frequency oscillatory ventilation and airway pressure release ventilation in acute lung injury and acute respiratory distress syndrome. *Clin Chest Med* 2008; 29: 265–275.

128. Habashi NM. Other approaches to open-lung ventilation: airway pressure release ventilation. *Crit Care Med* 2005; 33: Suppl. 3, S228–S240.

129. Kaplan LJ, Bailey H, Formosa V. Airway pressure release ventilation increases cardiac performance in patients with acute lung injury/adult respiratory distress syndrome. *Crit Care* 2001; 5: 221–226.

130. Putensen C, Zech S, Wrigge H, *et al.* Long-term effects of spontaneous breathing during ventilatory support in patients with acute lung injury. *Am J Respir Crit Care Med* 2001; 164: 43–49.

131. Putensen C, Muders T, Varelmann D, *et al.* The impact of spontaneous breathing during mechanical ventilation. *Curr Opin Crit Care* 2006; 12: 13–18.

132. Putensen C, Mutz NJ, Putensen-Himmer G, *et al.* Spontaneous breathing during ventilatory support improves ventilation-perfusion distributions in patients with acute respiratory distress syndrome. *Am J Respir Crit Care Med* 1999; 159: 1241–1248.

133. Yoshida T, Rinka H, Kaji A, *et al.* The impact of spontaneous ventilation on distribution of lung aeration in patients with acute respiratory distress syndrome: airway pressure release ventilation *versus* pressure support ventilation. *Anesth Analg* 2009; 109: 1892–1900.

134. Dart BW 4th, Maxwell RA, Richart CM, et al. Preliminary experience with airway pressure release ventilation in a trauma/surgical intensive care unit. *J Trauma* 2005; 59: 71–76.

135. Cane RD, Peruzzi WT, Shapiro BA. Airway pressure release ventilation in severe acute respiratory failure. *Chest* 1991; 100: 460–463.

136. Rasanen J, Cane RD, Downs JB, *et al.* Airway pressure release ventilation during acute lung injury: a prospective multicenter trial. *Crit Care Med* 1991; 19: 1234–1241.

137. Sydow M, Burchardi H, Ephraim E, *et al.* Long-term effects of two different ventilatory modes on oxygenation in acute lung injury. Comparison of airway pressure release ventilation and volume-controlled inverse ratio ventilation. *Am J Respir Crit Care Med* 1994; 149: 1550–1556.

138. Maxwell RA, Green JM, Waldrop J, *et al.* A randomized prospective trial of airway pressure release ventilation and low tidal volume ventilation in adult trauma patients with acute respiratory failure. *J Trauma* 2010; 69: 501–510.

139. Varpula T, Jousela I, Niemi R, *et al.* Combined effects of prone positioning and airway pressure release ventilation on gas exchange in patients with acute lung injury. *Acta Anaesthesiol Scand* 2003; 47: 516–524.

140. Varpula T, Valta P, Niemi R, *et al.* Airway pressure release ventilation as a primary ventilatory mode in acute respiratory distress syndrome. *Acta Anaesthesiol Scand* 2004; 48: 722–731.

141. Krishnan JA, Brower RG. High-frequency ventilation for acute lung injury and ARDS. *Chest* 2000; 118: 795–807.

142. Fessler HE, Hess DR. Respiratory controversies in the critical care setting. Does high-frequency ventilation offer benefits over conventional ventilation in adult patients with acute respiratory distress syndrome? *Respir Care* 2007; 52: 595–605.

143. Sud S, Sud M, Friedrich JO, *et al.* High frequency oscillation in patients with acute lung injury and acute respiratory distress syndrome (ARDS): systematic review and meta-analysis. *BMJ* 2010; 340: c2327.

144. Slutsky AS, Drazen JM. Ventilation with small tidal volumes. *N Engl J Med* 2002; 347: 630–631.

145. dos Santos CC, Slutsky AS. Overview of high-frequency ventilation modes, clinical rationale, and gas transport mechanisms. *Respir Care Clin N Am* 2001; 7: 549–575.

146. Chang HK. Mechanisms of gas transport during ventilation by high-frequency oscillation. *J Appl Physiol* 1984; 56: 553–563.

147. Fessler HE, Hager DN, Brower RG. Feasibility of very high-frequency ventilation in adults with acute respiratory distress syndrome. *Crit Care Med* 2008; 36: 1043–1048.
148. Ritacca FV, Stewart TE. Clinical review: high-frequency oscillatory ventilation in adults – a review of the literature and practical applications. *Crit Care* 2003; 7: 385–390.
149. Chan KP, Stewart TE, Mehta S. High-frequency oscillatory ventilation for adult patients with ARDS. *Chest* 2007; 131: 1907–1916.
150. Kao KC, Tsai YH, Wu YK, *et al.* High frequency oscillatory ventilation for surgical patients with acute respiratory distress syndrome. *J Trauma* 2006; 61: 837–843.
151. Andersen FA, Guttormsen AB, Flaatten HK. High frequency oscillatory ventilation in adult patients with acute respiratory distress syndrome–a retrospective study. *Acta Anaesthesiol Scand* 2002; 46: 1082–1088.
152. Ferguson ND, Chiche JD, Kacmarek RM, *et al.* Combining high-frequency oscillatory ventilation and recruitment maneuvers in adults with early acute respiratory distress syndrome: the Treatment with Oscillation and an Open Lung Strategy (TOOLS) Trial pilot study. *Crit Care Med* 2005; 33: 479–486.
153. Mehta S, Granton J, MacDonald RJ, *et al.* High-frequency oscillatory ventilation in adults: the Toronto experience. *Chest* 2004; 126: 518–527.
154. David M, Weiler N, Heinrichs W, *et al.* High-frequency oscillatory ventilation in adult acute respiratory distress syndrome. *Intensive Care Med* 2003; 29: 1656–1665.
155. Fort P, Farmer C, Westerman J, *et al.* High-frequency oscillatory ventilation for adult respiratory distress syndrome – a pilot study. *Crit Care Med* 1997; 25: 937–947.
156. Mehta S, Lapinsky SE, Hallett DC, *et al.* Prospective trial of high-frequency oscillation in adults with acute respiratory distress syndrome. *Crit Care Med* 2001; 29: 1360–1369.
157. Cartotto R, Cooper AB, Esmond JR, *et al.* Early clinical experience with high-frequency oscillatory ventilation for ARDS in adult burn patients. *J Burn Care Rehabil* 2001; 22: 325–333.
158. Cartotto R, Ellis S, Gomez M, *et al.* High frequency oscillatory ventilation in burn patients with the acute respiratory distress syndrome. *Burns* 2004; 30: 453–463.
159. Claridge JA, Hostetter RG, Lowson SM, *et al.* High-frequency oscillatory ventilation can be effective as rescue therapy for refractory acute lung dysfunction. *Am Surg* 1999; 65: 1092–1096.
160. Finkielman JD, Gajic O, Farmer JC, *et al.* The initial Mayo Clinic experience using high-frequency oscillatory ventilation for adult patients: a retrospective study. *BMC Emerg Med* 2006; 6: 2.
161. Mehta S, MacDonald R, Hallett DC, *et al.* Acute oxygenation response to inhaled nitric oxide when combined with high-frequency oscillatory ventilation in adults with acute respiratory distress syndrome. *Crit Care Med* 2003; 31: 383–389.
162. Demory D, Michelet P, Arnal JM, *et al.* High-frequency oscillatory ventilation following prone positioning prevents a further impairment in oxygenation. *Crit Care Med* 2007; 35: 106–111.
163. Derdak S, Mehta S, Stewart TE, *et al.* High-frequency oscillatory ventilation for acute respiratory distress syndrome in adults: a randomized, controlled trial. *Am J Respir Crit Care Med* 2002; 166: 801–808.
164. Bollen CW, van Well GT, Sherry T, *et al.* High frequency oscillatory ventilation compared with conventional mechanical ventilation in adult respiratory distress syndrome: a randomized controlled trial [ISRCTN24242669]. *Crit Care* 2005; 9: R430–R439.
165. Wunsch H, Mapstone J. High-frequency ventilation *versus* conventional ventilation for treatment of acute lung injury and acute respiratory distress syndrome. *Cochrane Database Syst Rev* 2004; 1: CD004085.
166. Allan PF, Osborn EC, Chung KK, *et al.* High-frequency percussive ventilation revisited. *J Burn Care Res* 2010; 31: 510–520.
167. Lucangelo U, Fontanesi L, Antonaglia V, *et al.* High frequency percussive ventilation (HFPV). Principles and technique. *Minerva Anestesiol* 2003; 69: 841–848.
168. Chung KK, Wolf SE, Renz EM, *et al.* High-frequency percussive ventilation and low tidal volume ventilation in burns: a randomized controlled trial. *Crit Care Med* 2010; 38: 1970–1977.
169. Salim A, Martin M. High-frequency percussive ventilation. *Crit Care Med* 2005; 33: Suppl. 3, S241–S245.
170. Lucangelo U, Zin WA, Antonaglia V, *et al.* High-frequency percussive ventilation during surgical bronchial repair in a patient with one lung. *Br J Anaesth* 2006; 96: 533–536.
171. Hurst JM, Branson RD, Davis K Jr, *et al.* Comparison of conventional mechanical ventilation and high-frequency ventilation. A prospective, randomized trial in patients with respiratory failure. *Ann Surg* 1990; 211: 486–491.
172. Velmahos GC, Chan LS, Tatevossian R, *et al.* High-frequency percussive ventilation improves oxygenation in patients with ARDS. *Chest* 1999; 116: 440–446.
173. Paulsen SM, Killyon GW, Barillo DJ. High-frequency percussive ventilation as a salvage modality in adult respiratory distress syndrome: a preliminary study. *Am Surg* 2002; 68: 852–856.
174. Gallagher TJ, Boysen PG, Davidson DD, *et al.* High-frequency percussive ventilation compared with conventional mechanical ventilation. *Crit Care Med* 1989; 17: 364–366.
175. Eastman A, Holland D, Higgins J, *et al.* High-frequency percussive ventilation improves oxygenation in trauma patients with acute respiratory distress syndrome: a retrospective review. *Am J Surg* 2006; 192: 191–195.

Chapter 3

Recruitment manoeuvres in patients with acute lung injury

T. Paterson and E. Fan

Summary

A pressure- and volume-limited ventilatory strategy has been shown to improve short-term mortality in patients with acute lung injury (ALI). However, such a strategy may lead to alveolar de-recruitment and atelectrauma. Recruitment manoeuvres (RMs) may be an important component of a lung protective strategy, leading to increased end-expiratory lung volume, with a subsequent improvement in oxygenation and respiratory mechanics. Furthermore, experimental data suggest that RMs may play an important role in preventing ventilator-associated lung injury. Clinical studies have yielded conflicting results, with some demonstrating a transient improvement in oxygenation following RMs, which has not translated into a significant survival advantage. Thus, despite a strong pathophysiological rationale, there is little evidence to support their routine use in unselected ALI populations. While serious complications may be uncommon, it is essential to monitor for barotrauma and hypotension. Further clinical trials are needed to confirm the safety and efficacy of RMs in ALI patients with recruitable disease, as well as to elucidate the optimal type, timing and frequency of RMs in these patients.

Keywords: Acute lung injury, acute respiratory distress syndrome, artificial respiration, intensive care unit, recruitment manoeuvres

Interdepartmental Division of Critical Care Medicine, University of Toronto and Mount Sinai Hospital, Toronto, ON, Canada.

Correspondence: E. Fan, Mount Sinai Hospital, 600 University Avenue, Room 18-232, Toronto, M5G 1X5, ON, Canada.
Email efan@mtsinai.on.ca

Eur Respir Mon 2012; 55: 40–53.
Printed in UK – all rights reserved
Copyright ERS 2012
European Respiratory Monograph
ISSN: 1025-448x
DOI: 10.1183/1025448x.10001511

Acute lung injury (ALI) is a syndrome of inflammatory, non-cardiogenic pulmonary oedema leading to hypoxaemic respiratory failure. At present, the ventilatory management of patients with ALI is characterised by a pressure- and volume-limited lung protective strategy [1], which may potentiate further alveolar de-recruitment, particularly if insufficient positive end-expiratory pressure (PEEP) is applied [2]. In addition to pressure and volume limitation, recruitment manoeuvres (RMs) may be an important component of a lung protective strategy. Recruitment refers to the dynamic process of opening collapsed, non-aerated lung units through a transient intentional increase in the transpulmonary pressure above that achieved by tidal ventilation. Recruitment is a continuous process occurring along the entire inflationary limb of the pressure–volume curve [3].

The concept of opening the injured lung is not new [4], with the goal of increasing end-expiratory lung volume (EELV), which may lead to an improvement in gas exchange and respiratory mechanics. Moreover, experimental data suggest that this intervention may play an important role in preventing ventilator-associated lung injury (VALI) [5], although this has not been uniformly supported by clinical studies. Clinical studies have yielded conflicting results, with a number of studies demonstrating a transient improvement in oxygenation following RMs, which has not translated into a significant survival advantage [6, 7]. Possible explanations for these discrepant results include the different types of RMs used, which may influence the results [8], along with difficulty in determining the population of ALI patients with recruitable disease. Finally, the optimal timing, duration and frequency of RMs have not been determined or tested in large clinical trials. The aim of this chapter is to describe the pathophysiological basis and clinical role for RMs in patients with ALI.

The rationale for lung recruitment

ALI is a heterogeneous syndrome characterised by de-recruitment

The acutely injured lung comprises a heterogeneous population of aerated and non-aerated lung, with the non-aerated lung consisting of collapsed or consolidated alveoli [9], resulting in reduced effective ventilatable volume (the so-called "baby lung") [10]. The injured lung is particularly susceptible to VALI, with positive-pressure ventilation generating stress at the boundaries between aerated and non-aerated lung, and repeated high-pressure inflations leading to damaging shear forces at these junctional interfaces. In addition, positive-pressure ventilation may induce atelectrauma, the cyclic opening and closing of alveoli in the presence of insufficient PEEP to maintain alveolar patency through the respiratory cycle. These mechanical stresses may have a number of effects, including epithelial and endothelial damage, cellular inflammatory damage and the release of cytokines leading to a systemic inflammatory response [11]. Pressure- and volume-limited ventilatory strategies have been introduced to limit these ventilator-induced stresses, but do not address the primary problem of inhomogeneous aeration of the lung. In fact, low tidal volume ventilation is probably responsible for de-recruitment of functional alveolar units and increased atelectrauma.

Safely and effectively ventilating a patient with ALI is challenging, as the fragile junctional regions need enough pressure to open and prevent cyclical collapse, while the open and/or hyperinflated lung units need reduced pressure to prevent overdistension. From a pathophysiological perspective, attempts to open the non-aerated lung units seem appropriate, bearing in mind that only collapsed, but not consolidated, alveoli are likely to respond. The injured lung has a wide range of alveolar opening and closing pressures [3, 12, 13], but not all lung units may be recruitable at safe pressures. In general, lung units can be kept open by airway pressures that are lower than those required to open them [3], leading to the concept of recruitment using periodic high-pressure RMs with sufficient levels of post-RM PEEP to maintain alveolar patency. The fact that alveolar opening pressure always exceeds closing pressure has a number of consequences: 1) more pressure is required to open a lung unit than to maintain its patency; and 2) pressure sufficient to maintain an open unit's patency will not open any units that are currently closed. The "open" lung is ventilated on the expiratory limb of the pressure–volume curve, rather than the underinflated lung on the inspiratory portion of the curve.

Consequences of pressure- and volume-limited ventilation

Functional residual capacity (FRC) is reduced by 60–75% in patients with ALI [14, 15]. The degree of FRC loss is related to the pattern of radiographic infiltration, with diffuse infiltrates being worse than both lobar and patchy infiltrates [14]. Pressure- and volume-limited ventilation attempts to reduce overdistension of open lung units, and evidence suggests that this strategy reduces mortality in patients with ALI [1, 16, 17]. However, the lower airway pressures that result from this technique minimise the role of tidal recruitment [12, 18]. Furthermore, the ensuing collapse of lung units may be amplified by high inspiratory oxygen fraction (FI,O_2) and/or frequent endotracheal suctioning. De-recruitment of the lung in patients with ALI may lead to a further reduction in total FRC (tissue and gas) by 20% [14]. The resulting reduction in compliance has a number of consequences: the lung will tend to collapse more than expand and a higher distending pressure is required to hold it open.

Increasing PEEP to maximise alveolar recruitment should minimise end-expiratory cyclical collapse of unstable alveoli, reducing the burden of VALI from atelectrauma in patients with ALI. Although physiologically intuitive and backed by promising data in several animal models, the body of clinical evidence supporting this strategy in unselected ALI patients is not strong [19–22]. There is also conflicting opinion as to the correct method for selecting "optimal" PEEP. Once collapsed, lung units require a higher opening pressure than maintenance pressure and, thus, using higher PEEP alone may not be the most efficient method of alveolar recruitment.

Potential benefits and adverse effects of RMs in patients with ALI

Oxygenation

Transpulmonary shunt through non-ventilated lung units is the primary cause of hypoxaemia in patients with ALI. Opening these units and thus increasing the surface area available for gas exchange should improve ventilation/perfusion (V'/Q') matching within the lung and decrease the amount of blood flowing through shunt regions, with a resulting improvement in arterial oxygenation. The use of RMs increases EELV in various animal models of ALI, with a subsequent improvement in hypoxaemia in a variety of experimental models, including during apnoeic [23] or oscillatory oxygenation [24]. The effect is greatest when PEEP is low, and is ablated by high tidal volume ventilation [25]. However, increasing EELV is not necessarily linked to an improvement in oxygenation [25]. This may reflect overdistension of open lung units, rather than recruitment of collapsed lung units, with subsequent redistribution of pulmonary blood flow to collapsed lung units.

Lung protection

Even with strict ventilation according to the Acute Respiratory Distress Syndrome (ARDS) Network low tidal volume protocol [17], up to a third of patients are exposed to end-expiratory alveolar overdistension [18]. This phenomenon predominantly occurs in patients with a larger proportion of non-aerated lung, presumably because the tidal volume is distributed into a much smaller aerated ("baby lung") compartment. Recruiting non-aerated lung may attenuate this over distension injury by distributing the tidal volume more homogeneously, into a larger volume of aerated lung.

The peak inspiratory pressure during an RM is typically higher than the pressure limits accepted as standard of care for continuous mechanical ventilation. It is not clear if RMs promote overdistension VALI. There is evidence from animal models that infrequent RMs do not promote alveolar epithelial damage to the same extent as injurious, high-pressure mechanical ventilation [26]. However, the volume of hyperinflated lung units does increase when an RM is performed (from 1% to 3% of lung volume) [27]. Indeed, the application of high transpulmonary pressures progressively increased the volume of open lung units that were hyperinflated, demonstrating the potential for worsening iatrogenic lung injury in a dose-dependent fashion [9]. Finally, laboratory studies have suggested that partial recruitment may aggravate cytokine production in the lung. The atelectatic lung has little cytokine production, which may be markedly increased by inadequate recruitment or repeated de-recruitment [28]. Thus, VALI may be further mitigated by opening, and keeping open, those unstable lung units that are cyclically collapsing, thus preventing atelectrauma.

Potential side-effects and complications

Although RMs are generally well tolerated with few adverse effects, several potential complications should be anticipated. Due to the transient increase in intrathoracic pressure and consequent reduction in venous return, cardiac output may be impaired producing hypotension, a complication that appears to be more common in those with poor chest wall compliance and limited oxygenation response from recruitment [29]. Generally, hypotension during an RM suggests relative volume depletion. A decrease in cerebral perfusion pressure has been noted, which may contraindicate this procedure in patients with head injury. Barotrauma, including pneumomediastinum and pneumothorax, has been described although, the exact risk remains unclear. Elevated pressure may alter the integrity of the alveolar–capillary membrane, increasing bacterial and cytokine translocation into the systemic circulation [26, 30].

In a systematic review of clinical studies evaluating adverse events associated with the use of RMs in patients with ALI (31 studies; 985 patients), the majority of these events occurred during an RM, with hypotension (12%) and desaturation (8%) being the most common complications [7]. Serious adverse events, such as barotrauma (1%) and arrhythmias (1%), were uncommon. Only 1% of patients were reported to have had their RMs terminated early due to an adverse event. Finally, 17 studies (287 patients) reported no adverse events from RMs. Ultimately, identifying the correct patients (*i.e.* with a high level of recruitability) is of paramount importance, as applying RMs to patients with low recruitability will probably expose these patients to unnecessary risks with little hope of any significant benefit [9].

Types of RMs

Sustained inflation

A sustained inflation is usually achieved by changing to a continuous positive airway pressure (CPAP) mode and setting the pressure to the desired level (*e.g.* 35–50 cmH$_2$O for 20–40 seconds), and is an extremely common type of RM (fig. 1) [7]. It is important to ensure that the pressure support level is set to zero to avoid additional pressure increases. It is possible that this technique does not expose the lung to a high enough transpulmonary pressure to achieve maximal recruitment. To that end, RMs may need to be individualised, with higher airway pressures required to generate an equivalent transpulmonary pressure in the patient with poor chest wall compliance (*e.g.* increased intra-abdominal pressure). Furthermore, some evidence suggests that the distribution of opening pressures is bimodal (fig. 2) [13, 31], suggesting that there is the potential for recruiting a significant proportion of atelectatic lung units at higher inflation pressures than are traditionally used with a single sustained

inflation. Paralysis is usually not required for sustained inflations, but additional short-acting sedation may be useful as there is no ventilatory support provided during this manoeuvre; thus, it may not be as well tolerated by the patient. The patient should be closely monitored during this short period for hypotension and hypoxaemia.

Sigh

Broadly, there are two main types of sighs that have been used as RMs in patients with ALI: 1) a number of independent or consecutive sighs to reach high inspiratory pressure in either the pressure- or volume-control mode; or 2) a periodic increase in PEEP for a few breaths [32]. Intermittent sighs have been demonstrated to achieve recruitment using three consecutive sighs

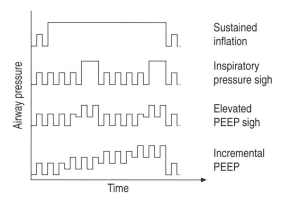

Figure 1. Schematic diagram showing typical airway pressure tracings during different types of recruitment manoeuvres. PEEP: positive end-expiratory pressure.

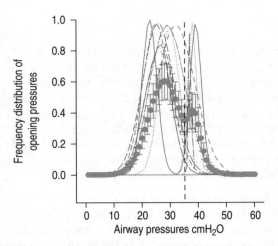

Figure 2. Frequency distribution of threshold opening pressures as a function of airway pressures. The distribution of opening pressures for individual patients (grey lines) and the average distribution across patients (red line) are shown. - - - -: airway pressure of 35 cmH₂O, showing that a substantial portion of lung may be recruited at higher airway pressure. Reproduced from [13] with permission from the publisher.

set at a pressure of 45 cmH₂O [33], or using an intermittent increase in PEEP for two breaths every minute [34]. An "extended sigh" has been described, involving a stepwise increase in PEEP and decrease in tidal volume over 2 minutes, to a CPAP level of 30 cmH₂O for 30 seconds [35].

Pressure-controlled ventilation

RMs using tidal recruitment with intermittent increases in airway pressure may reduce the haemodynamic compromise and VALI associated with sustained inflation RMs. Typically, a high starting PEEP is used (*e.g.* 20–25 cmH₂O) in the pressure-control mode, and may be associated with incremental increases over the duration of the manoeuvre (*e.g.* in increments of 5 cmH₂O every 30 seconds, up to 40–45 cmH₂O). The peak airway pressures achieved exceed the opening pressure of most collapsed lung units (*e.g.* 40–50 cmH₂O) [32]. The supported tidal ventilation may also ease the dyssynchrony seen during other RMs, with tidal breathing above an increased level of PEEP augmenting alveolar recruitment [27].

An incremental recruitment strategy employing plateau pressures up to 60 cmH₂O allowed near maximal recruitment in the majority of patients studied, allowing further gains in oxygenation and lung recruitment over a single sustained inflation technique in a recent study [13]. The additional recruitment achieved with ventilatory pressure >35–40 cmH₂O reflects the bimodal distribution of alveolar opening pressures in the injured lung [31]. Without the use of these higher recruitment pressures, up to a quarter of the lung may remain atelectatic [9, 36]. The effect of recruitment may not be sustained unless adequate PEEP is applied to prevent de-recruitment [9, 36–39]. In a recent study, the use of moderate levels of PEEP (15 cmH₂O) was only able to maintain 50% of recruited lung following sustained inflation at a plateau pressure of 45 cmH₂O [9].

Sustained recruitment with alternative ventilatory strategies

In addition to discrete RMs performed during conventional mechanical ventilation of ALI patients, several recent innovations may provide their benefit largely through progressive lung recruitment. These include high-frequency oscillatory ventilation (HFOV) and airway pressure release ventilation (APRV) [40]. Both these modalities use high, constant mean airway pressures to recruit and maintain adequate end-expiratory pressure while attenuating VALI. Similar to higher levels of PEEP, HFOV has been shown to maintain the oxygenation benefit from lung recruitment achieved with prone positioning [41]. Like RMs, both HFOV and APRV have been shown to improve oxygenation but lack a significant mortality benefit in the small number of clinical studies performed to date [40]. Future studies will be required to identify the role of these ventilation strategies in the therapeutic armamentarium for ALI patients.

Prone positioning

Prone positioning recruits lung volume in the dorsal areas and reduces the antero-posterior intrathoracic pressure gradient. However, the pressure required to achieve recruitment is lower and the effect is more sustained [36, 42]. Thus, RMs performed in the prone position may be more effective and durable than in the supine position. Indeed, a recent prospective study in patients with early ARDS demonstrated that an RM (45 cmH₂O extended sigh) combined with prone positioning led to a significant and durable improvement in oxygenation, as compared to the same RM in the supine position [43]. A more detailed discussion regarding the rationale, risks and benefits of prone positioning in patients with ALI is beyond the scope of the present discussion, but has recently been the subject of a number of systematic reviews and meta-analyses [44–46].

Which is the optimal type of RM?

Despite the increasing literature on recruitment, few studies have compared these various methods in terms of efficacy and adverse effects (table 1). Sustained high pressure may cause transient hypotension, and may be less well tolerated than methods using pressure-controlled ventilation. Sustained or intermittent increases in peak pressure also carry the risk of barotrauma. The choice of RM may depend on the baseline ventilatory mode: a spontaneously breathing patient may not tolerate a sustained (high-pressure) inflation. A transient increase in PEEP and peak pressure may be more appropriate in this situation. There is some evidence that the aetiology of ALI (i.e. pulmonary versus extra-pulmonary) may affect tolerance and efficacy for various recruitment modalities [36]. The frequency with which RMs need be applied is also unknown. This probably depends on the underlying disease, the level of PEEP and procedures such as endotracheal suctioning [38]. Other than the study by AMATO et al. [47], no outcome data exist to suggest a mortality benefit of RMs in patients with ALI.

Monitoring the effect of RMs

A number of different modalities have been proposed to evaluate lung recruitment in ALI patients, including imaging techniques (e.g. lung ultrasound, computed tomography (CT) scanning and electric impedance tomography (EIT)), lung mechanics (e.g. using pressure–volume curves) and physiological parameters (e.g. arterial oxygen tension (P_{a,O_2}) and/or arterial carbon dioxide tension (P_{a,CO_2})). While CT scanning can be useful in the comprehensive evaluation of ALI patients, including lung recruitment, disadvantages of this technique include repeated radiation exposure, the need for

Table 1. Potential advantages and disadvantages of different types of recruitment manoeuvres

Manoeuvre	Advantages	Disadvantages
Sustained inflation	Simple	Requires sedation and/or paralysis during manoeuvre (i.e. no spontaneous breathing)
	Single intervention of short duration (e.g. 30–40 seconds)	Moderate-to-high risk for hypotension, particularly if hypovolemic prior to manoeuvre
	Requires the use of moderate-to-high airway pressure	Moderate-to-high risk for desaturation during manoeuvre
		Typically only modest amount of lung recruitment
Sigh	Simple	Low-to-moderate risk of hypotension
	Single intervention of short duration, which may be repeated (e.g. two breaths every 2 minutes)	Low-to-moderate risk of desaturation
	Can be incorporated and well tolerated in spontaneous breathing modes	Typically only modest amount of lung recruitment
	Requires the use of moderate airway pressure	
Pressure-controlled ventilation	Single intervention	Complex intervention typically requiring progressive adjustment of ventilator settings
	Typically good amount of lung recruitment	Relatively longer duration manoeuvre
		May require sedation and/or paralysis during manoeuvre
		Typically requires high airway pressure
		Moderate risk of hypotension
		Moderate risk of desaturation

intrafacility transport to the CT scanner (not available at the bedside) and cost. Lung ultrasound and EIT are promising techniques that may allow effective bedside assessment and monitoring of lung recruitment, but require further study. EIT is a noninvasive technique that allows real-time, bedside monitoring of regional ventilation in both normal patients and patients with ALI [48, 49]. The generation of pressure–volume curves typically requires an interruption in mechanical ventilation, leading to controversy regarding the interpretation of the lower inflection point [50]; there are problems with reproducibility and interobserver reliability [51], and the lack of a lower inflection point does not necessarily imply a low potential for recruitability [32].

From a practical perspective, improved oxygenation with a reduction in Pa,CO_2 indicates lung recruitment. Pressure effects may redirect blood flow and improve oxygenation in the absence of recruitment, but this would not be associated with a reduced Pa,CO_2. BORGES et al. [13] recently correlated a blood gas index of $Pa,O_2 + Pa,CO_2 \geqslant 400$ mmHg (on 100% oxygen) as an indicator of maximal lung recruitment in early ALI, corresponding to $\geqslant 95\%$ lung recruitment as seen on a quantitative CT scan (85% sensitivity, 82% specificity) [13]. Oxygenation at PEEP 5 cmH$_2$O [9] has also been suggested, but neither of these methods have been confirmed in prospective trials.

Clinical indications for RMs in patients with ALI

Which ALI patients are recruitable?

Although there are no strong clinical data to support a clear role for RMs, they may be utilised in a number of clinical situations. While most studies have evaluated RMs in the context of ALI, this intervention may be of value in patients with atelectasis related to general anaesthesia, during post-operative ventilation [52], following suctioning [38], after endotracheal intubation [53] or in other conditions producing hypoxaemia, including heart failure.

As outlined previously, ALI is a highly heterogeneous disease process with a range of potential "recruitability" across patients. Response to RMs does not occur in all patients with ALI [29, 54], with non-responders having more pronounced side-effects [55]. Thus, identifying those patients who will respond to an RM is important, and several studies have identified characteristics that may predict a response, in terms of oxygenation or improved lung mechanics. GATTINONI et al. [9] performed CT measurements of lung volumes at three different levels of PEEP (5, 15 and 45 cmH$_2$O) amongst 68 ALI patients, and correlated the lung findings with a variety of variables. A broad range of potentially recruitable lung was seen, from 0% to nearly 60% with an average of 13% of total lung weight. On average, 24% of lung volume remained unrecruited despite 45 cmH$_2$O PEEP. Factors indicating a higher severity of ALI (as measured by oxygenation, lung compliance, amount of dead space and rate of death) correlated with higher recruitable volumes [9].

The duration of ALI appears to be an important factor, with a higher response rate noted in patients early in their disease course (e.g. <72 hours) compared with later [29]. This probably relates to the change in the disease from an exudative to a fibroproliferative process. Moreover, lung mechanics in ARDS vary with time [51] and it remains unknown whether the recruitment response varies through the day, or is related to changes in patient position or spontaneous ventilatory effort. While a response is more likely early in the course of disease, these studies have only been performed at a single time-period.

Similarly, the underlying pulmonary process may impact on responsiveness to recruitment attempts. Patients with extra-pulmonary ALI (e.g. secondary to sepsis) tend to have a higher response rate than those with pulmonary ALI (e.g. pneumonia) [15, 33], although recent studies have shown conflicting results [9, 13]. Patients with pneumonia may have a limited amount of recruitable lung tissue and the higher pressure may overinflate normal lung rather than aerating the consolidated tissue [3]. Similarly, radiological appearance may also predict response to an RM. Patients with focal lung pathology have a limited recruitment response when compared to patients with diffuse or patchy lung pathology [53]. Focal lung pathology also predisposes to significant hyperinflation during an RM.

Poorer compliance was also found in the more- compared to less-recruitable patients (40 *versus* 49 mL·cmH$_2$O^{-1}) [9]. Conversely, a recent systematic review of RMs suggested a lack of a significant oxygenation benefit in patients with extremely poor compliance (<30 mL·cmH$_2$O^{-1}) [7]. These discrepant results may be explained by a U-shaped relationship between lung compliance and recruitment efficacy. Healthy lungs gain no benefit from RMs because they are already maximally recruited and are only exposed to the potential adverse effects of an RM. Critically injured lungs may have a larger volume of inflammatory atelectasis and more severe aberrations in pulmonary mechanics, making them unrecruitable at clinically relevant levels of transpulmonary pressure. This leaves a group of patients with moderately decreased compliance as those with the most potential benefit from a RM. Furthermore, the effect of RMs may be limited by the ability of the chest wall to expand. Patients with poor chest wall compliance were less likely to benefit from RMs than those with compliant chest walls [29]. Patients with ALI who are ventilated with high tidal volumes or higher levels of PEEP are less apt to de-recruitment and may not show a response to RMs [34, 56]. Finally, the F_1,O_2 may affect lung recruitment, due to absorption atelectasis, with the recruitment effect rapidly lost in patients ventilated on 100% oxygen [57].

RMs and decremental PEEP trials

The best method of determining "optimal" PEEP in patients with ALI is controversial. Another potential role for RMs is in the evaluation of the appropriate PEEP and tidal volume combination for a patient, and to gauge responsiveness to PEEP. In patients with a clear response to a RM, the PEEP level required to prevent de-recruitment can be assessed by a decrement PEEP trial. Following the RM, PEEP is gradually reduced (*e.g.* 2 cmH$_2$O every 1–2 minutes) while monitoring oxygen saturation. The PEEP at which oxygen desaturation occurs (*e.g.* arterial oxygen saturation measured by pulse oximetry (S_p,O_2) ≤90%) is noted, and PEEP is set 2 cmH$_2$O above this level following a further RM. This strategy can identify the optimal PEEP level required to maintain the oxygenation benefit from a RM [31]. In a small series of critically ill surgical patients with early ALI, this strategy has been shown to be effective in identifying the "optimal" PEEP level required to maintain the oxygenation benefit accrued by a series of sustained inflation RMs [31]. Alternatively, respiratory mechanics can be used during a decrement PEEP trial following an RM, with "optimal" PEEP being set 2 cmH$_2$O above the PEEP level at which the best compliance is identified [58, 59]. The utility and efficacy of RMs and decrement PEEP trials require confirmation in large, prospective clinical trials.

Routine incorporation and after circuit disconnection

RMs can be regularly incorporated into a ventilation prescription as a "sigh" breath. A large tidal volume breath is programmed, typically once or twice per minute. One exploratory study with four patients per treatment arm found an improvement in oxygenation at 60 minutes with the use of "sigh" breaths, when compared to a single RM or no RMs [60]. Static compliance was marginally better in the "sigh" group. Low tidal volume and open lung ventilation strategies were used in all arms. The medium- and long-term effects of this technique (especially the potential for worsening VALI) are unknown.

An open circuit, if it persists for long enough, can result in total pulmonary depressurisation. Intra-alveolar pressure equilibrates with the atmosphere, and in patients dependent on mechanical ventilation this can result in significant de-recruitment. This application has been used in some studies [19, 47].

Refractory hypoxaemia

There are no randomised controlled trials specifically evaluating the use of RMs in patients with ALI and refractory hypoxemia [61]. However, it is interesting to note that there was a decreased risk of refractory hypoxaemia requiring "rescue ventilation" without an added risk of barotrauma in the Lung Open Ventilation (LOV) study [19], and a subsequent patient level meta-analysis confirmed a significantly decreased risk of requiring rescue therapies for (relative risk (RR) 0.61, 95% CI 0.38–0.99) and death from (RR 0.56, 95% CI 0.34–0.93), refractory hypoxaemia in ALI patients receiving a lung recruitment ventilation strategy using higher PEEP [21]. Thus, in ALI patients with life-threatening hypoxaemia, the use of an RM may be appropriate to improve oxygenation, even transiently, particularly if there is evidence for a significant amount of non-aerated lung that is potentially available for recruitment.

Clinical evidence for the use of RMs in patients with ALI

Clinical studies of RMs in patients with ALI have yielded variable results. This may relate to heterogeneity of the patients studied in terms of their underlying lung disease, duration of ALI and method of recruitment. Several studies have demonstrated a beneficial effect on oxygenation, which may be sustained in the presence of adequate PEEP. Patients ventilated in the supine position benefit more than when in the prone position, which is probably related to the presence of more dependent, collapsed lung. Similarly, the oxygenation benefit of RMs in patients ventilated with a higher PEEP strategy is only modest, suggesting the benefit from RMs is probably greatest in those patients who are not already recruited (*e.g.* by high PEEP or tidal volume) [25]. For instance, a study of a moderate sustained inflation RM (35 cmH_2O for 30 seconds) in patients on a relatively high PEEP ventilation protocol demonstrated only a small and variable improvement in oxygenation that was not sustained [54].

Oxygenation

RMs are associated with an improvement in oxygenation, at least transiently. There have been three randomised controlled trials (table 2) that evaluated the use of RMs in patients with ALI [19, 54, 62]. Following a PEEP trial in 30 consecutive patients with extra-pulmonary ALI, OCZENSKI *et al.* [62] randomised them to undergo a sustained inflation RM (50 cmH_2O for 30 seconds) or not. Compared to baseline, both oxygenation ($Pa,O_2/FI,O_2$ 139 *versus* 246; $p<0.001$) and venous admixture (Qs/Qt 30.8% *versus* 21.5%; $p<0.005$) improved significantly 3 minutes after the RM, but returned to baseline within 30 minutes. There were no significant differences in oxygenation or venous admixture between the RM group and the control group at baseline or at 30 minutes. In an ancillary multicentre study of RMs in ALI patients, the ARDS Network examined 43 patients who had received at least one RM (35–40 cmH_2O for 30 seconds) and one sham RM as a part of a higher PEEP ventilation strategy (ALVEOLI) [54]. Oxygenation improved significantly 10 minutes after RMs compared to sham RMs, but the magnitude of change was small (change in Sp,O_2 1.7 *versus* 0.6%; $p<0.01$) and the initial response was highly variable across patients. There was no significant effect of RMs on requirements for FI,O_2/PEEP at any time-point. Finally, in a randomised controlled trial of a total of 983 ALI patients randomised to an open lung strategy that included higher PEEP and RMs (40 cmH_2O for 40 seconds), oxygenation improved significantly in the intervention group compared to the control group at day 1 ($Pa,O_2/FI,O_2$ 187 *versus* 149; $p<0.001$), day 3 ($Pa,O_2/FI,O_2$ 197 *versus* 164; $p<0.001$) and day 7 ($Pa,O_2/FI,O_2$ 213 *versus* 181; $p<0.001$) [19]. It is important to note that all three trials also employed higher PEEP, making it difficult to ascertain the specific effect, if any, of RMs on oxygenation in these patients.

Finally, a systematic review of RMs in ALI patients encompassing 40 studies (1,185 patients), including case series, observational studies and randomised trials, found a significant improvement in oxygenation after an RM (mean $Pa,O_2/FI,O_2$ from 139 to 251; $p<0.001$) [7]. This increase was observed across a broad range of initial ALI severity, as measured by baseline $Pa,O_2/FI,O_2$ ratio. Although the specific RM technique used did vary, 45% of included studies used a single sustained inflation technique. Oxygenation gains were generally short-lived, with most studies showing return to baseline oxygenation within 24 hours (and many within 30 minutes).

Mortality

There are few randomised controlled trials incorporating RMs. Greater proportions of non-aerated lung correlate with increased mortality [9]. However, there is no evidence that recruiting this non-aerated lung produces a clinically significant alteration in mortality [7]. This may be because measures of baseline oxygenation do not clearly predict mortality in ALI, and it is recognised that the majority of patients with ALI do not usually die from hypoxaemia [63–66]. Thus, treatment modalities (*e.g.* inhaled nitric oxide and prone positioning) that focus on oxygenation may never show a mortality benefit [44, 67].

Table 2. Randomised controlled trials of recruitment manoeuvres (RMs)

First author [ref.]	Subjects n	Type of RM used	Frequency of RM	Main outcome measures	Adverse events
BROWER [54]	43	Sustained inflation (CPAP 35–40 cmH$_2$O for 30 seconds)	Every other day (alternating with sham RMs)	Greater increase in Sp,O_2 with RM *versus* sham RM (1.7±0.2% *versus* 0.6±0.3%; $p<0.01$) Changes in FI,O_2/PEEP requirements were not significantly different up to 8 hours from RM or sham RM	Greater decrease in SBP with RM *versus* sham RM (-9.4±1.1 *versus* -3.1±1.1 mmHg; $p<0.01$) Three RMs terminated early due to transient hypotension or desaturation New barotraumas following one RM and one sham RM
OCZENSKI [62]	30	Sustained inflation (CPAP 50 cmH$_2$O for 30 seconds)	Once	Significant increase in P/F ratio at 3 minutes post-RM (139±46 *versus* 246±111 mmHg; $p<0.001$) with return to baseline values by 30 minutes No significant differences in P/F ratio between RM and control group at baseline and after 30 minutes	No change in any haemodynamic variables at 3 minutes post-RM compared to baseline values No significant differences between groups in any haemodynamic variables detected at 30 minutes compared to baseline values
MEADE [19]	366	Sustained inflation (CPAP 40 cmH$_2$O for 40 seconds)	Up to four times daily	Significant improvement in P/F ratio over the course of 7 days from randomisation: day 1 (187 *versus* 149; $p<0.001$), day 3 (197 *versus* 164; $p<0.001$), day 7 (213 *versus* 181; $p<0.001$)	81 (22%) patients with complications from 151 (11%) RMs: hypotension (n=61, 5%), desaturation (n=58, 4%), tachycardia/bradycardia (n=24, 2%), new air leak (n=4, 0.3%) and new arrhythmia (n=4, 0.3%)

CPAP: continuous positive airway pressure; Sp,O_2: arterial oxygen saturation measured by pulse oximetry; FI,O_2: inspiratory oxygen fraction; PEEP: positive end-expiratory pressure; SBP: systolic blood pressure; P/F: ratio of partial pressure of arterial oxygen to FI,O_2.

In contrast, attenuating VALI and subsequent multiple organ dysfunction has a clear mortality benefit. However, it remains unknown whether this is associated with a reduction in VALI in humans, as has been demonstrated in animal models. Some trials of ventilation strategies incorporating RMs have shown a mortality benefit, but this benefit may be attributed to the other lung protective components in the intervention arm and it is difficult to determine the beneficial effect of the recruitment component given the other significant differences in ventilatory strategy [47]. There have been two randomised controlled trials incorporating RMs in their ventilation strategy that examined mortality [19, 54]. An ARDS Network study (ALVEOLI) comparing an open-lung strategy with a pressure-limited strategy was discontinued early due to a lack of benefit [54]. Similarly, the large multicentre LOV study, incorporating RMs into a lung protective strategy using pressure-controlled ventilation with high PEEP levels, did not confer a significant survival benefit as compared to a conventional lung protective ventilation strategy [19].

Future directions

Determining the efficacy and optimal type of RM

Unfortunately, there have been no prospective, randomised controlled trials demonstrating the efficacy of RMs on patient-important outcomes in ALI, such as mortality. As a result, it is impossible to determine the comparative effectiveness of two or more different types of RMs on patient-important outcomes in ALI patients. However, experimental data suggest that sustained inflation RMs may be associated with more VALI as compared to progressive recruitment with more gradual inflation methods, resulting in a more homogeneous distribution of pressure in the injured lung [68]. In addition to patient-important outcomes (*e.g.* mortality), future studies should also examine the potential effect of different RMs on VALI (*e.g.* lung and systemic inflammatory mediators), lung morphology (*e.g.* CT scans and EIT) and respiratory mechanics.

Which ALI patients should receive RMs?

The current definition of ALI [69] results in a heterogeneous population of patients with variable response to interventions, including lung recruitment. A number of studies have suggested a differential response to RMs depending on a number of patient and disease factors, including: the nature of their lung injury, *e.g.* pulmonary *versus* extra-pulmonary; the radiographic appearance of their disease, *e.g.* focal *versus* diffuse; and the timing of RM use, *e.g.* early *versus* late ALI. Thus, the application of RMs to unselected patients with ALI would probably result in a balance between potential benefits in recruitable patients, offset by potential harm in non-recruitable patients. Therefore, ongoing research into readily available, noninvasive methods of identifying recruitable patients at the bedside (*e.g.* lung ultrasound and EIT) will be of great importance in determining potential candidates for RMs in ALI.

Conclusions

Despite strong pathophysiological rationale and supportive pre-clinical and observational data for lung recruitment in patients with ALI, there are limited data from clinical trials to advocate for the routine use of RMs in unselected populations. Although there are no data demonstrating that an RM will improve outcome, it may be reasonable to attempt this approach to improve oxygenation early in the course of patients with ALI and evidence of recruitability. While sustained inflation RMs are common, recent evidence suggests that tidal recruitment using pressure-controlled ventilation, or incremental PEEP strategies, may be more efficacious and have a better safety profile. Those who respond may accrue the additional benefit of reduced VALI, and this may be an important component of a lung protective ventilation strategy in these patients. While serious complications may be uncommon, it is essential to avoid harm by monitoring for barotrauma and adverse effects on cardiac output. Further randomised clinical trials are needed to confirm the safety and efficacy of RMs in a selected group of ALI patients with recruitable disease, as well as to elucidate the optimal type, timing and frequency of RMs in these patients.

Statement of interest

None declared.

References

1. Fan E, Needham DM, Stewart TE. Ventilatory management of acute lung injury and acute respiratory distress syndrome. *JAMA* 2005; 294: 2889–2896.
2. Muscedere JG, Mullen JB, Gan K, *et al.* Tidal ventilation at low airway pressures can augment lung injury. *Am J Respir Crit Care Med* 1994; 149: 1327–1334.

3. Crotti S, Mascheroni D, Caironi P, *et al.* Recruitment and derecruitment during acute respiratory failure: a clinical study. *Am J Respir Crit Care Med* 2001; 164: 131–140.
4. Lachmann B. Open up the lung and keep the lung open. *Intensive Care Med* 1992; 18: 319–321.
5. Dos Santos CC, Slutsky AS. Invited review: mechanisms of ventilator-induced lung injury: a perspective. *J Appl Physiol* 2000; 89: 1645–1655.
6. Hodgson C, Keating JL, Holland AE, *et al.* Recruitment manoeuvres for adults with acute lung injury receiving mechanical ventilation. *Cochrane Database Syst Rev* 2009; 2: CD006667.
7. Fan E, Wilcox ME, Brower RG, *et al.* Recruitment maneuvers for acute lung injury: a systematic review. *Am J Respir Crit Care Med* 2008; 178: 1156–1163.
8. Lim S-C, Adams AB, Simonson DA, *et al.* Intercomparison of recruitment maneuver efficacy in three models of acute lung injury. *Crit Care Med* 2004; 32: 2371–2377.
9. Gattinoni L, Caironi P, Cressoni M, *et al.* Lung recruitment in patients with the acute respiratory distress syndrome. *N Engl J Med* 2006; 354: 1775–1786.
10. Gattinoni L, Pesenti A. The concept of "baby lung". *Intensive Care Med* 2005; 31: 776–784.
11. Tremblay LN, Slutsky AS. Ventilator-induced lung injury: from the bench to the bedside. *Intensive Care Med* 2006; 32: 24–33.
12. Pelosi P, Goldner M, McKibben A, *et al.* Recruitment and derecruitment during acute respiratory failure: an experimental study. *Am J Respir Crit Care Med* 2001; 164: 122–130.
13. Borges JB, Okamoto VN, Matos GFJ, *et al.* Reversibility of lung collapse and hypoxemia in early acute respiratory distress syndrome. *Am J Respir Crit Care Med* 2006; 174: 268–278.
14. Puybasset L, Cluzel P, Gusman P, *et al.* Regional distribution of gas and tissue in acute respiratory distress syndrome. I. Consequences for lung morphology. CT Scan ARDS Study Group. *Intensive Care Med* 2000; 26: 857–869.
15. Gattinoni L, Pelosi P, Suter PM, *et al.* Acute respiratory distress syndrome caused by pulmonary and extrapulmonary disease. Different syndromes? *Am J Respir Crit Care Med* 1998; 158: 3–11.
16. Putensen C, Theuerkauf N, Zinserling J, *et al.* Meta-analysis: ventilation strategies and outcomes of the acute respiratory distress syndrome and acute lung injury. *Ann Intern Med* 2009; 151: 566–576.
17. Ventilation with lower tidal volumes as compared with traditional tidal volumes for acute lung injury and the acute respiratory distress syndrome. The Acute Respiratory Distress Syndrome Network. *N Engl J Med* 2000; 342: 1301–1308.
18. Terragni PP, Rosboch G, Tealdi A, *et al.* Tidal hyperinflation during low tidal volume ventilation in acute respiratory distress syndrome. *Am J Respir Crit Care Med* 2007; 175: 160–166.
19. Meade MO, Cook DJ, Guyatt GH, *et al.* Ventilation strategy using low tidal volumes, recruitment maneuvers, and high positive end-expiratory pressure for acute lung injury and acute respiratory distress syndrome: a randomized controlled trial. *JAMA* 2008; 299: 637–645.
20. Mercat A, Richard JC, Vielle B, *et al.* Positive end-expiratory pressure setting in adults with acute lung injury and acute respiratory distress syndrome: a randomized controlled trial. *JAMA* 2008; 299: 646–655.
21. Briel M, Meade M, Mercat A, *et al.* Higher *vs* lower positive end-expiratory pressure in patients with acute lung injury and acute respiratory distress syndrome: systematic review and meta-analysis. *JAMA* 2010; 303: 865–873.
22. Brower RG, Lanken PN, MacIntyre N, *et al.* Higher *versus* lower positive end-expiratory pressures in patients with the acute respiratory distress syndrome. *N Engl J Med* 2004; 351: 327–336.
23. Dorrington KL, Radcliffe FM. Effect of a single inflation of the lungs on oxygenation during total extracorporeal carbon dioxide removal in experimental respiratory distress syndrome. *Intensive Care Med* 1991; 17: 469–474.
24. Kolton M, Cattran CB, Kent G, *et al.* Oxygenation during high-frequency ventilation compared with conventional mechanical ventilation in two models of lung injury. *Anesth Analg* 1982; 61: 323–332.
25. Kloot TE, Blanch L, Melynne Youngblood A, *et al.* Recruitment maneuvers in three experimental models of acute lung injury. Effect on lung volume and gas exchange. *Am J Respir Crit Care Med* 2000; 161: 1485–1494.
26. Cakar N, Akinci O, Tugrul S, *et al.* Recruitment maneuver: does it promote bacterial translocation? *Crit Care Med* 2002; 30: 2103–2106.
27. Bugedo G, Bruhn A, Hernández G, *et al.* Lung computed tomography during a lung recruitment maneuver in patients with acute lung injury. *Intensive Care Med* 2003; 29: 218–225.
28. Chu EK, Whitehead T, Slutsky AS. Effects of cyclic opening and closing at low- and high-volume ventilation on bronchoalveolar lavage cytokines. *Crit Care Med* 2004; 32: 168–174.
29. Grasso S, Mascia L, del Turco M, *et al.* Effects of recruiting maneuvers in patients with acute respiratory distress syndrome ventilated with protective ventilatory strategy. *Anesthesiology* 2002; 96: 795–802.
30. Halbertsma FJ, Vaneker M, Pickkers P, *et al.* A single recruitment maneuver in ventilated critically ill children can translocate pulmonary cytokines into the circulation. *J Crit Care* 2010; 25: 10–15.
31. Girgis K, Hamed H, Khater Y, *et al.* A decremental PEEP trial identifies the PEEP level that maintains oxygenation after lung recruitment. *Respir Care* 2006; 51: 1132–1139.
32. Rocco PR, Pelosi P, de Abreu MG. Pros and cons of recruitment maneuvers in acute lung injury and acute respiratory distress syndrome. *Expert Rev Respir Med* 2010; 4: 479–489.
33. Pelosi P, Cadringher P, Bottino N, *et al.* Sigh in acute respiratory distress syndrome. *Am J Respir Crit Care Med* 1999; 159: 872–880.

34. Foti G, Cereda M, Sparacino ME, *et al.* Effects of periodic lung recruitment maneuvers on gas exchange and respiratory mechanics in mechanically ventilated acute respiratory distress syndrome (ARDS) patients. *Intensive Care Med* 2000; 26: 501–507.

35. Lim CM, Koh Y, Park W, *et al.* Mechanistic scheme and effect of "extended sigh" as a recruitment maneuver in patients with acute respiratory distress syndrome: a preliminary study. *Crit Care Med* 2001; 29: 1255–1260.

36. Lim C-M, Jung H, Koh Y, *et al.* Effect of alveolar recruitment maneuver in early acute respiratory distress syndrome according to antiderecruitment strategy, etiological category of diffuse lung injury, and body position of the patient. *Crit Care Med* 2003; 31: 411–418.

37. Maggiore SM, Lellouche F, Pigeot J, *et al.* Prevention of endotracheal suctioning-induced alveolar derecruitment in acute lung injury. *Am J Respir Crit Care Med* 2003; 167: 1215–1224.

38. Lapinsky SE, Aubin M, Mehta S, *et al.* Safety and efficacy of a sustained inflation for alveolar recruitment in adults with respiratory failure. *Intensive Care Med* 1999; 25: 1297–1301.

39. Hickling KG. Best compliance during a decremental, but not incremental, positive end-expiratory pressure trial is related to open-lung positive end-expiratory pressure: a mathematical model of acute respiratory distress syndrome lungs. *Am J Respir Crit Care Med* 2001; 163: 69–78.

40. Fan E, Stewart TE. New modalities of mechanical ventilation: high-frequency oscillatory ventilation and airway pressure release ventilation. *Clin Chest Med* 2006; 27: 615–625.

41. Demory D, Michelet P, Arnal J-M, *et al.* High-frequency oscillatory ventilation following prone positioning prevents a further impairment in oxygenation. *Crit Care Med* 2007; 35: 106–111.

42. Pelosi P, Bottino N, Chiumello D, *et al.* Sigh in supine and prone position during acute respiratory distress syndrome. *Am J Respir Crit Care Med* 2003; 167: 521–527.

43. Rival G, Patry C, Floret N, *et al.* Prone position and recruitment maneuver: the combined effect improves oxygenation. *Crit Care* 2011; 15: R125.

44. Sud S, Sud M, Friedrich JO, *et al.* Effect of mechanical ventilation in the prone position on clinical outcomes in patients with acute hypoxemic respiratory failure: a systematic review and meta-analysis. *CMAJ* 2008; 178: 1153–1161.

45. Sud S, Friedrich JO, Taccone P, *et al.* Prone ventilation reduces mortality in patients with acute respiratory failure and severe hypoxemia: systematic review and meta-analysis. *Intensive Care Med* 2010; 36: 585–599.

46. Guerin C, Gaillard S, Lemasson S, *et al.* Effects of systematic prone positioning in hypoxemic acute respiratory failure: a randomized controlled trial. *JAMA* 2004; 292: 2379–2387.

47. Amato MB, Barbas CS, Medeiros DM, *et al.* Effect of a protective-ventilation strategy on mortality in the acute respiratory distress syndrome. *N Engl J Med* 1998; 338: 347–354.

48. Wrigge H, Zinserling J, Muders T, *et al.* Electrical impedance tomography compared with thoracic computed tomography during a slow inflation maneuver in experimental models of lung injury. *Crit Care Med* 2008; 36: 903–909.

49. Costa ELV, Borges JB, Melo A, *et al.* Bedside estimation of recruitable alveolar collapse and hyperdistension by electrical impedance tomography. *Intensive Care Med* 2009; 35: 1132–1137.

50. Vieira SR, Puybasset L, Lu Q, *et al.* A scanographic assessment of pulmonary morphology in acute lung injury. Significance of the lower inflection point detected on the lung pressure–volume curve. *Am J Respir Crit Care Med* 1999; 159: 1612–1623.

51. Mehta S, Stewart TE, Macdonald R, *et al.* Temporal change, reproducibility, and interobserver variability in pressure–volume curves in adults with acute lung injury and acute respiratory distress syndrome. *Crit Care Med* 2003; 31: 2118–2125.

52. Dyhr T, Laursen N, Larsson A. Effects of lung recruitment maneuver and positive end-expiratory pressure on lung volume, respiratory mechanics and alveolar gas mixing in patients ventilated after cardiac surgery. *Acta Anaesthesiol Scand* 2002; 46: 717–725.

53. Constantin J-M, Futier E, Cherprenet A-L, *et al.* A recruitment maneuver increases oxygenation after intubation of hypoxemic intensive care unit patients: a randomized controlled study. *Crit Care* 2010; 14: R76.

54. Brower RG, Morris A, MacIntyre N, *et al.* Effects of recruitment maneuvers in patients with acute lung injury and acute respiratory distress syndrome ventilated with high positive end-expiratory pressure. *Crit Care Med* 2003; 31: 2592–2597.

55. Constantin J-M, Cayot-Constantin S, Roszyk L, *et al.* Response to recruitment maneuver influences net alveolar fluid clearance in acute respiratory distress syndrome. *Anesthesiology* 2007; 106: 944–951.

56. Richard JC, Maggiore SM, Jonson B, *et al.* Influence of tidal volume on alveolar recruitment. Respective role of PEEP and a recruitment maneuver. *Am J Respir Crit Care Med* 2001; 163: 1609–1613.

57. Rothen HU, Sporre B, Engberg G, *et al.* Influence of gas composition on recurrence of atelectasis after a reexpansion maneuver during general anesthesia. *Anesthesiology* 1995; 82: 832–842.

58. Suárez-Sipmann F, Böhm SH, Tusman G, *et al.* Use of dynamic compliance for open lung positive end-expiratory pressure titration in an experimental study. *Crit Care Med* 2007; 35: 214–221.

59. Kacmarek RM, Villar J. Lung recruitment maneuvers during acute respiratory distress syndrome: is it useful? *Minerva Anestesiol* 2011; 77: 85–89.

60. Badet M, Bayle F, Richard J-C, *et al.* Comparison of optimal positive end-expiratory pressure and recruitment maneuvers during lung-protective mechanical ventilation in patients with acute lung injury/acute respiratory distress syndrome. *Respir Care* 2009; 54: 847–854.

61. Pipeling MR, Fan E. Therapies for refractory hypoxemia in acute respiratory distress syndrome. *JAMA* 2010; 304: 2521–2527.

62. Oczenski W, Hörmann C, Keller C, *et al.* Recruitment maneuvers after a positive end-expiratory pressure trial do not induce sustained effects in early adult respiratory distress syndrome. *Anesthesiology* 2004; 101: 620–625.

63. Stapleton RD, Wang BM, Hudson LD, *et al.* Causes and timing of death in patients with ARDS. *Chest* 2005; 128: 525–532.

64. Ware LB. Prognostic determinants of acute respiratory distress syndrome in adults: impact on clinical trial design. *Crit Care Med* 2005; 33: Suppl. 3, S217–S222.

65. Phua J, Badia JR, Adhikari NK, *et al.* Has mortality from acute respiratory distress syndrome decreased over time? A systematic review. *Am J Respir Crit Care Med* 2009; 179: 220–227.

66. Bersten AD, Edibam C, Hunt T, *et al.* Incidence and mortality of acute lung injury and the acute respiratory distress syndrome in three Australian States. *Am J Respir Crit Care Med* 2002; 165: 443–448.

67. Adhikari NK, Burns KE, Friedrich JO, *et al.* Effect of nitric oxide on oxygenation and mortality in acute lung injury: systematic review and meta-analysis. *BMJ* 2007; 334: 779.

68. Riva DR, Contador RS, Baez-Garcia CSN, *et al.* Recruitment maneuver: RAMP *versus* CPAP pressure profile in a model of acute lung injury. *Respir Physiol Neurobiol* 2009; 169: 62–68.

69. Bernard GR, Artigas A, Brigham KL, *et al.* The American–European Consensus Conference on ARDS. Definitions, mechanisms, relevant outcomes, and clinical trial coordination. *Am J Respir Crit Care Med* 1994; 149: 818–824.

Chapter 4

Surfactant therapy in acute lung injury/acute respiratory distress syndrome

J. Kesecioglu and M.M.J. van Eijk

Summary

Acute lung injury (ALI) and acute respiratory distress syndrome (ARDS) occur after diverse pulmonary or systemic insults. Although necessary for keeping the patient alive, mechanical ventilation has been implicated in the associated high morbidity and mortality. New therapies have attempted to improve oxygenation and ventilation, while providing lung protection. A multitude of causes can lead to ALI/ARDS. However, the dysfunction of the endogenous surfactant system is a shared characteristic. It has been suggested to use surfactant replacement therapy in patients with ARDS in order to overcome the ongoing inactivation of endogenous surfactants by plasma proteins entering the alveolar spaces. The evidence regarding surfactant replacement therapy in ARDS patients is discussed in this chapter.

Although some small studies have shown beneficial effects of surfactant replacement therapy, larger studies failed to establish this effect. Therefore, exogenous surfactants are not recommended for routine use in patients with ALI/ARDS.

Keywords: Acute lung injury, acute respiratory distress syndrome, critical care, evidence-based medicine, mechanical ventilation, surfactant therapy

Dept of Intensive Care Medicine, University Medical Center Utrecht, Utrecht, The Netherlands.

Correspondence: J. Kesecioglu, Dept of Intensive Care, Room F06.149, University Medical Center Utrecht, Heidelberlaan 100, 3584 CX, Utrecht, The Netherlands.
Email J.Kesecioglu@umcutrecht.nl

Eur Respir Mon 2012; 55: 54–64.
Printed in UK – all rights reserved
Copyright ERS 2012
European Respiratory Monograph
ISSN: 1025-448x
DOI: 10.1183/1025448x.10001611

Acute lung injury (ALI) and acute respiratory distress syndrome (ARDS) represent common clinical syndromes that can occur after diverse pulmonary or systemic insults [1, 2]. The primary feature of these syndromes is the acute onset of severe hypoxaemia that is associated with diffuse, non-cardiogenic pulmonary infiltrates. Although necessary for keeping the patient alive, mechanical ventilation has been implicated in the associated high morbidity and mortality rate of patients with such syndromes [3]. Therefore, new therapies have been attempted to improve oxygenation and ventilation, while providing lung protection [4].

In spite of great improvements in supportive therapy within intensive care units (ICUs) in the past decades, recent epidemiological studies have shown that ALI/ARDS still have a high mortality rate of 40–50% [2, 5]. This highlights the necessity of new therapies directed at the cause of the pathology. A multitude of causes can lead to ALI/ARDS. However, the dysfunction of the endogenous surfactant system is a shared characteristic [6]. The composition of surfactants changes with various disease states [7]. Changes in surfactant composition may lead to alveolar instability, alveolar flooding and alveolar collapse. Both qualitative and quantitative changes of the surfactant occur in patients with ARDS [8–10] and in patients at risk for ARDS [10], respectively.

These alterations of the surfactant system have been documented in several diseases and prolonged mechanical ventilation has been found to induce these changes [11]. Therefore, it has been suggested to use surfactant replacement therapy in patients with ARDS, in order to overcome any ongoing inactivation of the endogenous surfactant by plasma proteins that enter the alveolar spaces.

Pulmonary surfactants consist of phospholipids (85%), different proteins, lipids and carbohydrates [12]. The pulmonary surfactant is synthesised by alveolar type II cells, stored in lamellar bodies and secreted to the alveolar space to cover the epithelial surface [13]. Surfactant protein (SP)-B and SP-C are small and extremely hydrophobic proteins that are important in surfactant dynamics within the terminal air spaces and are an essential part in the reduction of surface tension [14]. SP-A regulates the secretion and the uptake of the surfactant from the type II cells. SP-B and SP-C enable the adsorption of the phospholipid molecules rapidly into the monolayer. SP-A and SP-D both play a role in the lung's defence against infection.

Surfactant therapy

A historical perspective

In 1929, VON NEERGAARD [15] was the first to suggest that surface tension played a role in lung elasticity. Some 25 years later, MACKLIN [16] described the presence of a thin aqueous mucoid microfilm on the pulmonary alveolar walls, which was in constant slow movement towards the phagocytic pneumocytes and bronchioles. In 1955, PATTLE [17] analysed the foam and bubbles taken from lung oedema and healthy lungs and found them both to be very stable. He thought that the walls of these bubbles contained materials that lowered the surface tension to zero. Then, in 1957, CLEMENTS [18] found evidence to show surface-active materials occurred in the lungs. This was followed in 1959 by AVERY and MEAD [19] who demonstrated that the lung extracts of premature infants and infants dying from hyaline membrane disease had much higher surface tension than normal lung extracts, due to a deficiency in the surface-active material. FUJIWARA et al. [20] were the first to treat respiratory failure in premature babies with an exogenous surfactant.

Since 1980, more than 100,000 premature infants suffering from respiratory failure have been treated with exogenous surfactants [21, 22]. However, until recently, only a few case reports, results from limited clinical pilot studies and a few randomised controlled studies were available in which patients with respiratory failure, other than neonates, were treated with exogenous surfactant [23]. This situation has changed dramatically within the last decade.

Surfactant therapy in ARDS

Since there are many similarities between premature babies with respiratory failure and ARDS, ASHBAUGH et al. [1] postulated that the surface-active material of the lung is abnormal in patients with ARDS. It has been well established that abnormalities of the surfactant system occurs in ARDS and that these abnormalities contribute to the pathophysiology of ARDS [7]. In premature infants, a deficiency in the surfactant is the initiating problem [21]. In ARDS patients, the biophysical and biochemical abnormalities in the pulmonary surfactant system have been observed alongside a deficiency in surfactant [14].

The rationale for surfactant replacement therapy in patients with ARDS is to restore the normal composition of the surfactant system, as well as to overcome the ongoing inactivation of the present surfactant by plasma proteins, which enter the alveolar spaces. Surfactant replacement therapy can normalise the composition of the surfactant system [24, 25] and restore its surface activity [26], which results in the restoration of the gas exchange [24, 27, 28].

Research on surfactant therapy in ARDS

In 1987, a child with near drowning and superimposed pneumonia was treated with exogenous surfactant, resulting in a dramatic improvement of gas exchange [29]. This was the first report on the treatment of an ARDS patient with an exogenous surfactant. RICHMAN et al. [30] described their initial experience with surfactant replacement in three patients in 1989, and HASLAM et al. [31] described four patients treated with surfactants in 1994. Since then several pilot studies, phase II studies and phase III studies have been performed to investigate the efficacy of surfactant replacement therapies in patients with ARDS.

Pilot and phase I studies on surfactant replacement therapy

WALMRATH et al. [27] and GÜNTHER et al. [25] investigated the impact of a bronchoscopic instillation of a natural bovine surfactant extract (Alveofact; Thomae, Biberach, Germany) on the biochemical and biophysical properties of surfactants in patients with severe and early ARDS and septic shock [25, 27]. The efficacy of bronchoscopic surfactant instillation on gas exchange was investigated in the same group of patients [24]. A total of 27 patients were described in three reports on this pilot study, which contained no control group (i.e. there were no patients with ARDS not receiving a surfactant). Severe surfactant abnormalities were demonstrated in the ARDS patients, compared with healthy subjects. Surfactant replacement resulted in a near normalisation of the surfactant properties and, within 12 hours, gas exchange was found to have improved in most patients. Patients with a relapse received a second instillation of the surfactant, which again resulted in an improvement of the arterial oxygenation.

WISWELL et al. [32] performed an open-label phase I trial to assess the safety and tolerability of sequential bronchopulmonary segmental lavage with a diluted synthetic surfactant (Surfaxin; Discovery Laboratories, Doylestown, PA, USA) in 12 adults with ARDS. Patients received one of three dosing regimens in which aliquots of Surfaxin were administered in each and all of the bronchopulmonary segments via a wedged bronchoscope. Similar to the studies by WALMRATH and co-workers [24, 27] and GÜNTHER et al. [25] mentioned earlier, there was no control group. Patients received: 1) one 30-mL aliquot of 2.5 mg·mL^{-1} Surfaxin in each segment followed by a second 30-mL aliquot of 10 mg·mL^{-1} (n=3); 2) two 30-mL aliquots of 2.5 mg·mL^{-1} followed by a third lavage with 10 mg·mL^{-1} (n=4); or 3) similar treatment as 2) plus a possible extra dose 6–24 hours later (n=5). Suctioning was performed 10–30 seconds after the instillation of the individual aliquots. During the 96 hours after treatment was initiated, inspiratory oxygen fraction (F_{I,O_2}) decreased from 0.80 to 0.52 and positive end expiratory pressure (PEEP) decreased from 10.3 to 7.6 cmH$_2$O.

In a study by SPRAGG et al. [28], six patients with ARDS were treated with a single dose of porcine surfactant (Curosurf; Chiesi Farmaceutici, Parma, Italy). The surfactant was delivered via a bronchoscope in aliquots into each of the lobar bronchi and was well tolerated, and caused a modest transient improvement in gas exchange. Bronchoalveolar lavage (BAL) phospholipid concentrations were elevated 3 hours after the surfactant was administrated compared with the pre-administered levels, and then fell within 24 hours. In addition, a reduced inhibition of the surfactant's function in BAL after surfactant replacement was observed in two patients.

Phase II studies on surfactant replacement therapy

Several phase II studies on surfactant replacement therapy have been conducted (table 1). To evaluate the safety and potential efficacy of an aerosolised lipid-based synthetic surfactant (Exosurf; Burroughs Wellcome, Quebec, QC, Canada) in patients with ARDS, WEG et al. [33] performed a prospective,

Table 1. Phase II studies on surfactant replacement therapy

First author [ref.]	Year	Surfactant	Instillation technique	Diagnosis ($P_{a,O_2}/F_{I,O_2}$ ratio)	Study details	Patients n	Main result	Phase III follow-up
WEG [33]	1994	Exosurf synthetic surfactant	Aerosolisation	ARDS (50–299)	Phase II study, prospective, multicentre, randomised trial	51	Surfactant administration was safe, dose-dependent trend in reduction of mortality	No
GREGORY [26]	1997	Survanta natural surfactant (bovine)	Intra-tracheal	ARDS (NA)	Phase II study, prospective, randomised trial	59	Surfactant administration was safe, decreased mortality	No
WALMRATH [34]	2000	Venticute synthetic surfactant + rSP-C	Intra-tracheal	ARDS (NA)	Phase II study, prospective, multicentre, randomised trial	41	Surfactant administration was safe, decreased ventilator-free days	Yes
SPRAGG [35]	2003	Venticute synthetic surfactant + rSP-C	Intra-tracheal	ARDS (NA)	Phase II study, prospective, multicentre, randomised trial	40	Surfactant administration was safe, decreased IL-6 levels in lavage	Yes
KESECIOGLU [36]	2001	HL-10 natural surfactant (porcine)	Intra-tracheal	ARDS/ALI (<300)	Phase II study, prospective, multicentre, randomised trial	36	Surfactant administration was safe, decreased mortality	Yes
KESECIOGLU [37]	2004	HL-10 natural surfactant (porcine)	Intra-tracheal	ARDS/ALI (<300)	Phase II study, prospective, randomised trial	23	Lower mortality in three dose regime compared with one dose	Yes

P_{a,O_2}: arterial oxygen tension; F_{I,O_2}: inspiratory oxygen fraction; ARDS: acute respiratory distress syndrome; NA: data not available; rSP-C: recombinant surfactant protein C; IL-6: interleukin-6; ALI: acute lung injury. Reproduced from [6] with permission from the publisher.

double-blind, placebo-controlled, randomised, parallel, multicentre pilot-dose clinical trial. A total of 51 patients with sepsis-induced ARDS were entered into this phase II study and were randomly assigned to four treatment groups: 1) 12 hours of surfactant per day (n=17); 2) 24 hours of surfactant per day (n=17); 3) 12 hours of 0.6% saline per day; and 4) 24 hours of 0.6% saline per day (controls combined: n=17). The surfactant and the saline were aerosolised continuously for up to 5 days using an in-line nebuliser. Surfactant administration was deemed safe. Although there were no differences in any physiological parameters between the treatment groups, there was a dose-dependent trend in the reduction of mortality from 47% in the placebo group to 41% and 35% in the groups treated with 12 hours and 24 hours of surfactant per day, respectively.

GREGORY et al. [26] performed a randomised, controlled, open-label clinical study of intra-tracheal administrated natural bovine surfactant (Survanta; Abbott Laboratories, Abbott Park, IL, USA) in 59 patients with ARDS to obtain information regarding its safety and efficacy. The F_{I,O_2} at 120 hours, after the instillation of the surfactant, was only significantly decreased for patients who had received up to four doses of 100 mg phospholipids per kg of surfactant when compared with control patients. Mortality in the same group of patients was 18.8%, compared with 43.8% in the control group (p=0.075).

In a multicentre, parallel-group controlled trial, WALMRATH et al. [34] randomised 41 patients with ARDS to receive standard therapy alone, or standard therapy plus a synthetic surfactant including recombinant (r) SP-C (Venticute; Atlanta Pharma, Konstanz, Germany). A total of 41 patients received standard therapy or standard therapy plus the surfactant. Intra-tracheal instillation of the surfactant resulted in an improved arterial oxygenation 24 hours after instillation when compared with the control group. Furthermore, more patients were weaned off the ventilator by day 28, compared with the patients in the control group.

SPRAGG et al. [35] also performed a study using rSP-C. Some 40 patients were prospectively randomised to receive standard therapy or standard therapy plus one of the two doses of an exogenous surfactant that was administered four times over a 24-hour period. They reported that the exogenous surfactant instillation was safe, but they could not show any improvement of arterial oxygenation due to the surfactant instillation. However, interleukin (IL)-6 concentrations were significantly lower in the BAL of the treated patients when compared with the control group, suggesting an anti-inflammatory treatment effect.

Table 2. Phase III studies on surfactant replacement therapy

First author [ref.]	Year	Surfactant	Installation technique	Diagnosis ($P_{a,O_2}/F_{I,O_2}$ ratio)	Study details	Patients n	Main result
Anzueto [38]	1996	Exosurf, synthetic surfactant	Aerosolisation	ARDS/ALI and sepsis (<250)	Phase III study, prospective, multicentre, randomised, placebo-controlled trial	725	No beneficial effects of surfactant administration
Spragg [39]	2004	Venticute, synthetic surfactant + rSP-C	Intra-tracheal	ARDS (<200)	Phase III study, prospective, multicentre, randomised trial	448	No beneficial effects of surfactant administration
Willson [40]	2005	Calfactant natural surfactant (bovine)	Intra-tracheal	ALI <18 years (<300)	Phase III study, prospective, multicentre, randomised trial	153	Surfactant decreased mortality (19% versus 27%) and improved oxygenation
Kesecioglu [41]	2009	HL-10, natural surfactant (porcine)	Intra-tracheal	ALI/ARDS (NA)	Phase III study, prospective, multicentre, randomised trial	418	No beneficial effects of surfactant administration and a trend towards increased mortality and adverse effects
Spragg [42]	2011	Synthetic surfactant + rSP-C	Intra-tracheal	ARDS/ALI (<170)	Phase III study, prospective, multicentre, randomised trial	843	No beneficial effects of surfactant administration

P_{a,O_2}: arterial oxygen tension; F_{I,O_2}: inspiratory oxygen fraction; ARDS: acute respiratory distress syndrome; ALI: acute lung injury; rSP-C: recombinant surfactant protein C; NA: data not available. Reproduced from [6] with permission from the publisher.

Lastly, Kesecioglu *et al.* [36] determined the efficacy and safety of the intra-tracheal instillation of the natural porcine surfactant HL-10 in patients with ALI/ARDS using a prospective, randomised, multicentre, open-label, phase II study in Europe. Patients (24 surfactant and 12 control) were randomised to receive standard therapy plus surfactant or standard therapy alone. Dosage was from 200 mg phospholipids per kg for ideal body weights (up to four doses in case of relapse). Efficacy variables were changes in arterial oxygen tension (P_{a,O_2})/F_{I,O_2}, length of hospital stay and the 28-day mortality rate. Measurements of oxygenation, duration of mechanical ventilation and length of stay in the ICU did not differ significantly between the two groups. However, the 28-day mortality rate in the surfactant group was 9% *versus* 43% in the control group (p=0.036). Based on these promising results, the group concluded that surfactant therapy might improve survival. In preparation for a phase III study, Kesecioglu *et al.* [37] determined the efficacy and safety of three doses of surfactant compared with one dose. The authors reported a mortality of 14.3% in the group receiving three doses *versus* 33.3% receiving one dose.

The aforementioned studies performed by Weg *et al.* [33], Walmrath *et al.* [34], Spragg *et al.* [35] and Kesecioglu and co-workers [36, 37] were followed by phase III studies due to the promising results obtained. No phase III study was performed with Survanta.

Phase III studies on surfactant replacement therapy

Four phase III studies in adults and one study in paediatrics with ARDS have been reported to date (table 2). 10 years, ago Anzueto *et al.* [38] used an aerosolised surfactant on adults with sepsis-induced ARDS. Using a multicentre, double-blind, placebo-controlled trial, they randomised the patients to receive either Exosurf (n=364) or 0.45% saline (n=361) for up to 5 days. Haemodynamic measurements, changes in oxygenation, duration of mechanical ventilation and length of stay in the ICU did not differ significantly between the two groups. Survival at 30 days was 60% for both groups. Survival was similar in both groups when analysed according to Acute Physiology and Chronic Health Evaluation (APACHE) III score, which established cause of death, time of onset, severity of ARDS, presence or absence of documented sepsis, and underlying disease. The investigators concluded that the continuous administration of an aerosolised synthetic surfactant to patients with sepsis induced ARDS had no beneficial effects.

SPRAGG *et al.* [39] performed two multicentre, randomised, double-blind, parallel-group controlled studies, which involved 448 patients with ARDS. The research group compared standard therapy alone with standard therapy plus up to four intra-tracheal doses of rSP-C based surfactant that was administered within a 24-hour period. Although there was a significant improvement of oxygenation in the first 24 hours, no improvement of survival was observed due to exogenous surfactant instillation. The combined data showed 68% survival in the control group and 64% in the surfactant group. They concluded that the routine use of a surfactant in the treatment of patients with ARDS is not justified. However, they have performed a *post hoc* analysis to see whether there were different treatment effects among patients with direct compared to indirect lung injury. All models for an interaction between treatment and the cause of ARDS (direct or indirect) were evaluated. There was a significant interaction (p=0.002) for the mortality analysis but not for the analysis on the number of ventilator-free days (p=0.14), indicating that among the patients where ARDS was caused by a direct lung injury, those who received the surfactant tended to have a higher survival rate than those who received standard therapy.

Encouraged by this *post hoc* analysis, SPRAGG *et al.* [42] performed another study to determine the clinical benefit of administering an rSP-C based synthetic surfactant to patients with severe direct lung injury due to pneumonia or aspiration. A prospective randomised blinded study was performed at 161 centres in 22 countries. Patients were randomly allocated to receive usual care plus up to eight doses of rSP-C surfactant, which was administered over a 96-hour period (n=419), or only usual care (n=424). Although it was planned to randomise 1,200 patients, the study was terminated due to futility after the second interim analysis of 800 patients. The study did not show a significantly reduced mortality rate at day 28 for patients receiving surfactant when compared with those receiving standard care, 22.7% *versus* 23.8%, respectively. Subgroup analysis showed no difference in mortality rates for groups defined by mechanism of direct lung injury (aspiration or pneumonia), presence of ARDS or geographic location. Patients alive at 3 and 6 months were similar between the groups (64.9% and 62.5% for surfactant plus usual care *versus* 65.6% and 63.9% for usual care alone). Both groups had improved oxygenation after randomisation; there was no significant difference of oxygenation between the administrations of the surfactant compared with usual care alone. Similarly, no significant difference in the median number of ventilator free days was observed at day 28 (9 days for surfactant plus usual care and 10 days for usual care alone). A shearing step was added to the surfactant preparation protocol in order to improve dispersion of the rSP-C surfactant during suspension. The authors concluded that shearing of the surfactant during re-suspension may have resulted in impairment of surface tension-lowering function and increased susceptibility to inhibition by plasma proteins, hence lack of clinical effect.

After the encouraging results of their phase II studies, KESECIOGLU *et al.* [41] conducted a phase III trial to determine whether the instillation of exogenous surfactant would improve the 28-day outcome of adult patients with ALI or ARDS. A total of 418 patients with ALI and ARDS were included in an international, multicentre, stratified, randomised, controlled, open, parallel-group study. They randomly assigned the patients to receive usual care either with or without instillation of the exogenous natural porcine surfactant HL-10 as large boluses. The sample size of 1,000 patients was needed to detect a 10% point absolute reduction in mortality from 40% to 30%. The study was prematurely terminated because a 300-patient safety analysis showed a trend toward higher mortality in the treatment group, even though the increased mortality signal was largely in the 60- to 90-day follow-up, but not at the 28-day time-point. In the study, the HL-10 group 28-day mortality rate was 28.8% and the mortality rate from usual care alone was 24.5%. However, given the trends in morbidity and mortality, a positive effect of intervention was highly unlikely and would, at best, indicate futility and at worst an adverse effect. No improvement related to HL-10 was observed either in the secondary study objective (mortality at day 180) or after the *post hoc* analysis of the 28-day and 180-day mortality rate in the direct and indirect lung injury groups. Days alive and out of ICU and days alive and out of ICU for the subgroup of patients alive at day 28 were significantly worse for patients receiving HL-10. No improvement of oxygenation was observed in the group who received HL-10. Analyses of secondary objectives support the conclusion of the primary objective, *i.e.* that patients receiving HL-10 have a trend towards an inferior outcome. The extent to which these adverse outcomes are directly related to the surfactant itself *versus* the installation procedure and/or the associated ventilation practice was not clear. KESECIOGLU *et al.* [41] speculated that neonatal or paediatric deaths often occurred as a result of respiratory failure, whereas adults with ALI/ARDS often die as a result of multiple organ failure. Therefore, it may not be surprising to find that surfactant alone is not effective in reducing the mortality rate in adult patients. Interestingly, LU *et al.* [43] performed computed tomography (CT) scans on a subgroup of 20 patients (10 treated with HL-10 and 10 controls) from the study by KESECIOGLU *et al.* [41]. They reported that intra-tracheal surfactant replacement induced a significant and prolonged lung re-aeration in the previously atelectatic areas. It also induced a significant increase in lung tissue in normally aerated lung areas whose mechanism was not clear. They concluded that benefit, in terms of aeration of poorly or non-aerated regions of the lung, was likely to be counteracted by a negative impact of HL-10 on aeration of the previously normally aerated lung.

In 2005, WILLSON *et al.* [40] reported their multicentre, randomised, blinded phase III trial which compared the use of natural lung surfactant (Calfactant; ONY Inc., Amherst, NY, USA) with a placebo in 153 infants, children and adolescents with respiratory failure from ALI. Patients were treated with intra-tracheal instillations of two doses of 80 mL·m^{-2} Calfactant or an equal volume of air placebo, both administered 12 hours apart. Although ventilator-free days did not differ, mortality was significantly greater in the placebo group 36% compared with 19% in the Calfactant group (27 out of 75 *versus* 15 out of 77, respectively). More patients in the placebo group did not respond to conventional mechanical ventilation. Calfactant acutely improved oxygenation and significantly decreased mortality in infants, children and adolescents with ALI.

All adult phase III trials on ALI/ARDS surfactant therapy failed to demonstrate any beneficial effect on outcome, either with respect to mortality or ventilator-free days. Only in a phase III trial in paediatric patients did the exogenous surfactant reduce mortality.

Comments on surfactant studies

Data from the phase II and phase III studies on surfactant replacement in patients with ARDS are contradictory: promising results from the studies by WEG *et al.* [33], WALMRATH *et al.* [24], SPRAGG *et al.* [35] and KESECIOGLU and co-workers [36, 37] were not reproduced in their follow-up studies, *i.e.* ANZUETO *et al.* [38], SPRAGG and co-workers [39, 42] and KESECIOGLU *et al.* [41], respectively. By contrast, two phase II studies showed a trend towards mortality reduction [26] or a significant improvement of survival [36]. One of the most important differences between the aforementioned studies is the sample size: "positive" phase II studies, showing potential benefit of surfactant instillation in patients with acute lung injury, were all on limited numbers of patients, while in the "negative" phase III studies larger patient groups were studied. In this chapter it is not our intention to extensively discuss differences between phase II and phase III studies in general. However, apart from the number of patients recruited in the published studies on surfactant instillation in patients with ARDS, there are some important differences, such as the type of surfactant used, the method of surfactant instillation, dosing of the surfactant and last, but not least, the mechanical ventilation strategies utilised.

Composition of surfactant

In studies of surfactant replacement therapy, different types of surfactants have been used. One can roughly divide the studies into those using natural surfactants (bovine or porcine), those containing the SP-B and SP-C [26, 36, 37, 41], and those using a synthetic surfactant without any surfactant proteins [33, 38], or only containing SP-C [34, 39, 42].

Although synthetic surfactants can be produced in larger quantities, both experimental and clinical data have demonstrated the superiority of natural surfactant preparations over synthetic products. Natural surfactants have been found to be more effective in increasing arterial oxygenation and alveolar stability [44]. Furthermore, the use of natural surfactants results in a more rapid improvement and natural surfactants are less sensitive to inhibition by serum proteins and other inflammatory mediators. Indeed, a recent study by AINSWORTH *et al.* [45] on premature neonates, which compared a natural surfactant with a synthetic surfactant, demonstrated a significant decrease in mortality when treated with the natural surfactant. These results might be a possible explanation for the lack of effect by the surfactant on the mortality rates in the previous studies, where investigators used synthetic exogenous surfactants [38, 39, 42]. Alternatively, exogenous natural porcine surfactant was used in the study by KESECIOGLU et al. [41] with no effect on mortality. The results reported in this study contradict the findings of AINSWORTH et al. [45].

Independent of the surfactant being natural or synthetic, each surfactant preparation has its own unique composition. Therefore, it does not necessarily mean that the results obtained with one surfactant preparation would be similar when another surfactant has been used.

Techniques for the delivery of surfactants

Different techniques have been used to instil surfactants into patients with ARDS. In two of the studies, described previously, the surfactants were instilled by means of aerosolisation [33, 38], whereas in other studies surfactant instillation was achieved by means of a bronchoscope [24, 25, 27, 28, 32]. Most of the reviewed studies used intra-tracheal instillation [26, 34, 36, 37, 39, 41, 42].

Although aerosolising the surfactant is a promising technique, its inadequacy to deliver sufficient amounts of surfactant to the terminal airways precludes this technique from being used nowadays. The aerosolisation system used in the studies by WEG et al. [33] and ANZUETO et al. [38] allowed the investigators to instil <5 mg·kg^{-1} of the required dose of 112 mg·kg^{-1} per day (i.e. only 4.5%). The amount of surfactant delivered with this technique is only a sixteenth of the dose that was delivered in the studies by GREGORY et al. [26] and KESECIOGLU et al. [37], which is an insufficient amount to overcome the inhibiting activities of plasma proteins present in the airways of patients with ARDS [46].

Other studies used a bronchoscopic lavage for the instillation of the surfactant into the lungs [24, 25, 27, 28, 32]. Investigators claimed that this instillation technique provided both "cleansing" of the airways, and enabled the instillation of the surfactant to occur in all segments of the lungs. Bronchoscopic lavages are expected to be efficient in patients with direct lung injury, because during this procedure inflammatory mediators are removed from the lung [32]. However, this procedure is very time consuming. In the study by WISWELL et al. [32] the median duration of the lavage procedure was more than 90 minutes, and in the reports by WALMRATH et al. [24] and GÜNTHER et al. [25] the bronchoscopic procedure lasted 45 minutes. This time consuming aspect may prohibit the treatment of many patients with ARDS who are all in one clinic at the same time.

In the majority of the reviewed studies, the surfactant was instilled as a bolus, either by means of a catheter installed via the endotracheal tube and advanced upwards to above the carina [26, 34, 39] or by means of a bolus through a syringe connected to the endotracheal tube [36, 37, 41]. Instillation of surfactants by this method is very simple to perform and less time consuming than instillation via a bronchoscope. Importantly, distribution of the surfactant in this way is adequate. It has been argued that this method of instillation may give rise to a problem with respect to the volume that is instilled into the lungs. However, it has been demonstrated that the volume of fluid that has to be instilled is rapidly absorbed [47].

Whatever method is used, the important requirements are that an adequate amount of surfactant is instilled and the instilled surfactant reaches as large an area as possible in the alveolar surface. These requirements were clearly not present in the studies where aerosolisation was used. Recently, RUPPERT et al. [48] reported the development and successful use of a new dry powder aerosolisation technique for the administration of surfactants. It has been questioned in an article whether this device will be the solution for optimal instillation [49].

Surfactant dosage

The dose of an exogenous surfactant must be large enough to overcome all the inhibitors present in the ALI/ARDS lung. It has been estimated that approximately 1 mg of surfactant is needed to overcome the inhibitory effect of 1 mg plasma proteins [46]. Furthermore, it may be necessary to administer surfactants more than once. GREGORY *et al.* [26] used four different doses of surfactant. They demonstrated that the maximum improvement in oxygenation, the minimum ventilator requirement, and the lowest mortality rate were obtained when four and eight doses of 100 mg·kg^{-1} of a natural surfactant (total amount of 400–800 mg·kg^1) were instilled. Similarly, KESECIOGLU *et al.* [37] observed a trend towards a reduced mortality rate when three doses of the surfactant were instilled when compared with one dose.

In the previous study, the dosing protocol used by KESECIOGLU *et al.* [36] allowed the investigators to repeat surfactant instillation several times until improvement in oxygenation was achieved. Furthermore, on each instillation sufficient amounts of surfactant was instilled to allow an optimal effectiveness of the therapy. However, the phase III study performed thereafter, using a similar dosing protocol did not show an improvement in survival, which suggests that the dose is not a determinant factor alone.

Mechanical ventilation strategies

The contradictory data from the randomised clinical trials, especially between the phase II and phase III studies may be caused, in part, by differences in the applied ventilation strategy between studies. Introduction of a more lung-protective ventilation strategy in ALI/ARDS patients improved patient outcome and decreased mortality in the last decade [4, 50]. In this respect the power analysis used for the phase III trial studies may have been underpowered and, therefore, unable to demonstrate a clear effect of surfactant replacement therapy on mortality. Furthermore, the definition of ALI/ARDS does not consider ventilator settings. Recent publications indicate the importance of these settings on the outcome of ALI/ARDS patients [51]. Investigating 41 patients with early ARDS ($Pa,O_2/FI,O_2$ baseline ⩽200), standardised ventilator settings were used (tidal volume 7–8 mL·kg^{-1}, PEEP 10 cmH$_2$O, FI,O_2 1.0) and the $Pa,O_2/FI,O_2$ was reassessed after 30 minutes. Persistent ARDS was present in 17 (41.5%) patients; however, in 24 (58.5%) patients the $Pa,O_2/FI,O_2$ increased above 200 mmHg within 30 minutes (transient ARDS). The ICU mortality rate for persistent ARDS patients was significantly greater and was 52.9% compared with 12.5% in the transient ARDS patients. This study suggests that in many ALI/ARDS trials inclusion of patients with lower than expected mortality resulted in under powering of these studies.

Conclusions

Compositional changes or decreased content of surfactants have been shown in the lungs of patients with or developing ALI/ARDS. Therefore, the instillation of exogenous surfactants may restore the normal composition of the surfactant system within the lung and restore its surface activity, which would result in improving lung compliance and gas exchange.

Natural surfactants are supposed to be more effective due to the availability of surfactant proteins in their composition. Confirming this, premature neonates show improvement in survival rates when natural surfactants are used in comparison with synthetic surfactants. No such data is available for adults with ALI/ARDS. The amount of surfactant instilled should be large enough, and maybe even repeated doses should be given, to overcome the ongoing inactivation of the surfactant. Furthermore, the instillation technique used should make optimal distribution of the surfactant in the lung. This is possible by either bolus or bronchoscopic administration of the surfactant. However, recent experimental data has shown promising results using an aerosolisation technique. Furthermore, inclusion criteria should be more stringent and incorporate ventilator guidelines. Many case reports, uncontrolled studies and phase II studies have shown beneficial effects of surfactants on oxygenation and mortality of patients with ALI/ARDS. However, recent randomised, controlled trials could not demonstrate any improvement of survival in these patients treated with a surfactant. Interestingly, exogenous surfactant instillation has improved survival in paediatric patients. This might be due to the lower incidence of multiple organ failure seen with these patients compared with adults, which may contribute to the mortality as an extrapulmonary component. Different surfactant preparations may show differing effects due to their different compositions. However, considering the present results, exogenous surfactants are not recommended for routine use in patients with ALI/ARDS.

Statement of interest

None declared.

References

1. Ashbaugh DG, Bigelow DB, Petty TL, *et al.* Acute respiratory distress in adults. *Lancet* 1967; 2: 319–323.
2. Ware LB, Matthay MA. The acute respiratory distress syndrome. *N Engl J Med* 2000; 342: 1334–1349.
3. Ranieri VM, Giunta F, Suter PM, *et al.* Mechanical ventilation as a mediator of multisystem organ failure in acute respiratory distress syndrome. *JAMA* 2000; 284: 43–44.
4. Ventilation with lower tidal volumes as compared with traditional tidal volumes for acute lung injury and the acute respiratory distress syndrome. The Acute Respiratory Distress Syndrome Network. *N Engl J Med* 2000; 342: 1301–1308.
5. Luhr OR, Antonsen K, Karlsson M, *et al.* Incidence and mortality after acute respiratory failure and acute respiratory distress syndrome in Sweden, Denmark, and Iceland. The ARF Study Group. *Am J Respir Crit Care Med* 1999; 159: 1849–1861.
6. Kesecioglu J, Haitsma JJ. Surfactant therapy in adults with acute lung injury/acute respiratory distress syndrome. *Curr Opin Crit Care* 2006; 12: 55–60.
7. Hallman M, Spragg R, Harrell JH, *et al.* Evidence of lung surfactant abnormality in respiratory failure. Study of bronchoalveolar lavage phospholipids, surface activity, phospholipase activity, and plasma myoinositol. *J Clin Invest* 1982; 70: 673–683.
8. Petty TL, Silvers GW, Paul GW, *et al.* Abnormalities in lung elastic properties and surfactant function in adult respiratory distress syndrome. *Chest* 1979; 75: 571–574.
9. Lewis JF, Jobe AH. Surfactant and the adult respiratory distress syndrome. *Am Rev Respir Dis* 1993; 147: 218–233.
10. Gregory TJ, Longmore WJ, Moxley MA, *et al.* Surfactant chemical composition and biophysical activity in acute respiratory distress syndrome. *J Clin Invest* 1991; 88: 1976–1981.
11. Tsangaris I, Lekka ME, Kitsiouli E, *et al.* Bronchoalveolar lavage alterations during prolonged ventilation of patients without acute lung injury. *Eur Respir J* 2003; 21: 495–501.
12. Jobe A, Ikegami M. Surfactant for the treatment of respiratory distress syndrome. *Am Rev Respir Dis* 1987; 136: 1256–1275.
13. King RJ, Clements JA. Surface active materials from dog lung. II. Composition and physiological correlations. *Am J Physiol* 1972; 223: 715–726.
14. Frerking I, Günther A, Seeger W, *et al.* Pulmonary surfactant: functions, abnormalities and therapeutic options. *Intensive Care Med* 2001; 27: 1699–1717.
15. von Neergaard K. Neue Auffassungen uber einen Grundbegriff der Atemmechanik. Die Retraktionskraft der Lunge, abhangig von der Oberflachenspannung in den Alveolen. *Z Gesamte Exp Med* 1929; 66: 373–394.
16. Macklin CC. The pulmonary alveolar mucoid film and the pneumonocytes. *Lancet* 1954; 266: 1099–1104.
17. Pattle RE. Properties, function and origin of the alveolar lining layer. *Nature* 1955; 175: 1125–1126.
18. Clements JA. Surface tension of lung extracts. *Proc Soc Exp Biol Med* 1957; 95: 170–172.
19. Avery ME, Mead J. Surface properties in relation to atelectasis and hyaline membrane disease. *AMA J Dis Child* 1959; 97: 517–523.
20. Fujiwara T, Maeta H, Chida S, *et al.* Artificial surfactant therapy in hyaline-membrane disease. *Lancet* 1980; 1: 55–59.
21. Engle WA, American Academy of Pediatrics Committee on Fetus and Newborn. Surfactant-replacement therapy for respiratory distress in the preterm and term neonate. *Pediatrics* 2008; 121: 419–432.
22. Jobe AH. Pulmonary surfactant therapy. *N Engl J Med* 1993; 328: 861–868.
23. Hartog A, Gommers D, Lachmann B. Role of surfactant in the pathophysiology of the acute respiratory distress syndrome (ARDS). *Monaldi Arch Chest Dis* 1995; 50: 372–377.
24. Walmrath D, Grimminger F, Pappert D, *et al.* Bronchoscopic administration of bovine natural surfactant in ARDS and septic shock: impact on gas exchange and haemodynamics. *Eur Respir J* 2002; 19: 805–810.
25. Günther A, Schmidt R, Harodt J, *et al.* Bronchoscopic administration of bovine natural surfactant in ARDS and septic shock: impact on biophysical and biochemical surfactant properties. *Eur Respir J* 2002; 19: 797–804.
26. Gregory TJ, Steinberg KP, Spragg R, *et al.* Bovine surfactant therapy for patients with acute respiratory distress syndrome. *Am J Respir Crit Care Med* 1997; 155: 1309–1315.
27. Walmrath D, Günther A, Ghofrani HA, *et al.* Bronchoscopic surfactant administration in patients with severe adult respiratory distress syndrome and sepsis. *Am J Respir Crit Care Med* 1996; 154: 57–62.
28. Spragg RG, Gilliard N, Richman P, *et al.* Acute effects of a single dose of porcine surfactant on patients with the adult respiratory distress syndrome. *Chest* 1994; 105: 195–202.

29. Lachmann B. The role of pulmonary surfactant in the pathogenesis and therapy of ARDS. *In:* Vincent JL, ed. Update In Intensive Care and Emergency Medicine. Berlin, Springer-Verlag, 1987; pp. 123–134.

30. Richman PS, Spragg RG, Robertson B, *et al.* The adult respiratory distress syndrome: first trials with surfactant replacement. *Eur Respir J* 1989; 1: Suppl. 3, 109s–111s.

31. Haslam PL, Hughes DA, MacNaughton PD, *et al.* Surfactant replacement therapy in late-stage adult respiratory distress syndrome. *Lancet* 1994; 343: 1009–1011.

32. Wiswell TE, Smith RM, Katz LB, *et al.* Bronchopulmonary segmental lavage with Surfaxin (KL(4)-surfactant) for acute respiratory distress syndrome. *Am J Respir Crit Care Med* 1999; 160: 1188–1195.

33. Weg JG, Balk RA, Tharratt RS, *et al.* Safety and potential efficacy of an aerosolized surfactant in human sepsis-induced adult respiratory distress syndrome. *JAMA* 1994; 272: 1433–1438.

34. Walmrath D, De Vaal JB, Bruining HA, *et al.* Treatment of ARDS with a recombinant SP-C (rSP-C) based synthetic surfactant. *Am J Respir Crit Care Med* 2000; 161: A379.

35. Spragg RG, Lewis JF, Wurst W, *et al.* Treatment of acute respiratory distress syndrome with recombinant surfactant protein C surfactant. *Am J Respir Crit Care Med* 2003; 167: 1562–1566.

36. Kesecioglu J, Schultz MJ, Lundberg D, *et al.* Treatment of acute lung injury (ALI/ARDS) with surfactant. *Am J Respir Crit Care Med* 2001; 163: A819.

37. Kesecioglu J, Schultz MJ, Maas JJ, *et al.* Treatment of acute lung injury and ARDS with surfactant is safe. *Am J Respir Crit Care Med* 2004; 169: A349.

38. Anzueto A, Baughman RP, Guntupalli KK, *et al.* Aerosolized surfactant in adults with sepsis-induced acute respiratory distress syndrome. Exosurf Acute Respiratory Distress Syndrome Sepsis Study Group. *N Engl J Med* 1996; 334: 1417–1421.

39. Spragg RG, Lewis JF, Walmrath HD, *et al.* Effect of recombinant surfactant protein C-based surfactant on the acute respiratory distress syndrome. *N Engl J Med* 2004; 351: 884–892.

40. Willson DF, Thomas NJ, Markovitz BP, *et al.* Effect of exogenous surfactant (calfactant) in pediatric acute lung injury: a randomized controlled trial. *JAMA* 2005; 293: 470–476.

41. Kesecioglu J, Beale R, Stewart TE, *et al.* Exogenous natural surfactant for treatment of acute lung injury and the acute respiratory distress syndrome. *Am J Respir Crit Care Med* 2009; 180: 989–994.

42. Spragg RG, Taut FJ, Lewis JF, *et al.* Recombinant surfactant protein C-based surfactant for patients with severe direct lung injury. *Am J Respir Crit Care Med* 2011; 183: 1055–1061.

43. Lu Q, Zhang M, Girardi C, *et al.* Computed tomography assessment of exogenous surfactant-induced lung reaeration in patients with acute lung injury. *Crit Care* 2010; 14: R135.

44. Gommers D, van 't Veen A, Verbrugge SJC, *et al.* Comparison of eight different surfactant preparations on improvement of blood gases in lung-lavaged rats. *Appl Cardiopulm Pathophysiol* 1998; 7: 95–102.

45. Ainsworth SB, Beresford MW, Milligan DW, *et al.* Pumactant and poractant alfa for treatment of respiratory distress syndrome in neonates born at 25–29 weeks' gestation: a randomised trial. *Lancet* 2000; 355: 1387–1392.

46. Lachmann B, Eijking EP, So KL, *et al. In vivo* evaluation of the inhibitory capacity of human plasma on exogenous surfactant function. *Intensive Care Med* 1994; 20: 6–11.

47. Gilliard N, Richman PM, Merritt TA, *et al.* Effect of volume and dose on the pulmonary distribution of exogenous surfactant administered to normal rabbits or to rabbits with oleic acid lung injury. *Am Rev Respir Dis* 1990; 141: 743–747.

48. Ruppert C, Kuchenbuch T, Boensch M, *et al.* Dry powder aerosolization of a recombinant surfactant protein-C-based surfactant for inhalative treatment of the acutely inflamed lung. *Crit Care Med* 2010; 38: 1584–1591.

49. Kesecioglu J. Farewell to exogenous surfactant therapy in acute lung injury/acute respiratory distress syndrome! Or, must we start all over again? *Crit Care Med* 2010; 38: 1606–1607.

50. Amato MB, Barbas CS, Medeiros DM, *et al.* Effect of a protective-ventilation strategy on mortality in the acute respiratory distress syndrome. *N Engl J Med* 1998; 338: 347–354.

51. Ferguson ND, Kacmarek RM, Chiche JD, *et al.* Screening of ARDS patients using standardized ventilator settings: influence on enrollment in a clinical trial. *Intensive Care Med* 2004; 30: 1111–1116.

Chapter 5

NIV in hypoxaemic acute respiratory failure

J-C. Lefebvre*,#, S. Dimassi* and L. Brochard*,¶

Summary

Physiological studies have clearly established the effectiveness of noninvasive ventilation (NIV) in patients with hypoxaemic acute respiratory failure (ARF). Patient selection is nevertheless crucial and the risk–benefit ratio should be carefully evaluated for each potential patient. It is essential to consider the use of NIV separately, based on the different aetiologies of hypoxaemic ARF, because the results vary accordingly. Use of NIV in the post-operative period emerges as an important indication that requires further studies. It is critical that NIV does not delay a necessary endotracheal intubation as this has been linked to the worst clinical outcomes. A practical approach for using NIV in hypoxaemic ARF patients will be proposed in this chapter.

Keywords: Acute lung injury, acute respiratory distress syndrome, acute respiratory failure, continuous positive airway pressure, hypoxaemia, noninvasive ventilation

*Intensive Care Dept, University Hospital,
¶University of Geneva, Geneva, Switzerland.
#Intensive Care Unit, Centre Hospitalier Universitaire de Québec, Québec, QC, Canada.

Correspondence: L. Brochard, Hopitaux Universitaires de Genève, Rue Gabrielle-Perret-Gentil 4, 1211 Geneva 14, Switzerland.
Email Laurent.brochard@hcuge.ch

Eur Respir Mon 2012; 55: 65–80.
Printed in UK – all rights reserved
Copyright ERS 2012
European Respiratory Monograph
ISSN: 1025-448x
DOI: 10.1183/1025448x.10001711

Noninvasive ventilation (NIV) refers to the application of artificial ventilation without an invasive airway device and primarily encompasses pressure support ventilation (PSV) plus positive end-expiratory pressure (PEEP), also referred to as bilevel positive airway pressure (BiPAP), and continuous positive airway pressure (CPAP). Even if there is no active inspiratory aid, CPAP can arguably be viewed as a form of NIV in the context of acute respiratory failure (ARF) [1]. In this chapter, we will specifically refer to CPAP when this was the technique used in a study.

The emergence of NIV in clinical practice was followed by the progressive generalisation of its use in the late 1990s and 2000s, such that NIV is now established as a standard of care in several forms of ARF [2]. The use of NIV for patients with acute exacerbation of chronic obstructive pulmonary disease (COPD) or cardiogenic pulmonary oedema (CPO) is supported by several randomised controlled trials (RCTs), making it a first-line intervention in these conditions [3–6]. By avoiding endotracheal intubation (ETI), NIV reduces complications related to tube insertion, sedation requirements and the loss of airway integrity induced by the tube itself. Maintenance of the natural airway barriers explains the lower rate of nosocomial pneumonia associated with NIV [7–9].

A reduction in nonrespiratory infections has also been shown, partly related to a lesser use of invasive monitoring and catheter devices [7]. Furthermore, NIV can increase comfort by allowing patients to drink, eat, cough and talk.

Theoretically, these advantageous effects of NIV can be expected in other categories of patients with ARF. NIV is still gaining popularity in the intensive care unit (ICU) and its use has been expanded beyond the indications supported by the strongest level of evidence (severe exacerbation of COPD and CPO) [2, 10, 11]. This chapter will focus exclusively on hypoxaemic ARF, one of the more debated indications for NIV. Post-operative use of NIV will also be discussed, since post-operative pulmonary complications are mostly hypoxaemic episodes of ARF. Respiratory failure exacerbating a chronic cardiac or lung insufficiency will not be discussed here and the use of NIV as an adjunct for mechanical ventilation withdrawal is addressed specifically in another chapter of this *Monograph* [12].

Pathophysiology of hypoxaemic ARF

Hypoxaemic ARF is characterised by acute severe hypoxaemia (arterial oxygen tension (P_{a,O_2})/inspiratory oxygen fraction (F_{I,O_2}) ratio $\leqslant 300$), usually accompanied by high-level activity of the respiratory muscles owing to the strong hypoxaemic drive and direct pulmonary receptor stimulation. There is a clear rationale for using NIV in hypoxaemic ARF because it addresses both the hypoxaemia (lung failure) and the high load imposed on the respiratory muscles (latent pump failure). NIV improves oxygenation by increasing functional residual capacity (FRC) while promoting alveolar recruitment of collapsed alveoli, which in turn reduces ventilation–perfusion mismatches and sometimes even true pulmonary shunt. Besides gas exchange correction, NIV can increase alveolar ventilation by synchronously increasing the transpulmonary pressure swings with consequential larger tidal volumes. This increase in alveolar ventilation is not at the expense of a greater work of breathing as the ventilator shares part of the work with the patient [13].

Regarding specific NIV settings in this population, the short-term effects of different combinations of PSV and PEEP were assessed in 10 patients with acute lung injury [14]. As expected, PSV level had no impact on oxygenation, and the highest level of PEEP studied (10 cmH$_2$O) resulted in the greatest oxygenation improvement. Otherwise, CPAP alone failed to unload the respiratory muscles, which could be done efficiently with provision of PSV. Inspiratory muscle efforts were reduced with PSV, irrespective of the level of PEEP, and dyspnoea relief was significantly better with the highest level of PSV (15 cmH$_2$O) [14]. Hence, to adequately handle the lung and pump failure with NIV, clinicians should provide a sufficient level of PEEP to improve oxygenation, while ensuring an optimal PSV to unload the respiratory muscles. These two additive pressures form the peak airway pressure, one of the major determinants of leaks, asynchrony and potential gastric air distension. As leaks can greatly reduce NIV efficiency, one must usually balance PSV and PEEP levels, while limiting peak airway pressure to under 20 cmH$_2$O [15, 16]. This implies that patients with severely restrictive respiratory mechanics, notably severe acute respiratory distress syndrome (ARDS), will not be favourable candidates for NIV due to the requirement of high airway pressures.

Should NIV be used in hypoxaemic ARF?

As often in intensive care medicine, this issue can be approached from an evidence-based perspective and by applying known physiological principles. Robust RCTs are scarce, explaining why the absence of specific recommendations often predominates in the evidence-based guidelines [11]. It is up to the clinician to reconcile the various studies and the pathophysiological principles to make patient-oriented decisions. A practical approach is therefore required and will be exposed in this chapter through a concise review of the literature correlated with the application of physiological concepts.

Unlike exacerbation of COPD or CPO, hypoxaemic ARF represents a heterogeneous group of diseases with different prognoses and treatments. This large heterogeneity can explain some of the literature's contradictory results, which suggest that outcomes vary depending on the study population [17, 18]. It is thus advisable to analyse the literature from the various subgroups of hypoxaemic ARF separately.

Acute lung injury/ARDS/pneumonia

One must first distinguish whether NIV is used as part of a strategy to prevent intubation or as an alternative to replace intubation. The subset of immunocompromised patients also deserves to be discussed separately.

NIV to prevent intubation in immunocompetent patients

The use of NIV in patients with mixed causes of hypoxaemic ARF remains controversial. This is because contrasting results exist between the benefits observed in short-term physiological studies and in a few RCTs on the one hand, and both the high rates of failure described in observational studies and the well-identified risk of delaying intubation on the other hand. Early uncontrolled studies evoked ambiguous results and the first RCT did not show any benefit [19–24]. In a large RCT of patients with diverse hypoxaemic ARF, Delclaux et al. [25] showed that the use of CPAP resulted in a greater subjective response and an increase in the $Pa,O_2/FI,O_2$ ratio at 1 hour; nevertheless, this physiological improvement neither reduced the need for ETI nor improved clinical outcomes. We can speculate that the absence of respiratory muscle unloading with CPAP could have contributed to these negative results [14]. In addition, an important concern was the significant increase in adverse events within the NIV group, including four cardiac arrests occurring at the time of ETI or with mask dislodgement [25]. A subsequent study performed in three centres by Ferrer et al. [26] included 105 nonhypercapnic patients with persistent hypoxaemic ARF, randomised between NIV or standard treatment with high-concentration oxygen. The strict patient selection was based on clinical cooperation, state of consciousness and the absence of concomitant organ dysfunctions. The study population was heterogeneous in terms of aetiologies, with around 30% CPO, a similar rate of pneumonia and 20% immunocompromised patients. NIV significantly reduced intubation rate (25% versus 52%; p=0.010), septic shock (12% versus 31%; p=0.028) and ICU mortality (18% versus 39%; p=0.028). These beneficial results were similar in the subgroup of patients with pneumonia [26]. Extrapolating these results to individual patients requires the application of the same careful selection process, with the exclusion of all patients with contraindications. This may explain in part why observational studies often failed to reproduce these benefits in everyday practice outside clinical trials (fig. 1) [27]. Also, reproducing these results is necessary because the outcomes of the control group could vary from one centre to another, making the difference with the NIV group more or less pronounced.

NIV in patients with ARDS

No published RCTs have focused exclusively on NIV in patients with ARDS. One trial reported a significantly lower intubation rate (40% versus 69%; p=0.02) with NIV in 84 patients with ARDS, but was published in abstract form only [28]. In contrast to these results, most observational studies and subgroup analysis of RCTs identified ARDS diagnosis as a strong predictor of NIV failure [18, 26, 29, 30–32]. The largest prospective survey of NIV in 147 ARDS patients confirmed a failure rate of around 50% [33]. The observational study design precludes any inference with respect to outcomes and it should be noted that the study centres had extensive experience with NIV. Even in these rigorously selected patients, the high mortality rate (54%) observed in patients intubated after failing NIV raises the issue that delaying intubation might have contributed to mortality. Conversely, it is not possible to determine whether the low mortality rate (19%) of patients who succeeded with NIV truly represents a beneficial effect or simply denotes that the patients were less sick [33]. Attempts have been made to better define predictors of NIV failure in

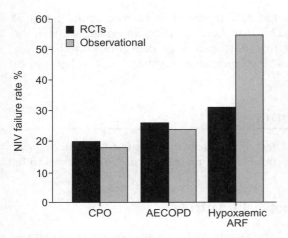

Figure 1. Examples of the failure rate of non-invasive ventilation (NIV) in randomised controlled trials (RCTs) as opposed to observational studies outside clinical trials. Results were presented separately depending on three diagnostic categories: cardiogenic pulmonary oedema (CPO), acute exacerbation of chronic obstructive pulmonary disease (AECOPD) and hypoxaemic acute respiratory failure (ARF). Good results from RCTs have not been reproduced for hypoxaemic patients in everyday clinical practice. This emphasises the necessity of following strict patient selection for these patients. References for RCTs: CPO [6], AECOPD [5] and hypoxaemic ARF [24, 25]; for observational studies: CPO and AECOPD [27] and hypoxaemic ARF [9, 18, 27].

ARDS patients [31]. Presence of shock was uniformly associated with failure and patients who failed were more likely to have metabolic acidosis, higher severity of illness scores and a greater degree of hypoxaemia [31, 34]. Overall, the risk–benefit ratio of NIV is still not defined in ARDS and current evidence does not support the routine use of NIV in these patients.

NIV in patients with hypoxaemic ARF secondary to pneumonia

Pneumonia has also been identified as a risk factor for NIV failure [18]. High failure rates were described in pneumonia-related ARF, sometimes reaching 100% [20, 31, 35–37]. Nonetheless, acute physiological response has been shown in non-COPD patients with severe community-acquired pneumonia (CAP) [38]. Notwithstanding this acute improvement, 66% of patients still required intubation over time [38]. Another study confirmed that, despite a similar degree of hypoxaemia and an equivalent initial response to NIV, patients with severe CAP failed significantly more often than patients with CPO [39]. Conversely, *post hoc* analysis of the study by FERRER *et al.* [26] revealed a significant reduction in ETI rate with NIV in the subset of patients with pneumonia. Likewise, in a trial directly focusing on patients with severe CAP, NIV reduced intubation rate (21% *versus* 50%; p=0.03) and ICU length of stay (1.8±0.7 *versus* 6±1.8 days; p=0.04), but this benefit was entirely driven by pneumonia occurring in hypercapnic COPD patients [40]. Inconsistencies among studies preclude recommending the routine use of NIV in all patients with pneumonia without underlying COPD. Haemodynamic instability, mental status alteration and inability to clear secretions should seriously be considered as contraindications to NIV in these patients.

NIV as an alternative to conventional invasive ventilation

Most studies to date have focused on NIV as a tool to prevent ETI, but it has also been used, albeit less frequently, as an alternative to conventional mechanical ventilation. ANTONELLI *et al.* [41] randomised 64 heterogeneous patients with hypoxaemic ARF and a predefined indication for mechanical ventilation between NIV and immediate conventional ventilation through an endotracheal tube. ETI was successfully avoided in 22 (69%) out of 32 patients in the NIV group. There was no significant difference in mortality, but periods of ventilation were shorter in the NIV group, as was the ICU length of stay (9±7 *versus* 16±17 days; p=0.04). This study has raised the question as to whether ETI was absolutely necessary in all patients from the conventional group. In a similar study, ETI was avoided in 42% of patients from the NIV group, but ICU mortality and complications did not differ [35]. It is worth noting that half of this study cohort presented with a diagnosis of COPD [35]. Despite these encouraging results, NIV should not be viewed as a first-line alternative to invasive mechanical ventilation. If used at all for this indication, NIV should be reserved to experienced teams, in strictly selected patients without organ dysfunction apart from ARF and with a level of hypoxaemia that is not too severe.

NIV to prevent intubation in immunocompromised patients

ARF remains the most common cause of ICU admission in immunocompromised patients, including patients with malignancies [42]. Once considered dismal, the prognosis of immunocompromised patients with ARF has dramatically improved in the last decade or so, at least for several categories of patients [42–44]. Nevertheless, invasive mechanical ventilation was repeatedly identified as an independent mortality predictor in this population [45]. The potential to reduce infectious complications, combined with promising early uncontrolled studies, suggest a strong rationale for NIV use in immunocompromised patients [46–49]. 10 years ago, NIV was already pointed out as a protective factor against death in cancer patients with ARF [42]. The first RCT on immunocompromised patients with hypoxaemic ARF randomised 40 patients with early hypoxaemic ARF after solid organ transplant [50]. NIV reduced intubation rate (20% *versus* 70%; p=0.002), ICU length of stay in survivors (5.5 *versus* 9 days; p=0.03) and ICU mortality (20% *versus* 50%; p=0.05), but no difference was noted in hospital mortality. The invasive devices present at study entry were used for a shorter period of time in the NIV group (5 *versus* 9 days; p=0.05). A second RCT confirmed the benefit of a sequential use of NIV in 52 mixed immunocompromised patients with hypoxaemic ARF, fever and pulmonary infiltrates [51]. Intubation rate was significantly reduced with NIV (46% *versus* 77%; p=0.03) as was ICU mortality (38% *versus* 69%; p=0.03). Interestingly, a longer delay between admission and NIV first use was identified as a predictor of NIV failure in patients with haematological malignancies [30]. Similarly, precocious use of CPAP in the haematological ward for neutropenic patients with early respiratory changes has been shown to prevent evolution to acute lung injury and consequential ICU admission and even ETI [52].

It has often been more difficult to show convincing positive results in observational studies than in RCTs [44, 53, 54]. This has led some authors to question the generalisability of the results issued by expert centres to the real-life practice of other centres [11]. Nevertheless, in a recently published observational study from Italy, NIV was used in 21% of patients with haematological malignancies and requiring ventilatory support for ARF [32]. Despite a high failure rate of 46%, NIV was associated with lower mortality than invasive mechanical ventilation after propensity-score adjustment (OR 0.73, 95% CI 0.53–1.00). This study raises an important flag, as even if patients intubated from the start had a higher SAPS II score (Simplified Acute Physiology Score), their mortality was lower than patients who had an unsuccessful trial of NIV (50% *versus* 61%; p=0.01). This should caution us against harmfully delaying ETI by continuing NIV until overt failure in hypoxaemic ARF. Even so, a trial of NIV as a first-line intervention in selected immunocompromised patients with hypoxaemic ARF, that endeavours to meet all the favourable conditions, including using NIV early in the process, still appears justified [32]. Even in these patients with a serious prognosis once intubated, ETI should not be viewed as a last-ditch option and some patients would probably benefit from earlier ETI.

NIV to pre-oxygenate patients before ETI

Conditions for ETI are frequently non-optimal in critically ill patients and several laryngoscopic attempts are commonly required [55–57]. Severe hypoxaemia during ETI is especially prevalent in these patients and the usual pre-oxygenation technique with a bag-mask system has proved marginally effective [56, 58]. When compared with a bag-mask device, pre-oxygenation with NIV provides higher oxygen saturation and reduces episodes of severe hypoxaemia in ICU patients requiring ETI [59]. Recruitment of collapsed alveoli with NIV probably explains most of the benefit by directly increasing the oxygen reserve and decreasing the pulmonary shunt. It should be borne in mind that positive airway pressure ventilation applied noninvasively may increase gastric air content and promote pulmonary aspiration. However, as insufflation pressure is probably more strictly controlled with NIV than with a bag-mask system, this can hardly be a definitive argument. In general, pressure higher than 20 cmH$_2$O needs to be reached at the glottis level to see

J-C. LEFEBVRE ET AL.

an increase in the risk of gastric insufflation [16]. Even if it requires further studies, pre-oxygenation of hypoxaemic patients with NIV appears to be a useful technique that can be integrated into an intubation management protocol [60].

NIV as an adjunct per-bronchoscopy

While flexible bronchoscopy is usually well tolerated in healthy subjects, it remains an invasive procedure with an increased risk of complications in critically ill patients [61]. Bronchoscopy is associated with extra work of breathing and usually a decrease in the $Pa_{,O_2}$ by 10–20 mmHg that can persist, or even worsen, for a few hours after the procedure [62–64]. Oxygenation can be further impeded by saline instillation for bronchoalveolar lavage and by suctioning with a concomitant reduction in end-expiratory lung volume. Several preliminary and feasibility studies suggested that NIV with different interfaces during bronchoscopy could prove useful in at-risk patients [65–69]. NIV can prevent de-recruitment and compensate for the extra work of breathing imposed by the procedure. In 30 hypoxaemic patients, CPAP effectively reduced the per-procedure desaturations and the incidence of respiratory failure necessitating ventilatory support (one *versus* seven patients in the oxygen-only group; p<0.03) [70]. In another RCT of 26 hypoxaemic patients, the $Pa_{,O_2}/Fi_{,O_2}$ ratio increased by 82% in the NIV group during bronchoscopy, contrasting with a 10% decrease in the conventional oxygen group [71]. Intubation rate following the procedure was low in both groups and did not differ. NIV can thus effectively maintain oxygenation in hypoxaemic patients undergoing bronchoscopy, but whether this can translate into a sustainable reduction of procedure-related ETI remains to be demonstrated [72].

NIV in the post-operative period

Taking pulmonary condition before surgery into account, ARF mortality is largely related to post-operative re-intubation and complications of mechanical ventilation [73, 74]. Ventilatory assistance is frequently provided by placement of an endotracheal tube, but NIV is increasingly popular for the treatment of post-operative ARF, as evidenced by a 69% utilisation rate by French intensivists for the treatment of post-operative ARF [75].

Pathophysiology: respiratory modifications after surgery

Various factors may precipitate respiratory failure during the post-operative period, including direct effects from thoracic or upper abdominal procedures, depression from residual anaesthetic drugs or the patient's underlying pulmonary condition. These modifications and the frequently observed hypoxaemia of the early post-operative period may be accentuated by other factors, such as excessive peri-operative fluid loading, transfusion-related acute lung injury, inflammation, sepsis and aspiration. Regardless of the aetiology, a reduction in FRC usually occurs in the immediate post-operative period. This reduced FRC also modifies the resistance and compliance of the respiratory system, increasing the work of breathing and potentially leading to hypoventilation and respiratory insufficiency, especially in patients with limited respiratory reserve. Most respiratory modifications are maximal in the first hours after surgery and generally recede after 1 or 2 weeks [76, 77]. Because it can restore FRC, CPAP has been used for a long time in post-operative patients [78]. As a consequence, some authors advocate the use of post-operative NIV (either CPAP or PSV plus PEEP) both for prophylactic and curative indications [11, 73, 79].

NIV use after thoracic surgery

In the post-operative period of lung resection, pulmonary complications are the leading cause of death and ARF is fatal in up to 60–80% of these patients [80, 81]. Post-operative invasive mechanical ventilation increases the risk of bronchial stump disruption, bronchopleural fistula, persistent air leakage and pulmonary infection [76, 81, 82]. The high morbidity and mortality of ARF after thoracic surgery has led to a major concern for the prevention and treatment of this condition.

Prophylactic use of NIV after thoracic surgery

NIV was proposed to prevent re-intubation, infection and atelectasis in the post-operative period after chest surgery. Despite the theoretical concern of increasing pleural air leaks, a small study of 10 patients suggested the feasibility, efficacy in improving oxygenation and apparent safety of NIV use after lung resection surgery [83]. Prophylactic use of NIV pre- and post-operatively (7 days at home and then 3 days after the surgery) was specifically studied in 32 patients at a higher risk of complications after lung resection surgery due to a forced expiratory volume in 1 second (FEV1) of <70% [84]. NIV improved pulmonary spirometric values at 2 hours and oxygenation status for the first 3 days after the surgery [84]. Mixed results have been obtained with prophylactic use of NIV following cardiac surgery [85–88]. Nevertheless, the largest study randomised 500 patients scheduled for elective cardiac surgery between nasal CPAP for at least 6 hours and standard treatment including 10 minutes of intermittent CPAP every 4 hours [87]. The composite end-point of pulmonary complications was significantly reduced within the intervention group, but the re-intubation rate was rather low (three *versus* six patients in the control group) [87]. Thoraco-abdominal aortic aneurysm repair is another procedure associated with a high incidence of respiratory complications [89]. Continuous use of CPAP for the first 24 hours after the surgery improved oxygenation status and resulted in a reduction in pulmonary complications in these patients [90]. Despite these encouraging physiological and preliminary clinical studies, prophylactic use of post-operative NIV still needs more evidence to be recommended for clinical practice. Please note that, in this indication, CPAP, the simplest form of support, may be useful.

Curative use of NIV for ARF after thoracic surgery

NIV has also been used for the treatment of ARF after thoracic surgery. Observational studies have reported an NIV failure rate of between 15% and 30% in these patients and the absence of an initial positive physiological response was significantly associated with failure [91–93]. AURIANT *et al.* [81] performed an RCT in which 48 patients with ARF after lung resection were randomly assigned to NIV or standard treatment. NIV significantly decreased the ETI rate (50% *versus* 21%; p=0.035) and hospital mortality (13% *versus* 38%; p=0.045), probably by preventing intubation-related complications such as tracheobronchial bacterial contamination, bronchopleural fistula and pyothorax [81]. NIV did not reduce ICU or hospital length of stay, which was attributed by the authors to the long duration of their weaning protocol [81]. Similarly, the beneficial effect of NIV was suggested in patients with ARF after oesophagectomy and no increase in anastomotic leakage was noted [94]. Despite the paucity of data, a trial of NIV is recommended in these patients at an extremely high risk of complications with invasive mechanical ventilation [11]. However, the risk of surgical complications induced by positive pressure ventilation is still poorly defined and it is probably wise to keep airway pressures at the lowest effective level [73].

NIV use after abdominal surgery

Numerous factors linked to anaesthetic and surgical consequences can explain the high incidence of post-operative hypoxaemia after abdominal surgery [73, 76, 95]. NIV can address many of these issues, especially by restoring FRC, preventing atelectasis, improving gas exchange and decreasing the work of breathing [73, 96].

Prophylactic use of NIV after abdominal surgery

It is well established that NIV, including CPAP, reduces the incidence of post-operative hypoxaemia, but the effect on clinical outcomes is more controversial [79]. An early study revealed an advantageous effect of CPAP compared with incentive spirometry in preventing post-operative atelectasis [97]. Additionally, several studies have confirmed the physiological benefits of CPAP or PSV plus PEEP in post-operative patients following bariatric surgery, in terms of oxygenation and lung volume preservation, but conclusive effects on clinical outcomes have not been shown yet [98–100]. Likewise, beyond the expected decrease in oxygenation disturbances, pulmonary complications and mortality were not reduced by prophylactic CPAP for the first post-operative night in 204 patients after major vascular surgery [101]. SQUADRONE et al. [102] studied the effect of early CPAP delivered by helmet in 209 patients with $P_{a,O_2}/F_{I,O_2}$ <300 at 1 hour after elective major abdominal surgery. Compared with standard oxygen therapy, the intubation rate was reduced (1% versus 10%; p=0.005), as were pneumonia and sepsis. Despite a positive trend, ICU and hospital length of stay did not significantly differ. Strictly speaking, this study was not about the prophylactic use of NIV but rather about early use, with the same intention of preventing overt deterioration and more serious complications. The evidence does not justify the routine post-operative use of NIV, but it should be considered in patients at a higher risk of pulmonary complications. Further studies are required to better define the patients who will benefit the most and optimal application modalities. The available data and general experience with NIV suggest that an early use, as soon as a mild deterioration occurs, is the best timing.

Curative use of NIV for ARF after abdominal surgery

Several patients with post-operative hypoxaemic ARF were included in previously described studies on NIV in ARF from various causes [18, 24, 41]. Nonetheless, probably due to the low patient number and large heterogeneity, results from this specific subgroup were usually not available separately. JABER et al. [103] reported that ETI was avoided in 48 (67%) out of 72 patients treated with NIV for ARF after abdominal surgery. Interestingly, the $P_{a,O_2}/F_{I,O_2}$ ratio increased and the respiratory rate decreased significantly only in patients who were successfully treated with NIV and then avoided ETI. A similar rate of NIV failure had also been reported in two other observational studies of ARF in post-operative patients [104, 105]. With respect to the most appropriate interface, a case-matched study of patients with ARF after abdominal surgery compared the use of NIV delivered by helmet or by face mask [106]. Use of the helmet was associated with a significant decrease in intubation rate, mainly related to better patient tolerance.

NIV in trauma patients

Trauma patients present a high risk of pulmonary dysfunction with consecutive hypoxaemic ARF and a significant proportion of these patients will require ETI. The physiological efficacy of NIV has already been suggested in trauma patients and the low failure rate of the technique repeatedly described [18, 26, 107–109]. Compared with a high-flow oxygen mask, the use of NIV significantly reduced intubation rate (three (12%) versus 10 (40%); p=0.02) and hospital length of stay in a single-centre RCT of 50 patients with persistent hypoxaemia within the first 48 hours after thoracic trauma [110]. There was a nonsignificant trend towards a higher pneumothorax rate within the NIV group [110]. Two RCTs focusing on the use of CPAP in patients with severe chest trauma have also suggested a benefit, but methodological limitations preclude formal recommendations, notably because patients from the control group were all intubated immediately [111, 112]. The paucity of RCTs makes recommendations on NIV use in trauma patients difficult. NIV is probably a useful adjunct to manage hypoxaemic patients with predominant chest trauma, but adequate analgesia, often including regional anaesthesia, must not be neglected.

Key concepts and safety thoughts

Uncertainties in the current literature do not allow firm and definitive recommendations concerning the use of NIV in hypoxaemic ARF. ETI still remains a standard of care for many cases of severe hypoxaemic ARF. Nonetheless, NIV is part of our armamentarium and some optimally selected patients clearly benefit from its use.

Since the effectiveness of NIV in preventing ETI and its complications varies greatly depending on the underlying diagnosis, the focus should be on patients with the highest success rate and the most favourable risk–benefit ratio [18]. It thus seems likely that NIV should be considered further in patients with a high-risk profile following ETI, such as immunocompromised or post-operative patients, particularly after lung resection. Conversely, the role of NIV is still unclear in patients with the highest risk of failure, such as ARDS and pneumonia with sepsis. A cautious trial may be attempted by expert teams and with a low trigger for ETI. It cannot be asserted that there is nothing to lose with an NIV trial, as failure was identified as being independently associated with mortality [9]. Contrary to what was observed in patients with COPD or CPO, NIV failure by itself was associated with a mortality excess in *de novo* ARF (mostly representing hypoxaemic ARF). This finding was also suggested by other studies of NIV in patients with hypoxaemic ARF [9, 19, 25]. This worrisome association between time to intubation and increased mortality was already shown in the post-extubation period [113]. It is plausible that there is an opportunity window for NIV use in these patients, beyond which the prognosis is adversely influenced by the undue continuation of NIV.

The main concern with hypoxaemic ARF frequently depends on the underlying causative condition rather than on the respiratory insufficiency *per se*. NIV does not correct the primary process, as may be the case with respiratory muscle fatigue in COPD exacerbation. It should be viewed as a tool to buy the time required to address the primary process. This is crucial because recovery time is generally longer and NIV failure rate much higher in hypoxaemic ARF patients. The initial evaluation must determine whether the cause is reversible in a time-frame realistically compatible with NIV, based on the natural history of the disease and sometimes with the assistance of the initial response to NIV. Patients in whom prolonged mehanical ventilation is anticipated with a high level of support or who can barely tolerate NIV are far from ideal candidates.

NIV is often as effective as conventional invasive ventilation for acutely correcting gas exchange in hypoxaemic ARF [41, 114]. The challenge is to maintain this benefit over time because most of the

Table 1. Practical approach for noninvasive ventilation (NIV) in hypoxaemic acute respiratory failure (ARF): patient selection

Focus on patients most likely to benefit
  Patients at risk of ETI
    Moderate to severe dyspnoea
    Respiratory rate >30–35 breaths·min^{-1}
    Accessory muscle use or paradoxical breathing
    $P_{a,O_2}/F_{I,O_2}$ <200 while breathing through a Venturi mask
    ($P_{a,O_2}/F_{I,O_2}$ <300 in patients at increased risk of complications, such as haematological and post-operative patients)
  Early in the evolution of ARF
  Underlying cause reversible in a reasonable time-frame
  Favourable global risk–benefit ratio
Rigorous patient selection
  No major organ dysfunction apart from ARF
  No decrease in consciousness
  Absence of haemodynamic instability (no shock)
  Severity illness score not too high (SAPS II <35)
  Caution if used in patients at high risk of failure (ARDS and pneumonia)
  Exclusion of patients with usual NIV contraindications
    Emergent intubation needed (CPR or respiratory arrest)
    Inadequate patient cooperation
    Severe arrhythmia or myocardial ischaemia
    Active upper gastrointestinal bleeding or vomiting
    Mask intolerance or fitting impossible
    Facial deformities or recent oral, oesophageal or gastric surgery
    Inability to clear secretions or protect the airway

ETI: endotracheal intubation; P_{a,O_2}: arterial oxygen tension; F_{I,O_2}: inspiratory oxygen fraction; SAPS: Simplified Acute Physiology Score; ARDS: acute respiratory distress syndrome; CPR: cardiopulmonary resuscitation.

Table 2. Practical approach for noninvasive ventilation (NIV) in hypoxaemic acute respiratory failure: the settings

Ventilator
  ICU ventilator (with NIV algorithm) or
  Dedicated NIV ventilator (with oxygen blender for precise F_IO_2 titration)
Mode
  Modes with inspiratory aid such as PSV and PEEP preferable over CPAP alone
Interface
  Oronasal mask
  Helmet could be an alternative
Settings
  PEEP and PSV levels must be balanced (keeping P_{peak} <20–25 cmH$_2$O)
  Titrate PSV aiming for exhaled V_T of 5–8 mL·kg^{-1} PBW and RR <30–35 breaths·min^{-1}
    (usual range 7–15 cmH$_2$O)
  Progressively increase PEEP to obtain S_{p,O_2} ⩾92% with F_IO_2 <60% (usual range 4–10 cmH$_2$O)
Protocol
  Maintain NIV continuously for the first few hours (ideally for the first 24 hours)
  Periods without NIV are then interspaced according to patient tolerance
  Progressively discontinuing use after clinical improvement
  Exact timing depends on patient tolerance with and without NIV
Monitoring
  Bedside surveillance mandatory
  Highly monitored environment (ICU)
  Subjective response to and tolerance of the technique
  Mask fitting, leaks and potential pressure sores
  Check for initial improvement in gas exchange (S_{p,O_2} and blood gas) and respiratory pattern
  Early recognition of failure
  Remain vigilant to promptly detect late failure
  Remain attentive to detect excessively high V_T
  Emergent ETI must be readily available at all times
  Always keep a safety margin for unexpected sudden deterioration

ICU: intensive care unit; F_IO_2: inspiratory oxygen fraction; PSV: pressure support ventilation; PEEP: positive end-expiratory pressure; CPAP: continuous positive airway pressure; P_{peak}: peak airway pressure; V_T: tidal volume; PBW: predicted body weight; RR: respiratory rate; S_{p,O_2}: arterial oxygen saturation measured by pulse oximetry; ETI: endotracheal intubation.

oxygenation improvement waned quickly after withdrawal of PEEP [38, 115]. Hence, brutal de-recruitment could happen in the advent of sudden loss of PEEP (as with mask removal) and jeopardise patient safety by aggravating an already severe hypoxaemia. The absence of a secure airway, as with an endotracheal tube, makes these patients vulnerable to even brief removal of the interface, either for nursing care or because of patient intolerance. Patients should not be fully dependent on NIV and it may therefore be prudent to avoid NIV in patients who are unable to transiently maintain acceptable oxygenation using a standard high-flow oxygen mask.

The risk of ventilator-induced lung injury (VILI) is still unclear with NIV. Most of the patients with hypoxaemic ARF have a high respiratory drive and it has been shown experimentally that even spontaneous breathing could lead to lung injury when coupled with a high respiratory drive [116]. It has also been demonstrated that patients who failed NIV had a higher ventilatory demand with larger tidal volumes than those who succeeded [31]. This theoretical risk for VILI associated with large tidal volumes resulting from large swings of transpulmonary pressure remains to be explored but could potentially explain part of the worse prognosis associated with failure of NIV.

Practical approach for NIV use in hypoxaemic ARF patients

As NIV exerts its benefit by preventing ETI, it is necessary to target patients at risk for such an outcome. Patients must be sick enough to require ventilatory support but at the same time be taken sufficiently early to prevent deterioration (table 1). As already stressed, the underlying

Table 3. Predictors of noninvasive ventilation (NIV) failure in hypoxaemic acute respiratory failure

Predictors of NIV failure
   Age >40 years [18]
   ARDS or community-acquired pneumonia [18]
   SAPS II score ⩾35 [18] or APACHE II score >17 [119]
   Respiratory rate >25 breaths·min^{-1} after 1 hour of NIV [119]
   Haemodynamic shock [31]
   Severe initial hypoxaemia [31]
   $P_{a,O_2}/F_{I,O_2}$ ⩽175 after 1 hour of NIV [33]
Criteria favouring NIV discontinuation and endotracheal intubation
   Failure to maintain a P_{a,O_2} >60 mmHg with an F_{I,O_2} ⩾60%
   Severe restrictive syndrome requiring high airway pressures (P_{peak} >20 cmH$_2$O)
   No significant improvement in dyspnoea or gas exchange
   Mask intolerance/lack of cooperation/poor adherence
   Difficulties with the management of secretions
   Occurrence of any NIV contraindication
   At any time if it is judged that the risk–benefit ratio has become unfavourable

ARDS: acute respiratory distress syndrome, SAPS: simplified acute physiology score; APACHE: acute physiology and chronic health evaluation; P_{a,O_2}: arterial oxygen tension; F_{I,O_2}: inspiratory oxygen fraction; P_{peak}: peak airway pressure.

aetiology must be reversible and addressed in a timely fashion to take advantage of the opportunity window. It is critical to meticulously assess eligibility based on several clinical aspects simultaneously (table 1). This is mainly to reproduce inclusion criteria from major NIV trials while adapting them specifically to hypoxaemic ARF. The limits and concerns mentioned previously regarding NIV use in hypoxaemic ARF must be kept in mind and patient safety must always be ensured.

Once an NIV trial was deemed appropriate, specific settings had to be chosen (table 2). The oronasal mask is adequate in most patients presenting with ARF, but the helmet is an interesting alternative, despite some pitfalls such as asynchrony and noise inside the gear [37, 115, 117, 118]. It is preferable to actively support the inspiratory muscles, and intermittent positive pressure ventilation, such as PSV, must be preferred over CPAP [14, 25]. The notable potential exception is in prophylaxis, when at-risk patients are taken before failure of the respiratory muscles, such as with post-operative or haematological patients [52, 102].

Beyond any particular settings, close monitoring must detect failure as early as possible. Some predictors of failure are fairly well recognised and must be known, bearing in mind that none were prospectively validated (table 3) [120]. The presence of these predictors does not necessarily mean that NIV should not be attempted, but that a low threshold for ETI should be adopted. The initial assessment should involve the patient's subjective response and the observed physiological benefits, particularly in terms of oxygenation and respiratory mechanics (table 3). In a self-fulfilling prophecy, the best predictor of failure is the absence of clinical response to NIV. Beyond early failure, little is known about late failure occurring hours or days after starting NIV. Clinical judgement and experience must prevail, considering the patient's overall condition rather than only the respiratory parameters.

Conclusions

There is a strong rationale for using NIV in hypoxaemic ARF. Nevertheless, the literature has yielded conflicting results that probably reflect, on the one hand, the large heterogeneity of underlying diagnoses and, on the other hand, some pitfalls of the technique in these patients. Patient selection is a crucial aspect and the focus should be on patients with the most favourable risk–benefit ratio, such as immunocompromised and post-operative patients. NIV must be initiated early on in the process of ARF and in patients with a reversible underlying condition.

Gaining some time with NIV must make sense from a global perspective. Failure of NIV must also be recognised early to avoid delaying intubation. The delay in ETI is the leading hypothesis to explain the mortality excess of hypoxaemic ARF patients who failed NIV. The use of NIV in hypoxaemic ARF patients is part of a calculated risk-taking strategy that must take into account the pathophysiological concepts, the risks and limitations of the technique (always ensuring patient safety) and assess the risk–benefit ratio for each patient. As already suggested, future studies must explicitly target specific subgroups of hypoxaemic ARF.

Statement of interest

L. Brochard's laboratory has received research grants in the years 2005–2011 for the support of specific clinical studies from several manufacturers, including Drager, Covidien, General Electric, Fisher Paykel and Phillips Respironics. J-C. Lefebvre has received a research grant from Conseil des médecins, dentistes et pharmaciens du Centre hospitalier universitaire de Québec.

References

1. Evans TW. International Consensus Conferences in Intensive Care Medicine: non-invasive positive pressure ventilation in acute respiratory failure. Organised jointly by the American Thoracic Society, the European Respiratory Society, the European Society of Intensive Care Medicine, and the Société de Réanimation de Langue Française, and approved by the ATS Board of Directors, December 2000. *Intensive Care Med* 2001; 27: 166–178.
2. Demoule A, Girou E, Richard JC, *et al.* Increased use of noninvasive ventilation in French intensive care units. *Intensive Care Med* 2006; 32: 1747–1755.
3. Keenan SP, Sinuff T, Cook DJ, *et al.* Which patients with acute exacerbation of chronic obstructive pulmonary disease benefit from noninvasive positive-pressure ventilation? A systematic review of the literature. *Ann Intern Med* 2003; 138: 861–870.
4. Weng CL, Zhao YT, Liu QH, *et al.* Meta-analysis: noninvasive ventilation in acute cardiogenic pulmonary edema. *Ann Intern Med* 2010; 152: 590–600.
5. Brochard L, Mancebo J, Wysocki M, *et al.* Noninvasive ventilation for acute exacerbations of chronic obstructive pulmonary disease. *N Engl J Med* 1995; 333: 817–822.
6. Nava S, Carbone G, DiBattista N, *et al.* Noninvasive ventilation in cardiogenic pulmonary edema: a multicenter randomized trial. *Am J Respir Crit Care Med* 2003; 168: 1432–1437.
7. Girou E, Schortgen F, Delclaux C, *et al.* Association of noninvasive ventilation with nosocomial infections and survival in critically ill patients. *JAMA* 2000; 284: 2361–2367.
8. Hess DR. Noninvasive positive-pressure ventilation and ventilator-associated pneumonia. *Respir Care* 2005; 50: 924–929.
9. Demoule A, Girou E, Richard JC, *et al.* Benefits and risks of success or failure of noninvasive ventilation. *Intensive Care Med* 2006; 32: 1756–1765.
10. Esteban A, Ferguson ND, Meade MO, *et al.* Evolution of mechanical ventilation in response to clinical research. *Am J Respir Crit Care Med* 2008; 177: 170–177.
11. Keenan SP, Sinuff T, Burns KE, *et al.* Clinical practice guidelines for the use of noninvasive positive-pressure ventilation and noninvasive continuous positive airway pressure in the acute care setting. *CMAJ* 2011; 183: E195–E214.
12. Ferrer M, Sellares J, Torres A. NIV in withdrawal from mechanical ventilation. *Eur Respir Mon* 2012; 55: 191–205.
13. Brochard L, Isabey D, Piquet J, *et al.* Reversal of acute exacerbations of chronic obstructive lung disease by inspiratory assistance with a face mask. *N Engl J Med* 1990; 323: 1523–1530.
14. L'Her E, Deye N, Lellouche F, *et al.* Physiologic effects of noninvasive ventilation during acute lung injury. *Am J Respir Crit Care Med* 2005; 172: 1112–1118.
15. Navalesi P, Fanfulla F, Frigerio P, *et al.* Physiologic evaluation of noninvasive mechanical ventilation delivered with three types of masks in patients with chronic hypercapnic respiratory failure. *Crit Care Med* 2000; 28: 1785–1790.
16. Weiler N, Latorre F, Eberle B, *et al.* Respiratory mechanics, gastric insufflation pressure, and air leakage of the laryngeal mask airway. *Anesth Analg* 1997; 84: 1025–1028.
17. Keenan SP, Sinuff T, Cook DJ, *et al.* Does noninvasive positive pressure ventilation improve outcome in acute hypoxemic respiratory failure? A systematic review. *Crit Care Med* 2004; 32: 2516–2523.
18. Antonelli M, Conti G, Moro ML, *et al.* Predictors of failure of noninvasive positive pressure ventilation in patients with acute hypoxemic respiratory failure: a multi-center study. *Intensive Care Med* 2001; 27: 1718–1728.
19. Wood KA, Lewis L, Von Harz B, *et al.* The use of noninvasive positive pressure ventilation in the emergency department: results of a randomized clinical trial. *Chest* 1998; 113: 1339–1346.

20. Wysocki M, Tric L, Wolff MA, *et al.* Noninvasive pressure support ventilation in patients with acute respiratory failure. *Chest* 1993; 103: 907–913.

21. Meduri GU. Noninvasive positive-pressure ventilation in patients with acute respiratory failure. *Clin Chest Med* 1996; 17: 513–553.

22. Patrick W, Webster K, Ludwig L, *et al.* Noninvasive positive-pressure ventilation in acute respiratory distress without prior chronic respiratory failure. *Am J Respir Crit Care Med* 1996; 153: 1005–1011.

23. Rocker GM. Noninvasive positive pressure ventilation: successful outcome in patients with acute lung injury/ARDS. *Chest* 1999; 115: 173–177.

24. Wysocki M, Tric L, Wolff MA, *et al.* Noninvasive pressure support ventilation in patients with acute respiratory failure: a randomized comparison with conventional therapy. *Chest* 1995; 107: 761–768.

25. Delclaux C, L'Her E, Alberti C, *et al.* Treatment of acute hypoxemic nonhypercapnic respiratory insufficiency with continuous positive airway pressure delivered by a face mask: a randomized controlled trial. *JAMA* 2000; 284: 2352–2360.

26. Ferrer M, Esquinas A, Leon M, *et al.* Noninvasive ventilation in severe hypoxemic respiratory failure: a randomized clinical trial. *Am J Respir Crit Care Med* 2003; 168: 1438–1444.

27. Schettino G, Altobelli N, Kacmarek RM. Noninvasive positive-pressure ventilation in acute respiratory failure outside clinical trials: experience at the Massachusetts General Hospital. *Crit Care Med* 2008; 36: 441–447.

28. Guisset O, Gruson D, Vargas F. Noninvasive ventilation in acute respiratory distress syndrome (ARDS) patients. *Intensive Care Med* 2003; 29: S124.

29. Agarwal R, Aggarwal AN, Gupta D. Role of noninvasive ventilation in acute lung injury/acute respiratory distress syndrome: a proportion meta-analysis. *Respir Care* 2010; 55: 1653–1660.

30. Adda M, Coquet I, Darmon M, *et al.* Predictors of noninvasive ventilation failure in patients with hematologic malignancy and acute respiratory failure. *Crit Care Med* 2008; 36: 2766–2772.

31. Rana S, Jenad H, Gay PC, *et al.* Failure of non-invasive ventilation in patients with acute lung injury: observational cohort study. *Crit Care* 2006; 10: R79.

32. Gristina GR, Antonelli M, Conti G, *et al.* Noninvasive *versus* invasive ventilation for acute respiratory failure in patients with hematologic malignancies: a 5-year multicenter observational survey. *Crit Care Med* 2011; 39: 2232–2239.

33. Antonelli M, Conti G, Esquinas A, *et al.* A multiple-center survey on the use in clinical practice of noninvasive ventilation as a first-line intervention for acute respiratory distress syndrome. *Crit Care Med* 2007; 35: 18–25.

34. Garpestad E, Hill NS. Noninvasive ventilation for acute lung injury: how often should we try, how often should we fail? *Crit Care* 2006; 10: 147.

35. Honrubia T, Garcia Lopez FJ, Franco N, *et al.* Noninvasive *vs* conventional mechanical ventilation in acute respiratory failure: a multicenter, randomized controlled trial. *Chest* 2005; 128: 3916–3924.

36. Antro C, Merico F, Urbino R, *et al.* Non-invasive ventilation as a first-line treatment for acute respiratory failure: "real life" experience in the emergency department. *Emerg Med J* 2005; 22: 772–777.

37. Carron M, Freo U, Zorzi M, *et al.* Predictors of failure of noninvasive ventilation in patients with severe community-acquired pneumonia. *J Crit Care* 2010; 25: 540.e9–e14.

38. Jolliet P, Abajo B, Pasquina P, *et al.* Non-invasive pressure support ventilation in severe community-acquired pneumonia. *Intensive Care Med* 2001; 27: 812–821.

39. Domenighetti G, Gayer R, Gentilini R. Noninvasive pressure support ventilation in non-COPD patients with acute cardiogenic pulmonary edema and severe community-acquired pneumonia: acute effects and outcome. *Intensive Care Med* 2002; 28: 1226–1232.

40. Confalonieri M, Potena A, Carbone G, *et al.* Acute respiratory failure in patients with severe community-acquired pneumonia. A prospective randomized evaluation of noninvasive ventilation. *Am J Respir Crit Care Med* 1999; 160: 1585–1591.

41. Antonelli M, Conti G, Rocco M, *et al.* A comparison of noninvasive positive-pressure ventilation and conventional mechanical ventilation in patients with acute respiratory failure. *N Engl J Med* 1998; 339: 429–435.

42. Azoulay E, Alberti C, Bornstain C, *et al.* Improved survival in cancer patients requiring mechanical ventilatory support: impact of noninvasive mechanical ventilatory support. *Crit Care Med* 2001; 29: 519–525.

43. Azoulay E, Thiery G, Chevret S, *et al.* The prognosis of acute respiratory failure in critically ill cancer patients. *Medicine (Baltimore)* 2004; 83: 360–370.

44. Soares M, Salluh JI, Spector N, *et al.* Characteristics and outcomes of cancer patients requiring mechanical ventilatory support for >24 hrs. *Crit Care Med* 2005; 33: 520–526.

45. Blot F, Guiguet M, Nitenberg G, *et al.* Prognostic factors for neutropenic patients in an intensive care unit: respective roles of underlying malignancies and acute organ failures. *Eur J Cancer* 1997; 33: 1031–1037.

46. Conti G, Marino P, Cogliati A, *et al.* Noninvasive ventilation for the treatment of acute respiratory failure in patients with hematologic malignancies: a pilot study. *Intensive Care Med* 1998; 24: 1283–1288.

47. Tognet E, Mercatello A, Polo P, *et al.* Treatment of acute respiratory failure with non-invasive intermittent positive pressure ventilation in haematological patients. *Clin Intensive Care* 1994; 5: 282–288.

48. Hilbert G, Gruson D, Vargas F, *et al.* Noninvasive continuous positive airway pressure in neutropenic patients with acute respiratory failure requiring intensive care unit admission. *Crit Care Med* 2000; 28: 3185–3190.

49. Confalonieri M, Calderini E, Terraciano S, *et al.* Noninvasive ventilation for treating acute respiratory failure in AIDS patients with *Pneumocystis carinii* pneumonia. *Intensive Care Med* 2002; 28: 1233–1238.

50. Antonelli M, Conti G, Bufi M, *et al.* Noninvasive ventilation for treatment of acute respiratory failure in patients undergoing solid organ transplantation: a randomized trial. *JAMA* 2000; 283: 235–241.

51. Hilbert G, Gruson D, Vargas F, *et al.* Noninvasive ventilation in immunosuppressed patients with pulmonary infiltrates, fever, and acute respiratory failure. *N Engl J Med* 2001; 344: 481–487.

52. Squadrone V, Massaia M, Bruno B, *et al.* Early CPAP prevents evolution of acute lung injury in patients with hematologic malignancy. *Intensive Care Med* 2010; 36: 1666–1674.

53. Depuydt PO, Benoit DD, Vandewoude KH, *et al.* Outcome in noninvasively and invasively ventilated hematologic patients with acute respiratory failure. *Chest* 2004; 126: 1299–1306.

54. Depuydt PO, Benoit DD, Roosens CD, *et al.* The impact of the initial ventilatory strategy on survival in hematological patients with acute hypoxemic respiratory failure. *J Crit Care* 2010; 25: 30–36.

55. Schwartz DE, Matthay MA, Cohen NH. Death and other complications of emergency airway management in critically ill adults. A prospective investigation of 297 tracheal intubations. *Anesthesiology* 1995; 82: 367–376.

56. Jaber S, Amraoui J, Lefrant JY, *et al.* Clinical practice and risk factors for immediate complications of endotracheal intubation in the intensive care unit: a prospective, multiple-center study. *Crit Care Med* 2006; 34: 2355–2361.

57. Mort TC. Emergency tracheal intubation: complications associated with repeated laryngoscopic attempts. *Anesth Analg* 2004; 99: 607–613.

58. Mort TC. Preoxygenation in critically ill patients requiring emergency tracheal intubation. *Crit Care Med* 2005; 33: 2672–2675.

59. Baillard C, Fosse JP, Sebbane M, *et al.* Noninvasive ventilation improves preoxygenation before intubation of hypoxic patients. *Am J Respir Crit Care Med* 2006; 174: 171–177.

60. Jaber S, Jung B, Corne P, *et al.* An intervention to decrease complications related to endotracheal intubation in the intensive care unit: a prospective, multiple-center study. *Intensive Care Med* 2010; 36: 248–255.

61. Facciolongo N, Patelli M, Gasparini S, *et al.* Incidence of complications in bronchoscopy. Multicentre prospective study of 20,986 bronchoscopies. *Monaldi Arch Chest Dis* 2009; 71: 8–14.

62. Lindholm C, Ollman B, Snyder J, *et al.* Cardiorespiratory effects of flexible fiberoptic bronchoscopy in critically ill patients. *Chest* 1978; 74: 362–368.

63. Matsushima Y, Jones R, King E, *et al.* Alterations in pulmonary mechanics and gas exchange during routine fiberoptic bronchoscopy. *Chest* 1984; 86: 184–188.

64. Trouillet J, Guiguet M, Gibert C, *et al.* Fiberoptic bronchoscopy in ventilated patients. Evaluation of cardiopulmonary risk under midazolam sedation. *Chest* 1990; 97: 927–933.

65. Antonelli M, Conti G, Riccioni L, *et al.* Noninvasive positive-pressure ventilation *via* face mask during bronchoscopy with BAL in high-risk hypoxemic patients. *Chest* 1996; 110: 724–728.

66. Da Conceiçao M, Genco G, Favier JC, *et al.* Fibroscopie bronchique sous ventilation non invasive chez des patients atteints de bronchopathie chronique obstructive avec hypoxemie et hypercapnie [Fiberoptic bronchoscopy during noninvasive positive-pressure ventilation in patients with chronic obstructive lung disease with hypoxemia and hypercapnia]. *Ann Fr Anesth Reanim* 2000; 19: 231–236.

67. Antonelli M, Pennisi MA, Conti G, *et al.* Fiberoptic bronchoscopy during noninvasive positive pressure ventilation delivered by helmet. *Intensive Care Med* 2003; 29: 126–129.

68. Heunks LM, de Bruin CJ, van der Hoeven JG, *et al.* Non-invasive mechanical ventilation for diagnostic bronchoscopy using a new face mask: an observational feasibility study. *Intensive Care Med* 2010; 36: 143–147.

69. Baumann HJ, Klose H, Simon M, *et al.* Fiber optic bronchoscopy in patients with acute hypoxemic respiratory failure requiring noninvasive ventilation – a feasibility study. *Crit Care* 2011; 15: R179.

70. Maitre B, Jaber S, Maggiore SM, *et al.* Continuous positive airway pressure during fiberoptic bronchoscopy in hypoxemic patients. A randomized double-blind study using a new device. *Am J Respir Crit Care Med* 2000; 162: 1063–1067.

71. Antonelli M, Conti G, Rocco M, *et al.* Noninvasive positive-pressure ventilation *vs* conventional oxygen supplementation in hypoxemic patients undergoing diagnostic bronchoscopy. *Chest* 2002; 121: 1149–1154.

72. Murgu SD, Pecson J, Colt HG. Bronchoscopy during noninvasive ventilation: indications and technique. *Respir Care* 2010; 55: 595–600.

73. Jaber S, Chanques G, Jung B. Postoperative noninvasive ventilation. *Anesthesiology* 2010; 112: 453–461.

74. Tobias JD. Noninvasive ventilation using bilevel positive airway pressure to treat impending respiratory failure in the postanesthesia care unit. *J Clin Anesth* 2000; 12: 409–412.

75. Chanques G, Jaber S, Delay JM, *et al.* Enquete telephonique sur la pratique postoperatoire de la ventilation non invasive et ses modalites d'application [Phoning study about postoperative practice and application of non-invasive ventilation]. *Ann Fr Anesth Reanim* 2003; 22: 879–885.

76. Warner DO. Preventing postoperative pulmonary complications: the role of the anesthesiologist. *Anesthesiology* 2000; 92: 1467–1472.

77. Simonneau G, Vivien A, Sartene R, *et al.* Diaphragm dysfunction induced by upper abdominal surgery. Role of postoperative pain. *Am Rev Respir Dis* 1983; 128: 899–903.

78. Lindner KH, Lotz P, Ahnefeld FW. Continuous positive airway pressure effect on functional residual capacity, vital capacity and its subdivisions. *Chest* 1987; 92: 66–70.
79. Ferreyra GP, Baussano I, Squadrone V, *et al*. Continuous positive airway pressure for treatment of respiratory complications after abdominal surgery: a systematic review and meta-analysis. *Ann Surg* 2008; 247: 617–626.
80. Kutlu CA, Williams EA, Evans TW, *et al*. Acute lung injury and acute respiratory distress syndrome after pulmonary resection. *Ann Thorac Surg* 2000; 69: 376–380.
81. Auriant I, Jallot A, Herve P, *et al*. Noninvasive ventilation reduces mortality in acute respiratory failure following lung resection. *Am J Respir Crit Care Med* 2001; 164: 1231–1235.
82. Wright CD, Wain JC, Mathisen DJ, *et al*. Postpneumonectomy bronchopleural fistula after sutured bronchial closure: incidence, risk factors, and management. *J Thorac Cardiovasc Surg* 1996; 112: 1367–1371.
83. Aguilo R, Togores B, Pons S, *et al*. Noninvasive ventilatory support after lung resectional surgery. *Chest* 1997; 112: 117–121.
84. Perrin C, Jullien V, Venissac N, *et al*. Prophylactic use of noninvasive ventilation in patients undergoing lung resectional surgery. *Respir Med* 2007; 101: 1572–1578.
85. Jousela I, Rasanen J, Verkkala K, *et al*. Continuous positive airway pressure by mask in patients after coronary surgery. *Acta Anaesthesiol Scand* 1994; 38: 311–316.
86. Pinilla JC, Oleniuk FH, Tan L, *et al*. Use of a nasal continuous positive airway pressure mask in the treatment of postoperative atelectasis in aortocoronary bypass surgery. *Crit Care Med* 1990; 18: 836–840.
87. Zarbock A, Mueller E, Netzer S, *et al*. Prophylactic nasal continuous positive airway pressure following cardiac surgery protects from postoperative pulmonary complications: a prospective, randomized, controlled trial in 500 patients. *Chest* 2009; 135: 1252–1259.
88. Matte P, Jacquet L, Van Dyck M, *et al*. Effects of conventional physiotherapy, continuous positive airway pressure and non-invasive ventilatory support with bilevel positive airway pressure after coronary artery bypass grafting. *Acta Anaesthesiol Scand* 2000; 44: 75–81.
89. Svensson LG, Hess KR, Coselli JS, *et al*. A prospective study of respiratory failure after high-risk surgery on the thoracoabdominal aorta. *J Vasc Surg* 1991; 14: 271–282.
90. Kindgen-Milles D, Muller E, Buhl R, *et al*. Nasal-continuous positive airway pressure reduces pulmonary morbidity and length of hospital stay following thoracoabdominal aortic surgery. *Chest* 2005; 128: 821–828.
91. Lefebvre A, Lorut C, Alifano M, *et al*. Noninvasive ventilation for acute respiratory failure after lung resection: an observational study. *Intensive Care Med* 2009; 35: 663–670.
92. Riviere S, Monconduit J, Zarka V, *et al*. Failure of noninvasive ventilation after lung surgery: a comprehensive analysis of incidence and possible risk factors. *Eur J Cardiothorac Surg* 2011; 39: 769–776.
93. Rocco M, Conti G, Antonelli M, *et al*. Non-invasive pressure support ventilation in patients with acute respiratory failure after bilateral lung transplantation. *Intensive Care Med* 2001; 27: 1622–1626.
94. Michelet P, D'Journo XB, Seinaye F, *et al*. Non-invasive ventilation for treatment of postoperative respiratory failure after oesophagectomy. *Br J Surg* 2009; 96: 54–60.
95. Arozullah AM, Daley J, Henderson WG, *et al*. Multifactorial risk index for predicting postoperative respiratory failure in men after major noncardiac surgery. The National Veterans Administration Surgical Quality Improvement Program. *Ann Surg* 2000; 232: 242–253.
96. Pasquina P, Merlani P, Granier JM, *et al*. Continuous positive airway pressure *versus* noninvasive pressure support ventilation to treat atelectasis after cardiac surgery. *Anesth Analg* 2004; 99: 1001–1008.
97. Stock MC, Downs JB, Gauer PK, *et al*. Prevention of postoperative pulmonary complications with CPAP, incentive spirometry, and conservative therapy. *Chest* 1985; 87: 151–157.
98. Joris JL, Sottiaux TM, Chiche JD, *et al*. Effect of bi-level positive airway pressure (BiPAP) nasal ventilation on the postoperative pulmonary restrictive syndrome in obese patients undergoing gastroplasty. *Chest* 1997; 111: 665–670.
99. Neligan PJ, Malhotra G, Fraser M, *et al*. Continuous positive airway pressure *via* the Boussignac system immediately after extubation improves lung function in morbidly obese patients with obstructive sleep apnea undergoing laparoscopic bariatric surgery. *Anesthesiology* 2009; 110: 878–884.
100. Gaszynski T, Tokarz A, Piotrowski D, *et al*. Boussignac CPAP in the postoperative period in morbidly obese patients. *Obes Surg* 2007; 17: 452–456.
101. Bohner H, Kindgen-Milles D, Grust A, *et al*. Prophylactic nasal continuous positive airway pressure after major vascular surgery: results of a prospective randomized trial. *Langenbecks Arch Surg* 2002; 387: 21–26.
102. Squadrone V, Coha M, Cerutti E, *et al*. Continuous positive airway pressure for treatment of postoperative hypoxemia: a randomized controlled trial. *JAMA* 2005; 293: 589–595.
103. Jaber S, Delay JM, Chanques G, *et al*. Outcomes of patients with acute respiratory failure after abdominal surgery treated with noninvasive positive pressure ventilation. *Chest* 2005; 128: 2688–2695.
104. Varon J, Walsh GL, Fromm RE Jr. Feasibility of noninvasive mechanical ventilation in the treatment of acute respiratory failure in postoperative cancer patients. *J Crit Care* 1998; 13: 55–57.
105. Wallet F, Schoeffler M, Reynaud M, *et al*. Factors associated with noninvasive ventilation failure in postoperative acute respiratory insufficiency: an observational study. *Eur J Anaesthesiol* 2010; 27: 270–274.
106. Conti G, Cavaliere F, Costa R, *et al*. Noninvasive positive-pressure ventilation with different interfaces in patients with respiratory failure after abdominal surgery: a matched-control study. *Respir Care* 2007; 52: 1463–1471.

107. Gregoretti C, Beltrame F, Lucangelo U, *et al.* Physiologic evaluation of non-invasive pressure support ventilation in trauma patients with acute respiratory failure. *Intensive Care Med* 1998; 24: 785–790.

108. Xirouchaki N, Kondoudaki E, Anastasaki M, *et al.* Noninvasive bilevel positive pressure ventilation in patients with blunt thoracic trauma. *Respiration* 2005; 72: 517–522.

109. Beltrame F, Lucangelo U, Gregori D, *et al.* Noninvasive positive pressure ventilation in trauma patients with acute respiratory failure. *Monaldi Arch Chest Dis* 1999; 54: 109–114.

110. Hernandez G, Fernandez R, Lopez-Reina P, *et al.* Noninvasive ventilation reduces intubation in chest trauma-related hypoxemia: a randomized clinical trial. *Chest* 2010; 137: 74–80.

111. Bolliger CT, Van Eeden SF. Treatment of multiple rib fractures. Randomized controlled trial comparing ventilatory with nonventilatory management. *Chest* 1990; 97: 943–948.

112. Gunduz M, Unlugenc H, Ozalevli M, *et al.* A comparative study of continuous positive airway pressure (CPAP) and intermittent positive pressure ventilation (IPPV) in patients with flail chest. *Emerg Med J* 2005; 22: 325–329.

113. Esteban A, Frutos-Vivar F, Ferguson ND, *et al.* Noninvasive positive-pressure ventilation for respiratory failure after extubation. *N Engl J Med* 2004; 350: 2452–2460.

114. Domenighetti G, Moccia A, Gayer R. Observational case–control study of non-invasive ventilation in patients with ARDS. *Monaldi Arch Chest Dis* 2008; 69: 5–10.

115. Cosentini R, Brambilla AM, Aliberti S, *et al.* Helmet continuous positive airway pressure *vs* oxygen therapy to improve oxygenation in community-acquired pneumonia: a randomized, controlled trial. *Chest* 2010; 138: 114–120.

116. Mascheroni D, Kolobow T, Fumagalli R, *et al.* Acute respiratory failure following pharmacologically induced hyperventilation: an experimental animal study. *Intensive Care Med* 1988; 15: 8–14.

117. Pelosi P, Severgnini P, Aspesi M, *et al.* Non-invasive ventilation delivered by conventional interfaces and helmet in the emergency department. *Eur J Emerg Med* 2003; 10: 79–86.

118. Cavaliere F, Conti G, Costa R, *et al.* Noise exposure during noninvasive ventilation with a helmet, a nasal mask, and a facial mask. *Intensive Care Med* 2004; 30: 1755–1760.

119. Yoshida Y, Takeda S, Akada S, *et al.* Factors predicting successful noninvasive ventilation in acute lung injury. *J Anesth* 2008; 22: 201–206.

120. Nava S, Ceriana P. Causes of failure of noninvasive mechanical ventilation. *Respir Care* 2004; 49: 295–303.

Chapter 6

Biphasic PAP/airway pressure release ventilation in ALI

A. Güldner*, N.C. Carvalho*, P. Pelosi# and M. Gama de Abreu*

Summary

Biphasic positive airway pressure (BIPAP)/airway pressure release ventilation (APRV) is a mechanical ventilation mode based on a high flow or demand-valve continuous positive airway pressure (CPAP) system, in which the level of CPAP is switched between a higher and a lower pressure in a time-dependent manner, generating time-cycled, pressure-limited ventilation. Supported and unsupported spontaneous breathing is possible at both levels of airway pressure, but the optimal level of spontaneous breathing has yet to be determined. BIPAP/APRV has proved efficient in increasing oxygenation compared with controlled mechanical ventilation in acute respiratory distress syndrome (ARDS). In addition, BIPAP/APRV with spontaneous breathing waives the need for muscle paralysis, and allows reduced sedation, as well as cardiovascular support with drugs. BIPAP/APRV with spontaneous breathing seems to be a useful ventilatory strategy for patients with less severe hypoxaemic respiratory failure, but caution is required in those patients with more severe lung injury, as reflected by an arterial oxygen tension(Pa,O_2)/inspiratory oxygen fraction (FI,O_2) of <120 mmHg.

Keywords: Acute lung injury, acute respiratory distress syndrome, gas exchange, mechanical ventilation, morbidity, mortality

*Pulmonary Engineering Group, Dept of Anesthesiology and Intensive Care Therapy, University Hospital Carl Gustav Carus, Dresden University of Technology, Dresden, Germany.
#Dept of Surgical Sciences and Integrated Diagnostics, University of Genoa, Genoa, Italy.

Correspondence: M. Gama de Abreu, Dept of Anesthesiology and Intensive Care Therapy, University Hospital Carl Gustav Carus, Dresden University of Technology, Fetscherstr. 74, 01307 Dresden, Germany. Email mgabreu@uniklinikum-dresden.de

Eur Respir Mon 2012; 55: 81–96.
Printed in UK – all rights reserved
Copyright ERS 2012
European Respiratory Monograph
ISSN: 1025-448x
DOI: 10.1183/1025448x.10001811

ALI/ARDS epidemiology and mortality

Acute lung injury (ALI) and its more severe form, acute respiratory distress syndrome (ARDS), represent major challenges for intensive care therapy worldwide [1]. The complex ALI/ARDS is characterised by a diffuse inflammatory reaction of the lung parenchyma, leading to an increased alveolar capillary permeability and resulting in clinical, radiological and physiological abnormalities [2]. ARDS can be induced by a direct insult to the alveolar epithelium (pulmonary ARDS) or indirect damage through the vascular endothelium (extrapulmonary ARDS), where lung injury is caused by circulating inflammatory mediators released from an extrapulmonary focus into the blood [3, 4].

The incidence of ALI and ARDS has been estimated to be between 13.5 and 78.9 per 100,000 inhabitants per year, depending on the studied population [5], while amongst mechanically ventilated patients an incidence of 20% has been reported [6]. In European countries, intensive care unit (ICU) and hospital mortalities due to ALI were 22.6% and 32.7%, respectively. In patients suffering from ARDS, the ICU mortality was 49.4%, while in-hospital mortality was as high as 57.9%. These numbers are in accordance with data from a worldwide observation, which reported ARDS-related mortality rates of 56% in ICU and 63% in hospital [7]. Although the incidence of ICU and hospital-acquired ARDS seems to decrease [8], mortality due to ARDS remained relatively unchanged in the last 15 years, despite improvements in critical care and mechanical ventilation strategies [1].

Importance of mechanical ventilation in ALI/ARDS

ARDS is a life-threatening condition. Severe hypoxaemia, refractory to supplemental oxygen, remains one of the most serious challenges in the management of this disease [9]. Until recently, mechanical ventilation has represented the best way to ensure sufficient gas exchange and maintain adequate tissue oxygenation, while reducing the work of breathing [10]. In addition to its acute life-saving benefits, mechanical ventilation strategy with low tidal volume (V_T; 4–6 mL·kg^{-1}) and limited airway pressure has been the only therapeutic approach proven to have beneficial effects on the mortality and morbidity associated with this syndrome [11]. Numerous investigations of different pharmacological approaches failed to show significant effects on the clinical outcome [12]. Therefore, besides the treatment of the underlying causative condition, mechanical ventilation remains a cornerstone in the management of ALI/ARDS.

However, as well as being a potentially life-saving intervention, mechanical ventilation itself is able to induce or aggravate pre-existing lung injury (ventilator-induced lung injury (VILI) and ventilator-associated lung injury (VALI)) [13]; it can therefore even contribute to the development of multi-organ failure, one of the main causes of the high mortality associated with ALI/ARDS [14]. Because of this ambivalence, the critical care community faces the challenge of keeping the balance between utilising the beneficial effects of mechanical ventilation, while minimising its deleterious impact on the patient during ALI/ARDS.

Scope of the chapter

Different mechanical ventilation modes have been proposed for the management of patients with ALI/ARDS [15–17]. Given the recent interest in the use of spontaneous breathing during ventilation of such patients [18], this chapter will focus on two modes that allow unassisted spontaneous breathing throughout the respiratory cycle, namely biphasic positive airway pressure (BIPAP) and airway pressure release ventilation (APRV). The reader will notice that after defining the main characteristics and work principles of each mode, we merge both abbreviations into a single abbreviation, namely BIPAP/APRV. Following that, this chapter describes the main effects of BIPAP/APRV on lung function and damage, and discusses the limitations and unknowns in the management of patients with ALI/ARDS.

General aspects

History

First described in 1987 [19], APRV followed three main objectives: 1) to maintain a desired level of continuous airway pressure; 2) to deliver mechanical breaths while avoiding excessive airway pressures; and 3) to allow unrestricted spontaneous breathing at any time during the ventilatory cycle, overcoming limitations such as ineffective triggering of the ventilator and high peak airway pressures, which were common to other assisted-ventilation modes available at that time; for example, inspiratory flow assist [20] and intermittent mandatory ventilation [21]. Independent from APRV, BIPAP was first described in 1989; it also aimed to facilitate spontaneous breathing throughout the respiratory cycle [22]. Although both modes were based on a similar working principle, differences in airway pressure and time settings enabled BIPAP to be used throughout the whole clinical course of mechanical ventilation, making changes to the ventilatory mode unnecessary [23], as compared with APRV. After implementation of these modes in commercially available ventilators, a large number of experimental and clinical studies followed [24, 25], describing their performance in clinical and experimental settings.

Working principles

Since their first description, some technical aspects of APRV and BIPAP have changed dramatically, but the basic working principle of both ventilatory modes has remained the same. APRV and BIPAP are based on a high-flow or demand-valve continuous positive airway pressure (CPAP) system, in which the level of CPAP is switched between high airway pressure (P_{high}) and low airway pressure (P_{low}) in a time-dependent manner, generating a time-cycled, pressure-limited ventilation. Therefore, in the absence of spontaneous breathing efforts, the delivered V_T depends mainly on the difference between P_{high} and P_{low}, besides the mechanical properties of the respiratory system. The duration of a mandatory respiratory cycle is calculated upon the time spent at P_{high} and P_{low} (T_{high} and T_{low}, respectively). In contrast to conventional ventilatory modes, the desired airway pressure during BIPAP and APRV is achieved with a relatively high airflow in an open or demand-valve system. Such high airflow is necessary to accomplish the needs of the patient during active inspiration and expiration. Spontaneous breathing efforts against closed valves in the ventilator system are therefore avoided.

The typical settings of T_{high} and T_{low}, as well as P_{high} and P_{low}, differ importantly in BIPAP and APRV. In APRV, P_{high} is released (*i.e.* reduced to P_{low}) for no longer than 1.5 seconds; during BIPAP, T_{low} lasts longer and P_{low} is higher in comparison with APRV, closely mimicking pressure-controlled ventilation (PCV) with positive end-expiratory pressure (PEEP) [19, 22, 26].

In subsequent technical developments, synchronisation of the pressure changes and the subject's effort was implemented in BIPAP ventilation. This feature is not usually embedded in APRV, even though the intermittent mandatory pressure release ventilation (IMPRV) mode, a mode somehow comparable with "synchronised" APRV ventilation, is available in some ventilators [27]. Another technical development was the implementation of augmented spontaneous breathing (ASB) at P_{low} in BIPAP ventilation. Thereby, in a similar manner to CPAP+ASB, a subject's effort is supported with a set pressure level. Although technically possible, this feature is not usually combined with APRV. In some ventilators, ASB is also possible at P_{high}, in the mode known as bi-level.

Nomenclature and abbreviations

Since their first description, a number of different abbreviations for BIPAP and APRV have been proposed. Although such abbreviations may effectively describe differences in implementation and extra features, they are sometimes driven solely by the marketing purposes of manufacturers. Table 1 summarises the most common abbreviations used for BIPAP and APRV, as well as some of their most important variants.

Common settings

Since a consensus on definitions has not been achieved, it is difficult to characterise common settings of BIPAP and APRV. In fact, a recent review reported that ventilator settings during BIPAP and APRV vary considerably in the literature, making it hard to separate both modes using typical settings of the ventilatory key parameters, namely T_{high}, T_{low}, P_{high} and P_{low} [29]. Besides that, when performed with modern ventilators, BIPAP and APRV usually differ in their ability to

Table 1. Variants and abbreviations of biphasic positive airway pressure (BIPAP) and airway pressure release ventilation (APRV) in commercially available mechanical ventilators

Classification criteria	Abbreviation	Description
Spontaneous breathing	CMV-BIPAP	Controlled mandatory ventilation BIPAP: BIPAP without spontaneous breathing activity, similar to pressure-controlled ventilation
	IMV-BIPAP	Intermittent mandatory ventilation BIPAP: spontaneous breathing activity occurs on the lower airway pressure level
	APRV-BIPAP	Spontaneous breathing activity occurs on the higher airway pressure level
	Genuine BIPAP	Spontaneous breathing activity occurs on both airway pressure levels
Manufacturer	BIPAP	Dräger Medical AG, Lübeck, Germany
	Bi-level	Covidien, Mansfield, MA, USA
	BiPhasic	Care Fusion, San Diego, CA, USA
	Bi-Vent	Maquet, Rastatt, Germany
	DuoPAP	Hamilton, Bonaduz, Switzerland
Ventilator setting	IR-BIPAP	Inverse ratio BIPAP: Thigh > Tlow, similar time settings to APRV
Level of assistance	BIPAP-ASB	BIPAP and augmented spontaneous breathing BIPAP combined with pressure support: patient's efforts are supported with a set pressure support level
	IMPRV	Intermittent mandatory pressure release ventilation: APRV with synchronisation of release events with the patient's expiratory effort

Thigh: time spent at high pressure; Tlow: time spent at low pressure. Data from [23, 24, 28].

synchronise with the patient's inspiratory and expiratory efforts, introducing further difficulty into the attempt to describe typical settings.

Common settings of APRV

Most publications on APRV have used higher ratios of Thigh to Tlow, resulting in an extreme inverse ratio of ventilation, *i.e.* inspiration:expiration ratios (I:E) $\geqslant 2$. From the 39 publications reporting APRV settings, a mean Thigh of 3.4 seconds and a mean Tlow of 1.4 seconds could be identified [29]. Nevertheless, some investigators have reported Thigh values as high as 4.5 seconds and Tlow values as low as 0.5 seconds [30].

The setting of Tlow is particularly interesting in APRV. On the one hand, a longer pressure release can cause derecruitment of unstable alveoli; on the other hand, a shorter release time may facilitate an early disruption of expiratory flow, inducing air trapping and the development of auto-PEEP. However, since Plow is usually set at zero during APRV, a certain level of auto-PEEP may be necessary to maintain the lungs recruited, which can be achieved with adequate Tlow values. In turn, to guide the setting of Tlow, the expiratory flow signal can be used. Values of Tlow that lead to interruption of expiratory flow at 40% of the peak value have been suggested [18]. Usually, this can be achieved with Tlow in the range 0.6–0.8 seconds. Nevertheless, since an adequate level of auto-PEEP to protect lung units from collapse may require Tlow <0.6 seconds [31], the use of external PEEP has become increasingly common in APRV [29].

When commencing APRV, Phigh is usually set at the same value of the inspiratory plateau pressure during conventional ventilation, and adjusted in accordance with the response in oxygenation [18].

Common BIPAP settings

In contrast to APRV, which is mainly used during ALI/ARDS, BIPAP is also applied in other situations, using a wide range of ventilator settings. Compared with APRV, a lower I:E ratio is used during BIPAP. On average, a mean Thigh of 2.4 seconds and a mean Tlow of 3.4 seconds have been used [29]. Longer

*T*low values decrease the mean airway pressure and increase the likelihood of spontaneous efforts, which occur predominantly during the *P*low phase of the ventilatory cycle. Such inspiratory efforts at the *P*low level are able to generate negative intra-thoracic pressures, which may result in increased venous return and improved cardiac performance [28].

Depending on the mechanical properties of the respiratory system, *P*high and *P*low are set to ensure adequate ventilation, maintaining satisfactory gas exchange, and lung stability at end-expiration. In patients with ALI/ARDS, *P*high and *P*low should be chosen to yield low tidal volume ventilation, *i.e.* 4–8 mL·kg^{-1}, whereby the principles guiding the adjustment of *P*low are the same as for PEEP [15, 32].

Most modern ventilators offer a pressure support (ASB) component that can be combined with BIPAP ventilation, in order to support spontaneous inspiratory efforts. This is most common at *P*low, but some ventilators also offer it during *P*high. Although this technical feature may contribute to the alleviation of respiratory pump effort, little is known about its advantages and disadvantages during BIPAP. If ASB is used at all, attention must be paid to avoid overstretching of lung units, especially at *P*high.

BIPAP/APRV

Although the abbreviations BIPAP and APRV denote modes of mechanical ventilation with different characteristics, they also share similar properties. To improve readership, they will be used together as BIPAP/APRV in the subsequent sections of this chapter. More specifically, the abbreviation BIPAP/APRV will be used to describe a mode in which the mechanical ventilator switches between *P*high and *P*low independently of the patient's efforts (as in APRV), with I:E ratios of 1:1 or lower (as in BIPAP), whereby spontaneous breathing is possible at both the higher and the lower levels of airway pressure (as both in BIPAP and APRV).

Types of respiratory cycles during BIPAP/APRV

The patient does not trigger the mechanical ventilator during BIPAP/APRV, but spontaneous breathing may occur throughout the whole respiratory cycle. Accordingly, at least three types of respiratory cycle may be found: 1) mandatory or controlled; 2) purely spontaneous; and 3) mixed spontaneous/controlled, when the inspiratory effort coincides with ventilator cycling from *P*low to *P*high. Figure 1 shows tracing records of airflow, pressure at airways and oesophageal pressure during BIPAP/APRV, illustrating the different respiratory cycles in this mode.

Theoretically, spontaneous breaths occurring at *P*high and *P*low can have different characteristics. However, spontaneous breathing at *P*high occurs less often. Thus, they will be considered together for simplicity.

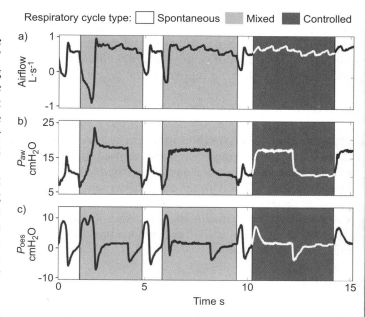

Figure 1. Types of respiratory cycle during mechanical ventilation with biphasic positive airway pressure airway pressure release ventilation. *P*aw: airway pressure; *P*oes: oesophageal pressure. Data from [33].

A. GÜLDNER ET AL.

Effects of BIPAP/APRV on lung function and damage

Table 2 depicts the most relevant effects of BIPAP/APRV on lung function and damage.

Lung aeration, ventilation and perfusion

Distribution of aeration

BIPAP/APRV results in higher mean airway pressure compared with both volume-controlled [36] and assisted ventilation with pressure support ventilation (PSV) [50, 51]. Computed tomography (CT) studies have shown that the total lung gas volume is increased when spontaneous breathing is superposed to BIPAP/APRV in experimental ALI [52, 53]. Such increase in gas volume is mainly due to a decrease in the amount of non-aerated and poorly aerated lung tissue, which is primarily localised in caudal and dependent lung zones, as shown both in experimental [54] and clinical studies [47].

The most likely explanation for the increased aeration in dependent lung zones is that spontaneous breathing, especially if not assisted by pressure support during BIPAP/APRV, generates transpulmonary pressures exceeding the critical opening pressures of those areas and, consequently, promotes lung recruitment.

Distribution of ventilation

In an experimental model of ALI, spontaneous breathing during BIPAP/APRV resulted in redistribution of ventilation from non-dependent to dependent lung zones [55]. According to preliminary results from our group, the redistribution of ventilation during this ventilatory strategy increases proportionally to the contribution of spontaneous breathing to total minute volume, becoming significant at >30%, as shown in figure 2 [33]. However, with the dynamic CT technique, our group could not show that BIPAP/APRV with spontaneous breathing was associated with increased ventilation of dependent lung zones compared with PSV [56]. Figure 3 shows the distribution of ventilation at the hilum during PSV and BIPAP/APRV with superposed spontaneous breathing in pigs with ALI.

Distribution of perfusion

NEUMANN *et al.* [55] have shown that perfusion is shifted to dependent lung zones during BIPAP/APRV when spontaneous breathing is allowed. In our experience, BIPAP/APRV with spontaneous breathing may also result in a shift of perfusion in the opposite direction, *i.e.* towards non-dependent zones [50]. This apparent discrepancy is explained by the fact that the distribution of perfusion usually accompanies the distribution of aeration and/or ventilation in the presence of preserved hypoxic vasoconstriction. Accordingly, perfusion will be more easily shifted to dependent lung zones if the spontaneous breathing during BIPAP/APRV effectively recruits the lung tissue in those areas.

Ventilation/perfusion matching

BIPAP/APRV with spontaneous breathing improved the global ventilation/perfusion (V'/Q') matching, assessed using the multiple gas elimination technique (MIGET), when compared with controlled mechanical ventilation and PSV both in experimental [57] and clinical [40] ALI. However, the regional V'/Q' matching of dependent lung zones, as determined by single photon emission tomography, was not changed in a model of lung injury [55]. Although apparently paradoxical, such an observation is explained by the fact that both V' and Q' increased in those areas, keeping their quotient approximately unchanged.

Table 2. Effects of biphasic positive airway pressure (BIPAP)/airway pressure release ventilation (APRV) on lung and distal organ function and clinical measures, compared with different ventilatory modes in adult patients with acute lung injury (ALI)/acute respiratory distress syndrome (ARDS)

First author [ref.]	Study design	Intervention/control	Patient population	Patients n	Spontaneous breathing	Lung function	Clinical measures
CANE [34]	Prospective, not randomised, crossover	VCV to APRV	Severe acute respiratory failure	18 (ARDS reported in 13 cases)	Not reported	Reduction of P_{peak} and V_T with APRV	NA
RASANEN [35]	Prospective, not randomised, crossover	CPAP and IMV to APRV	Severe acute respiratory failure	50	During APRV/CPAP and IMV	Reduction of P_{peak} and V_T, increase in P_{mean} with APRV	NA
DAVIS [36]	Prospective, not randomised, crossover	IMV to APRV	ARDS	15	During APRV/IMV	Reduction of P_{peak} and V_T, increase in P_{mean} with APRV	NA
SYDOW [37]	Prospective, randomised, crossover, 24 h	APRV/IR-VCV	ALI/ARDS	18	During APRV; muscle relaxation during IR-VCV	Reduction of P_{peak} and V_T, reduction in $P_{A-a,O_2}/F_{I,O_2}$ and venous admixture with APRV	NA
KIEHL [38]	Prospective, consecutively alternating assignment, two arm	BIPAP/VCV	ARDS	20	No spontaneous breathing during BIPAP/VCV	Reduction in P_{peak}, PEEP and F_{I,O_2} with comparable gas exchange with BIPAP	NA
HÖRMANN [39]	Prospective, not randomised, crossover	IR-BIPAP to IR-PCV to IR-BIPAP	ARDS	19	During IR-BIPAP	Reduction of dead space ventilation, venous admixture and P_{a,CO_2}, improved oxygenation with IR-BIPAP	NA
PUTENSEN [40]	Prospective, randomised, crossover	APRV/PSV/PCV (APRV without spontaneous breathing)	ARDS	24	During APRV/PSV	Reduction of P_{peak}, increase in DO_2, improvement in V/Q matching and oxygenation with APRV compared with PSV and PCV	NA
KAPLAN [41]	Prospective, not randomised, crossover	IR-PCV to APRV	ALI/ARDS	12	During APRV in majority of patients; muscle relaxation during IR-PCV in 74% of patients	Reduction of P_{peak} and P_{mean}, increase in CI, DO_2 and urine output with APRV	Reduction in use of vasopressors, sedatives and muscle relaxants
PUTENSEN [42]	Prospective, randomised, two arm	APRV/PCV (APRV without spontaneous breathing)	ALI/ARDS	30	During APRV (10–35% of total minute ventilation) muscle relaxation during PCV	Reduction of P_{peak}, increase in CI and compliance, improved oxygenation with APRV (with spontaneous breathing)	Reduction in use of vasopressors and sedatives, and length of ventilatory support and ICU stay

Table 2. Continued.

First author [ref.]	Study design	Intervention/control	Patient population	Patients n	Spontaneous breathing	Lung function	Clinical measures
HERING [43]	Prospective, randomised, crossover	APRV/PCV (APRV without spontaneous breathing)	ALI	12	During APRV (38% of total minute ventilation); muscle relaxation during PCV	Improved oxygenation, GFR and renal blood flow with APRV (with spontaneous breathing)	NA
VARPULA [44]	Prospective, randomised, two arm	APRV/SIMV-PS	ARDS (indicated for prone positioning)	28	During APRV (spontaneous V_T >10% of mandatory V_T) not reported for SIMV-PS	Improvement in oxygenation response to prone position with APRV	NA
VARPULA [45]	Prospective, randomised, two arm	APRV/SIMV-PS	ARDS	58	During APRV not reported for SIMV-PC/PS	Reduction of P_{peak} with APRV	No difference in clinical outcome
DART [46]	Retrospective cohort analysis, crossover	SIMV/PSV/AC to APRV	Patients at risk or with established ALI/ARDS	46	Not reported	Reduction of P_{peak}, improved oxygenation with APRV	NA
YOSHIDA [47]	Retrospective cohort analysis, two arm	APRV/PSV	ALI/ARDS	18	During APRV/PSV	Improved oxygenation and lung aeration with APRV	NA
GONZALEZ [48]	Propensity score-based case match analysis	APRV/AC-VCV	Various	234	Not reported	Reduction of P_{peak}, increase in PEEP, improved oxygenation	Higher rate of tracheostomy; no difference in length of ventilatory support, ICU stay and mortality
MAXWELL [49]	Prospective, randomised, two arm	APRV/SIMV-PS	Acute respiratory failure	ALI/ARDS in 45% (APRV) and 34% (SIMV-PS)	During APRV/SIMV-PS	Increase in P_{mean} with APRV	No difference in clinical outcome

VCV: volume-controlled ventilation; P_{peak}: peak airway pressure; V_T: tidal volume; NA: not applicable; CPAP: continuous positive airway pressure; IMV: intermittent mandatory ventilation; P_{mean}: mean airway pressure; IR: inverse ratio; P_{A-a,O_2}: alveolar-arterial oxygen tension difference; F_{I,O_2}: inspiratory oxygen fraction; PEEP: positive end-expiratory pressure; PCV: pressure-controlled ventilation; P_{a,CO_2}: arterial carbon dioxide tension; PSV: pressure support ventilation; D_{O_2}: oxygen delivery; V'/Q': ventilation/perfusion; CI: cardiac index; ICU: intensive care unit; GFR: glomerular filtration rate; SIMV: synchronised intermittent mandatory ventilation; PS: pressure support; PC: pressure control; AC: assist control. Data from [28].

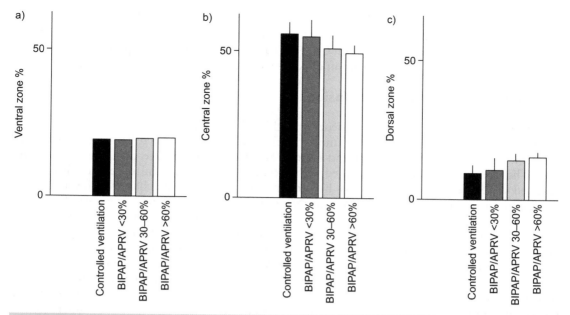

Figure 2. Distribution of relative ventilation during mechanical ventilation biphasic positive airway pressure (BIPAP)/airway pressure release ventilation (APRV) combined with different proportions of spontaneous breathing in total minute ventilation (<30%, 30–60% and >60%) in experimental lung injury (dorsal represents dependent zones). Note the redistribution of ventilation from the central to dorsal lung zones. Data from [33].

Gas exchange

In ALI/ARDS, BIPAP/APRV combined with spontaneous breathing seems to result in improved gas exchange, as compared with controlled mechanical ventilation. An increase in arterial oxygenation and a decrease in intrapulmonary shunt during BIPAP/APRV with superposed spontaneous breathing has been reported both in experimental [52, 57, 58] and clinical [40, 39, 42] settings. Furthermore, compared with pressure-controlled, synchronised intermittent mandatory ventilation (SIMV) with pressure support, BIPAP/APRV with spontaneous breathing after 24 hours increased the response of arterial oxygen tension (P_{a,O_2}) to prone position in patients with ALI [44]. Less is known about the effects of BIPAP/APRV on carbon dioxide elimination. BIPAP/APRV with superposed spontaneous breathing resulted in higher carbon dioxide arterial tension (P_{a,CO_2}) than PSV in two experimental studies at comparable minute ventilation [50, 51]. The likely explanation is that the relatively small V_T (<3 mL·kg^{-1}), as well as the relatively high proportion of minute ventilation, originating from spontaneous breath (>50%) in those investigations resulted in dead space ventilation and increased carbon dioxide retention. Theoretically, different ventilator settings in BIPAP/APRV could

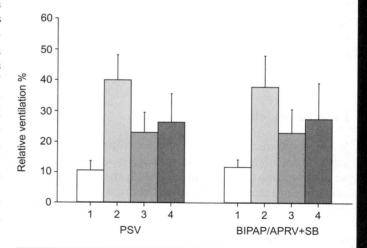

Figure 3. Distribution of relative ventilation at the hilum during pressure support ventilation (PSV) and biphasic positive airway pressure (BIPAP)/airway pressure release ventilation (APRV) with superposed spontaneous breathing (BIPAP/APRV+SB) in pigs with acute lung injury. Numbers 1–4 represent ventral, mid-ventral, mid-dorsal and dorsal lung zones, respectively. Data from [56].

A. GÜLDNER ET AL.

lead to better carbon dioxide elimination, at least comparable with other modes of assisted mechanical ventilation. In line with this hypothesis, RÄSÄNEN et al. [35] showed that BIPAP/APRV was able to reduce Pa,CO_2 compared with CPAP in patients suffering from respiratory failure; other studies could not detect improved carbon dioxide elimination compared with PCV [40, 42].

Haemodynamics and organ perfusion

BIPAP/APRV combined with spontaneous breathing has important effects on global haemodynamics and organ perfusion. In a canine model of ALI, controlled ventilation was associated with impairment of cardiac output and systolic arterial blood pressure compared with CPAP [59]. The use of BIPAP/APRV combined with spontaneous breathing in those animals partially reversed these effects, improving global haemodynamics. Similar results have also been observed in clinical trials. In ALI/ARDS patients, cardiac output increased by approximately 20% when switching from controlled ventilation to BIPAP/APRV combined with spontaneous breathing [42]. Interestingly, cardiac output not only remained higher during the treatment period of 3 days, but also 7 days thereafter, when spontaneous breathing was resumed in the controlled-ventilation group. The positive effects of BIPAP/APRV combined with spontaneous breathing on global haemodynamics have been ascribed to a decrease in intra-thoracic pressure, which in turn increases the venous return and cardiac preload. In addition, it can be postulated that a release of endogenous catecholamines during spontaneous breathing may have contributed to these effects.

The distribution of peripheral perfusion seems to be altered during BIPAP/APRV combined with spontaneous breathing. In 12 patients with ALI, the effective renal blood flow, the renal fraction of cardiac output, the renal vascular resistance index and the glomerular filtration rate were higher during BIPAP/APRV with superposed spontaneous breathing, as compared with controlled ventilation at the same mean airway pressure [43]. However, respiratory acidosis was present during controlled ventilation, possibly impairing renal function. In addition, cardiac output was higher during controlled ventilation, which may have been caused by differences in the infusion of drugs which impaired the renal perfusion. Nevertheless, positive effects in renal perfusion were still present when controlled ventilation and BIPAP/APRV with spontaneous breathing were matched for minute ventilation.

In a model of ALI, BIPAP/APRV with spontaneous breathing significantly increased the perfusion of the stomach, intestines and pancreas, compared with controlled ventilation. Moreover, a similar trend was observed with regard to spleen and liver perfusion. It is noteworthy that pre-portal blood flow during BIPAP/APRV with spontaneous breathing increased in excess of the improvement in cardiac output and intra-thoracic blood volume, as compared with controlled ventilation [60].

Respiratory effort

When spontaneous breathing is not supported by pressure during BIPAP/APRV, the energy expenditure of respiratory muscles is expected to be higher than with other modes of assisted ventilation. In a porcine model of ALI, the oesophageal pressure time product (PTP), which is a surrogate of inspiratory breathing effort, and the work of breathing (WOB) were higher during BIPAP/APRV with spontaneous breathing compared with PSV and pressure-assisted/controlled ventilation P-ACV [61]. In our experience, BIPAP/APRV with spontaneous breathing yields higher PTP than PSV, PSV combined with sighs, and variable PSV [51, 56]. In a similar manner to PTP, the mouth occlusion pressure at 100 milliseconds ($P0.1$), which is a surrogate of the inspiratory drive, was increased with BIPAP/APRV combined with spontaneous breathing, indicating that the respiratory centre became primed to an expected increased inspiratory WOB. To our knowledge, there is no data on the expiratory effort during BIPAP/APRV. However, it is conceivable that some expiratory cycles may be not entirely passive, especially if they occur at the higher level of airway pressure.

Subject–ventilator interaction

The basic concept underlying BIPAP/APRV is the total uncoupling of spontaneous breathing and mandatory cycles, which may generate a variety of breathing environments. Therefore, BIPAP/APRV should not be expected to result in enhanced subject–ventilator interaction. In line with this rationale, the synchrony between subject and mechanical ventilator decreased proportionally to $P0.1$ in an experimental model of ALI induced by oleic acid [61]. Since $P0.1$ was higher during BIPAP/APRV, this ventilation mode led to important subject–ventilator asynchrony. Our group confirmed such findings in another model of ALI. According to our data, BIPAP/APRV combined with spontaneous breathing is associated with lower comfort of breathing than different forms of PSV, mainly due to impaired subject–ventilator interaction [51]. Certainly, adequate levels of sedation can improve synchrony during mechanical ventilation. However, objective data on patient–ventilator interaction during BIPAP/APRV are lacking.

Lung damage and inflammation

Proportionally high transpulmonary pressures may occur if inspiratory breathing activity takes place simultaneously with switching of Plow to Phigh in BIPAP/APRV, during the so-called mixed respiratory cycles. Accordingly, VT greater than the protective range may result in such cycles, possibly overstretching the lung tissue. Thus, BIPAP/APRV with spontaneous breathing theoretically has the potential to injure the lungs, i.e. to result in VALI. However, due to the fact that spontaneous breathing is not supported by pressure, the resulting VT is usually lower during those cycles compared with mandatory ones.

An investigation on experimental ALI using dynamic CT showed that the phenomena of tidal re-aeration and tidal hyper-aeration, which may be associated with atelectrauma and volutrauma, respectively, are less pronounced during BIPAP/APRV with spontaneous breathing than PSV [56]. As suggested in that study, low VT generated by unsupported pressure could protect the lungs from further injury. Similar results have been reported by other investigators, who found that BIPAP/APRV with spontaneous breathing reduced the cyclic closing and reopening in dependent lung zones compared with controlled ventilation in oleic acid-induced ALI [53].

Preliminary results from a comprehensive investigation performed by our group on BIPAP/APRV with superposed spontaneous breathing suggest that the net effect of this mode of ventilation is a decrease in histologic lung damage and a release of markers of inflammation in a saline lung lavage model of ALI [33]. However, such a protective effect only seems to be significant if spontaneous breathing responds for more than 30% of total minute ventilation. Interestingly, such protective effects were observed despite the occurrence of mixed respiratory cycles with transpulmonary pressures as high as 30 cmH_2O.

Recently, the beneficial effects of spontaneous breathing activity in ARDS have been questioned. Papazian et al. [62] showed that the continuous administration of neuromuscular blocking agents (NMBAs) during the first 48 hours of mechanical ventilation, reduced the incidence of pneumothorax, increased the number of ventilator and ICU-free days, and even reduced mortality in patients with severe ARDS (Pa,O_2/inspiratory oxygen fraction (FI,O_2) <120 mmHg). It is possible that spontaneous breathing in those patients worsened lung injury, but beneficial effects of the paralysing agent (cis-atracurium) on lung inflammation cannot be ruled out. Furthermore, as the authors used volume assist-control ventilation, which supports spontaneous breathing efforts with fixed VT and is known to be prone to breath-stacking, it is unclear whether those findings can be extrapolated to BIPAP/APRV and other modes of assisted ventilation.

Clinical impact of BIPAP/APRV

Table 2 depicts the most relevant clinical studies on BIPAP/APRV.

Sedation

Based on its unique technical characteristic of a demand-valve CPAP system, allowing unrestricted spontaneous breathing, it has been proposed that during BIPAP/APRV, the need for sedatives and NMBAs can be reduced [23]. Several clinical studies confirmed this claim, showing reduced use of sedatives and NMBAs during BIPAP/APRV compared with controlled mechanical ventilation. In post-operative cardiac surgery patients [63], as well as in ALI/ARDS patients [41, 42], the total amount of sedatives could be reduced during ventilation with BIPAP/APRV. In addition, fewer NMBAs were needed during BIPAP/APRV, as compared with inverse ratio PCV (IR-PCV) [41] and APRV without spontaneous breathing [42]. However, NMBAs were used as part of the protocol for controlled ventilation in the latter study [42]. When comparing BIPAP/APRV with different assisted ventilatory modes, no clear picture can be drawn regarding the amount of sedative agents needed. While RATHGEBER et al. [63] found a reduction in the amount of benzodiazepines with BIPAP compared with SIMV, VARPULA et al. [45] were not able to confirm this finding with pressure support.

Cardiovascular active drugs

The cyclic reduction in intra-thoracic pressure, which occurs during unassisted spontaneous inspiratory efforts, may enhance the venous return into the heart, improving cardiac output and reducing the need for vasoactive and inotropic agents. Indeed, different clinical studies were able to show a respective reduction in the amount of these agents, comparing BIPAP/APRV with spontaneous breathing to different types of controlled und assisted mechanical ventilation [40, 42]. Despite the physiological mechanism, the reduction in sedation might play an important role in explaining these differences in cardiac performance. Interestingly, in their study, which maintained well-balanced sedation regimens, VARPULA et al. [45] could not detect any differences in the cardiac index between APRV and SIMV/pressure support.

Weaning and ICU-free days

Although several clinical investigations on BIPAP/APRV have been conducted in patients with ALI/ARDS, only a few of them were powered to show the differences in weaning and ICU-free days [28]. PUTENSEN et al. [42] showed a reduction in the mean ± SEM duration of ventilatory support (15 ± 2 versus 21 ± 2) and the length of ICU stay (23 ± 2 versus 30 ± 2) when BIPAP/APRV combined with spontaneous breathing was used during the first 3 days of treatment, as compared with controlled mechanical ventilation in the same period followed by BIPAP/APRV. In contrast, MAXWELL et al. [49] could not confirm an advantage of BIPAP/APRV over a low V_T strategy using SIMV or PCV in terms of weaning. However, in that study, patients in the BIPAP/APRV group had a higher Acute Physiology and Chronic Health Evaluation (APACHE) score at baseline, and the presence of spontaneous breathing was not reported, making the interpretation of results difficult. Despite the weaknesses in the study design of MAXWELL et al. [49], a recent observational study confirmed their results, failing to detect a difference in duration of ventilatory support and length of ICU stay between BIPAP/APRV and assist control ventilation [48]. In addition, VARPULA et al. [45] were unable to find differences in ventilator-free days when comparing BIPAP/APRV with SIMV pressure control/pressure support. Clearly, further clinical studies avoiding imbalances in baseline characteristics and using BIPAP/APRV combined with a well-defined target for the amount of spontaneous breathing, are needed to determine the impact of different assisted ventilatory modes on ventilator and ICU-free days in ALI/ARDS patients.

Mortality

Despite the beneficial effects of BIPAP/APRV with superposed spontaneous breathing on lung function and even outcome variables in patients with ALI/ARDS, it has thus far not been possible to show improvement in mortality [28]. It is possible that previous studies were underpowered to detect such an effect. In our opinion, a large prospective, randomised clinical trial using BIPAP/APRV combined with spontaneous breathing is justified. However, before such a trial can begin, the optimal set up of BIPAP/APRV regarding time and pressure settings and the amount of spontaneous breathing need to be defined.

Important unknowns in BIPAP/APRV

Although BIPAP/APRV has been used worldwide to ventilate patients with ALI/ARDS successfully, the settings used vary importantly among centres. While some intensive care givers prefer the use of inverse I:E ratios, *i.e.* genuine APRV, others use I:E values near to 1:1, which is closer to the setting used in BIPAP. Theoretically, higher I:E results in higher mean airway pressures, allowing increased functional residual capacity (FRC), while lower I:E may result in increased spontaneous breathing, which is more pronounced at P_{low}. Algorithms on how to set I:E would certainly be useful.

A perhaps unsolved issue in BIPAP/APRV regards the amount of spontaneous breathing to be used or allowed. Currently, 10–30% of total minute ventilation originating from spontaneous breathing is recommended. However, experimental studies have used as much as 50%. Our group's preliminary data in an animal model of ALI suggest that gas exchange improves when spontaneous breathing generates 10–30% of total minute ventilation; however, positive effects in lung damage and inflammation are detectable only when this percentage exceeds 30% [33]. In addition, there is uncertainty regarding the use of pressure support during BIPAP/APRV. Even though mechanical ventilators are able to support spontaneous breathing at P_{high} and P_{low}, most data has been obtained from settings without support.

Last but not least, the allowance of spontaneous breathing during BIPAP/APRV in the early phase of severe ARDS may be controversial. Recent data has shown that muscle paralysis results in reduced morbidity and mortality in ARDS patients, suggesting that spontaneous breathing may increase mechanical stress and inflammation in the lungs. At present, we do not know whether these data also apply to this mode, but given the new evidence, BIPAP/APRV with spontaneous breathing would be better avoided in severe ARDS until further clinical trials clarify this issue.

Statement of interest

M. Gama de Abreu has received lecture and consultation fees from Dräger Medical AG (Lübeck, Germany) and grants for investigations in biphasic positive airway pressure/airway pressure release ventilation.

References

1. Phua J, Badia JR, Adhikari NK, *et al.* Has mortality from acute respiratory distress syndrome decreased over time? A systematic review. *Am J Respir Crit Care Med* 2009; 179: 220–227.
2. Bernard GR, Artigas A, Brigham KL, *et al.* The American-European Consensus Conference on ARDS. Definitions, mechanisms, relevant outcomes, and clinical trial coordination. *Am J Respir Crit Care Med* 1994; 149: 818–224.
3. Menezes SL, Bozza PT, Neto HC, *et al.* Pulmonary and extrapulmonary acute lung injury: inflammatory and ultrastructural analyses. *J Appl Physiol* 2005; 98: 1777–1783.
4. Ware LB. Pathophysiology of acute lung injury and the acute respiratory distress syndrome. *Semin Respir Crit Care Med* 2006; 27: 337–349.
5. Rubenfeld GD, Herridge MS. Epidemiology and outcomes of acute lung injury. *Chest* 2007; 131: 554–562.
6. Estenssoro E, Dubin A, Laffaire E, *et al.* Incidence, clinical course, and outcome in 217 patients with acute respiratory distress syndrome. *Crit Care Med* 2002; 30: 2450–2456.
7. Esteban A, Ferguson ND, Meade MO, *et al.* Evolution of mechanical ventilation in response to clinical research. *Am J Respir Crit Care Med* 2008; 177: 170–177.

8. Li G, Malinchoc M, Cartin-Ceba R, *et al.* Eight-year trend of acute respiratory distress syndrome: a population-based study in Olmsted County, Minnesota. *Am J Respir Crit Care Med* 2011; 183: 59–66.
9. Ware LB, Matthay MA. The acute respiratory distress syndrome. *N Engl J Med* 2000; 342: 1334–1349.
10. Girard TD, Bernard GR. Mechanical ventilation in ARDS. *Chest* 2007; 131: 921–929.
11. Ventilation with lower tidal volumes as compared with traditional tidal volumes for acute lung injury and the acute respiratory distress syndrome. The Acute Respiratory Distress Syndrome Network. *N Engl J Med* 2000; 342: 1301–1308.
12. Calfee CS, Matthay MA. Nonventilatory treatments for acute lung injury and ARDS. *Chest* 2007; 131: 913–920.
13. Terragni PP, Rosboch GL, Lisi A, *et al.* How respiratory system mechanics may help in minimising ventilator-induced lung injury in ARDS patients. *Eur Respir J* 2003; 22: Suppl. 42, 15s–21s.
14. Slutsky AS, Tremblay LN. Multiple system organ failure. Is mechanical ventilation a contributing factor? *Am J Respir Crit Care Med* 1998; 157: 1721–1725.
15. Briel M, Meade M, Mercat A, *et al.* Higher *vs* lower positive end-expiratory pressure in patients with acute lung injury and acute respiratory distress syndrome: systematic review and meta-analysis. *JAMA* 2010; 303: 865–873.
16. Hodgson C, Keating JL, Holland AE, *et al.* Recruitment manoeuvres for adults with acute lung injury receiving mechanical ventilation. *Cochrane Database Syst Rev* 2009; 2: CD006667.
17. Wunsch H, Mapstone J. High-frequency ventilation *versus* conventional ventilation for treatment of acute lung injury and acute respiratory distress syndrome. *Cochrane Database Syst Rev* 2004; 1: CD004085.
18. Modrykamien A, Chatburn RL, Ashton RW. Airway pressure release ventilation: an alternative mode of mechanical ventilation in acute respiratory distress syndrome. *Cleve Clin J Med* 2011; 78: 101–110.
19. Stock MC, Downs JB, Frolicher DA. Airway pressure release ventilation. *Crit Care Med* 1987; 15: 462–466.
20. Hansen J, Wendt M, Lawin P. Ein neues weaning-Verfahren (Inspiratory Flow Assistance-IFA-) [A new weaning procedure (inspiratory flow assistance)]. *Anaesthesist* 1984; 33: 428–432.
21. Downs JB, Klein EF Jr, Desautels D, *et al.* Intermittent mandatory ventilation: a new approach to weaning patients from mechanical ventilators. *Chest* 1973; 64: 331–335.
22. Baum M, Benzer H, Putensen C, *et al.* Biphasic positive airway pressure (BIPAP) - eine neue Form der augmentierenden Beatmung [Biphasic positive airway pressure (BIPAP) – a new form of augmented ventilation]. *Anaesthesist* 1989; 38: 452–458.
23. Hormann C, Baum M, Putensen C, *et al.* Biphasic positive airway pressure (BIPAP) – a new mode of ventilatory support. *Eur J Anaesthesiol* 1994; 11: 37–42.
24. Frawley PM, Habashi N. Airway pressure release ventilation: theory and practice. *AACN Clinical Issues* 2001; 12: 234–246.
25. Myers TR, MacIntyre NR. Respiratory controversies in the critical care setting. Does airway pressure release ventilation offer important new advantages in mechanical ventilator support? *Respir Care* 2007; 52: 452–458.
26. Putensen C, Wrigge H. Clinical review: biphasic positive airway pressure and airway pressure release ventilation. *Crit Care* 2004; 8: 492–497.
27. Rouby JJ, Ben AM, Jawish D, *et al.* Continuous positive airway pressure (CPAP) *vs.* intermittent mandatory pressure release ventilation (IMPRV) in patients with acute respiratory failure. *Intensive Care Med* 1992; 18: 69–75.
28. Seymour CW, Frazer M, Reilly PM, *et al.* Airway pressure release and biphasic intermittent positive airway pressure ventilation: are they ready for prime time? *J Trauma* 2007; 62: 1298–1308.
29. Rose L, Hawkins M. Airway pressure release ventilation and biphasic positive airway pressure: a systematic review of definitional criteria. *Intensive Care Med* 2008; 34: 1766–1773.
30. Neumann P, Golisch W, Strohmeyer A, *et al.* Influence of different release times on spontaneous breathing pattern during airway pressure release ventilation. *Intensive Care Med* 2002; 28: 1742–1749.
31. Yoshida T, Uchiyama A, Mashimo T, *et al.* The effect of ventilator performance on airway pressure release ventilation: a model lung study. *Anesth Analg* 2011; 113: 529–533.
32. Burns KE, Adhikari NK, Slutsky AS, *et al.* Pressure and volume limited ventilation for the ventilatory management of patients with acute lung injury: a systematic review and meta-analysis. *PLoS One* 2011; 6: e14623.
33. Beda A, Carvalho NS, Güldner A, *et al.* Effects of different levels of spontaneous breathing activity during biphasic positive airway pressure ventilation on lung function and inflammation in experimental lung injury. *Am J Respir Crit Care Med* 2011; 183: A6233.
34. Cane RD, Peruzzi WT, Shapiro BA. Airway pressure release ventilation in severe acute respiratory failure. *Chest* 1991; 100: 460–463.
35. Räsänen J, Cane RD, Downs JB, *et al.* Airway pressure release ventilation during acute lung injury: a prospective multicenter trial. *Crit Care Med* 1991; 19: 1234–1241.
36. Davis K Jr, Johnson DJ, Branson RD, *et al.* Airway pressure release ventilation. *Arch Surg* 1993; 128: 1348–1352.

37. Sydow M, Burchardi H, Ephraim E, *et al.* Long-term effects of two different ventilatory modes on oxygenation in acute lung injury. Comparison of airway pressure release ventilation and volume-controlled inverse ratio ventilation. *Am J Respir Crit Care Med* 1994; 149: 1550–1556.

38. Kiehl M, Schiele C, Stenzinger W, *et al.* Volume-controlled *versus* biphasic positive airway pressure ventilation in leukopenic patients with severe respiratory failure. *Crit Care Med* 1996; 24: 780–784.

39. Hörmann C, Baum M, Putensen C, *et al.* Effects of spontaneous breathing with BIPAP on pulmonary gas exchange in patients with ARDS. *Acta Anaesthesiol Scand Suppl* 1997; 111: 152–155.

40. Putensen C, Mutz NJ, Putensen-Himmer G, *et al.* Spontaneous breathing during ventilatory support improves ventilation-perfusion distributions in patients with acute respiratory distress syndrome. *Am J Respir Crit Care Med* 1999; 159: 1241–1248.

41. Kaplan LJ, Bailey H, Formosa V. Airway pressure release ventilation increases cardiac performance in patients with acute lung injury/adult respiratory distress syndrome. *Crit Care* 2001; 5: 221–226.

42. Putensen C, Zech S, Wrigge H, *et al.* Long-term effects of spontaneous breathing during ventilatory support in patients with acute lung injury. *Am J Respir Crit Care Med* 2001; 164: 43–49.

43. Hering R, Peters D, Zinserling J, *et al.* Effects of spontaneous breathing during airway pressure release ventilation on renal perfusion and function in patients with acute lung injury. *Intensive Care Med* 2002; 28: 1426–1433.

44. Varpula T, Jousela I, Niemi R, *et al.* Combined effects of prone positioning and airway pressure release ventilation on gas exchange in patients with acute lung injury. *Acta Anaesthesiol Scand* 2003; 47: 516–524.

45. Varpula T, Valta P, Niemi R, *et al.* Airway pressure release ventilation as a primary ventilatory mode in acute respiratory distress syndrome. *Acta Anaesthesiol Scand* 2004; 48: 722–731.

46. Dart BW, Maxwell RA, Richart CM, *et al.* Preliminary experience with airway pressure release ventilation in a trauma/surgical intensive care unit. *J Trauma* 2005; 59: 71–76.

47. Yoshida T, Rinka H, Kaji A, *et al.* The impact of spontaneous ventilation on distribution of lung aeration in patients with acute respiratory distress syndrome: airway pressure release ventilation *versus* pressure support ventilation. *Anesth Analg* 2009; 109: 1892–1900.

48. Gonzalez M, Arroliga AC, Frutos-Vivar F, *et al.* Airway pressure release ventilation *versus* assist-control ventilation: a comparative propensity score and international cohort study. *Intensive Care Med* 2010; 36: 817–827.

49. Maxwell RA, Green JM, Waldrop J, *et al.* A randomized prospective trial of airway pressure release ventilation and low tidal volume ventilation in adult trauma patients with acute respiratory failure. *J Trauma* 2010; 69: 501–510.

50. Carvalho AR, Spieth PM, Pelosi P, *et al.* Pressure support ventilation and biphasic positive airway pressure improve oxygenation by redistribution of pulmonary blood flow. *Anesth Analg* 2009; 109: 856–865.

51. Gama de Abreu M, Spieth PM, Pelosi P, *et al.* Noisy pressure support ventilation: a pilot study on a new assisted ventilation mode in experimental lung injury. *Crit Care Med* 2008; 36: 818–827.

52. Wrigge H, Zinserling J, Neumann P, *et al.* Spontaneous breathing improves lung aeration in oleic acid-induced lung injury. *Anesthesiology* 2003; 99: 376–384.

53. Wrigge H, Zinserling J, Neumann P, *et al.* Spontaneous breathing with airway pressure release ventilation favors ventilation in dependent lung regions and counters cyclic alveolar collapse in oleic-acid-induced lung injury: a randomized controlled computed tomography trial. *Crit Care* 2005; 9: R780–R789.

54. Carvalho AR, Spieth PM, Guldner A, *et al.* Distribution of regional lung aeration and perfusion during conventional and noisy pressure support ventilation in experimental lung injury. *J Appl Physiol* 2011; 110: 1083–1092.

55. Neumann P, Wrigge H, Zinserling J, *et al.* Spontaneous breathing affects the spatial ventilation and perfusion distribution during mechanical ventilatory support. *Crit Care Med* 2005; 33: 1090–1095.

56. Gama de Abreu M, Cuevas M, Spieth PM, *et al.* Regional lung aeration and ventilation during pressure support and biphasic positive airway pressure ventilation in experimental lung injury. *Crit Care* 2010; 14: R34.

57. Putensen C, Rasanen J, Lopez FA. Ventilation-perfusion distributions during mechanical ventilation with superimposed spontaneous breathing in canine lung injury. *Am J Respir Crit Care Med* 1994; 150: 101–108.

58. Henzler D, Dembinski R, Bensberg R, *et al.* Ventilation with biphasic positive airway pressure in experimental lung injury. Influence of transpulmonary pressure on gas exchange and haemodynamics. *Intensive Care Med* 2004; 30: 935–943.

59. Räsänen J, Downs JB, Stock MC. Cardiovascular effects of conventional positive pressure ventilation and airway pressure release ventilation. *Chest* 1988; 93: 911–915.

60. Hering R, Viehofer A, Zinserling J, *et al.* Effects of spontaneous breathing during airway pressure release ventilation on intestinal blood flow in experimental lung injury. *Anesthesiology* 2003; 99: 1137–1144.

61. Henzler D, Pelosi P, Bensberg R, *et al.* Effects of partial ventilatory support modalities on respiratory function in severe hypoxemic lung injury. *Crit Care Med* 2006; 34: 1738–1745.

62. Papazian L, Forel JM, Gacouin A, *et al*. Neuromuscular blockers in early acute respiratory distress syndrome. *N Engl J Med* 2010; 363: 1107–1116.

63. Rathgeber J, Schorn B, Falk V, *et al*. The influence of controlled mandatory ventilation (CMV), intermittent mandatory ventilation (IMV) and biphasic intermittent positive airway pressure (BIPAP) on duration of intubation and consumption of analgesics and sedatives. A prospective analysis in 596 patients following adult cardiac surgery. *Eur J Anaesthesiol* 1997; 14: 576–582.

Chapter 7

Proportional assist ventilation

E. Akoumianaki, E. Kondili and D. Georgopoulos

Summary

Proportional assist ventilation (PAV) is a new mode of partially assisted mechanical ventilation, born from the growing demand for improvements in existing modes with respect to patient–ventilator interaction and physician facility. It differs radically in comparison with conventional modes (pressure support ventilation or assisted-controlled ventilation) in the way that, after triggering, mechanical support follows patient effort both in terms of timing and magnitude. Patient effort is represented by muscle pressure estimated by the equation of motion after measurement of elastance and resistance. Recently, with PAV+ (an updated version of PAV), these measurements are performed noninvasively and semi-continuously from the ventilator, eliminating errors and liberating the physician from extra workload. Studies performed with PAV+ have revealed that, compared with conventional modes, its application is simple and time saving, while it may more effectively reduce patient–ventilator dyssynchrony, facilitate weaning and improve sleep quality in critically ill adults. It can also be used as an alternative mode of noninvasive mechanical ventilation. However, further improvements are still needed in the field of triggering, especially in patients with flow limitation, since the presence of dynamic hyperinflation may counterbalance the advantages of PAV+. Meanwhile, following well-designed algorithms and bearing in mind specific limitations, PAV+ could be a valuable tool in the hands of experienced physicians.

Keywords: Assisted mechanical ventilation, patient–ventilator interaction, proportional assist ventilation

Dept of Intensive Care Medicine, University Hospital of Heraklion, Medical School, University of Crete, Heraklion, Crete, Greece.

Correspondence: D. Georgopoulos, Intensive Care Unit, University Hospital of Heraklion, Heraklion, 71110, Greece. Email georgop@med.uoc.gr

Eur Respir Mon 2012; 55: 97–115.
Printed in UK – all rights reserved
Copyright ERS 2012
European Respiratory Monograph
ISSN: 1025-448x
DOI: 10.1183/1025448x.10001911

Until the early 1980s, assisted mechanical ventilation was essentially employed only as an intermediate, short-term path between controlled mechanical ventilation and patient extubation. In the case of a weaning trial failure, the patient was usually re-sedated and controlled mechanical ventilation was re-applied. Allowing the patient to undertake part of their necessary ventilation over a period longer than a few minutes, or even over a few days, gained wide acceptance over the last two decades when several advantages of this approach became apparent:

reduced effects of prolonged sedation [1, 2], avoidance of ventilator-induced diaphragmatic dysfunction [3, 4], elimination of neuropathy associated with neuromuscular blocking agents [5, 6] and gas exchange improvement [7].

As the use of assisted mechanical ventilation spread, issues regarding the quality of patient–ventilator interaction and its potential consequences began to emerge. Pressure support ventilation (PSV) was introduced in 1985, permitting, for the first time, partial control of the ventilator rate, inspiratory assist time, inspiratory flow and delivered tidal volume (V_T) by the patient [8]. It was a major step forward in the field of patient–ventilator interaction and soon became a common mode of ventilator assist. However, due to inherent problems regarding its function profile, PSV does not guarantee patient–ventilator synchrony. Indeed, delayed triggering, ineffective efforts, auto-triggering, delayed or premature cycling off and multiple cycles are common during PSV [9, 10]. Furthermore, the amount of pressure delivered was predetermined and constant, independent of the patient's needs and variability in work of breathing.

A mode that could closely follow the patient's efforts throughout inspiration, continuously adapting its support accordingly would, theoretically, avert the aforementioned disadvantages of assisted mechanical support. Indeed, M. Younes presented, in 1992, proportional assist ventilation (PAV), a mode in which the magnitude of ventilator assistance (flow, volume or pressure) was neither predetermined nor constant but adjusted to the patient's respiratory drive and mechanical obstacles to its output (i.e. resistance and elastance) [11, 12]. PAV permits the patient to attain any breathing pattern, up to a limit, without constraints imposed by the ventilator and, theoretically, ensures harmonious cooperation between the ventilator machine and the patient. However, soon after the introduction of PAV, sophisticated, time-consuming and often inaccurate measurements of respiratory system mechanics (mandatory for proper application of PAV; see later in this chapter) limited its use, despite numerous publications supporting its superiority over PSV [13–20]. A crucial step towards the diffusion of PAV into daily clinical practice was made with PAV+, the evolution of the original mode in which an integrated software allowed automatic and noninvasive measurement of respiratory system mechanics, greatly simplifying its application [21, 22]. Currently, PAV+ is available in the Puritan-Bennett 840 ventilator (Tyco, Gosport, UK).

The aim of this chapter is to describe the basic operational principles of PAV function, potential advantages and drawbacks in comparison with other modes of assisted ventilation, focusing primarily on evidence derived from published studies. At the end of the chapter, a stepwise approach for applying PAV+ in daily intensive care unit (ICU) practice is provided.

Operational principles of PAV

With PAV, the equation of motion (the well-known mathematical approach to breath generation) forms the basis of the pressure delivery phase. In summary, flow and volume insertion into the lungs requires the exercise of a power, which, irrespective of its origin (inspiratory muscles, ventilator machine or both), can overcome the two main opposing forces: resistance of the respiratory system (R_{rs}) and elastance of the respiratory system (E_{rs}). Thus:

$$P_{tot} = V' \times R_{rs} + V \times E_{rs} + PEEPi \tag{1}$$

where P_{tot} (total pressure) is instantaneous pressure applied to the respiratory system, V' is instantaneous flow, V is instantaneous volume above end-expiratory lung volume and PEEPi (intrinsic positive end-expiratory pressure) is elastic recoil pressure at end-expiration (PEEPi is zero if end-expiratory lung volume is at functional residual capacity) [10, 23]. P_{tot} might be delivered entirely by inspiratory muscle pressure (P_{mus}) in spontaneously breathing patients ($P_{tot} = P_{mus}$), by the ventilator (i.e. by airway pressure (P_{aw})) in controlled mechanical ventilation ($P_{tot} = P_{aw}$), or the sum of these in assisted mechanical ventilation ($P_{tot} = P_{aw} + P_{mus}$). Consequently, during assisted modes of support, equation 1 is modified as follows:

$$P_{tot} = P_{mus} + P_{aw} = V' \times R_{rs} + V \times E_{rs} + PEEPi \tag{2}$$

Table 1. Main operational differences between the most popular modes of assisted mechanical ventilation

	AVC	PSV	PAV	PAV+
Triggering	Time or patient initiated	Patient initiated	Patient initiated	Patient initiated
Delivery phase	Preset amount of volume	Preset amount of pressure	Pressure proportional to instantaneous flow and volume	Pressure proportional to instantaneous flow and volume
Dependent variables	P_{aw}	Volume, flow	P_{aw}, flow, volume	P_{aw}, flow, volume
Cycling off	Time	Decrease of flow to percentage of peak inspiratory value	Decrease of flow to a predetermined value	Decrease of flow to a predetermined value
Respiratory mechanics estimation	No	No	No	Yes
P_{aw}–P_{mus} relationship	Negative	No relationship	Proportional	Proportional

AVC: assist volume control; PSV: pressure support ventilation; PAV: proportional assist ventilation; PAV+: updated version of PAV; P_{aw}: airway pressure; P_{mus}: muscle pressure.

With PAV, however, P_{aw} is not a standard value as in PSV (table 1). Instead, immediately after triggering, in an identical manner to PSV, the ventilator monitors inspiratory flow and volume and generates pressure (P_{aw}), which is, at any time during inspiration, the sum of instantaneous flow and volume multiplied by a predetermined gain factor (fig. 1).

$$P_{aw} = VA \times V + FA \times V' \tag{3}$$

where VA and FA are preset values of volume and flow assist (gain factors), expressed in $cmH_2O \cdot L^{-1}$ and $cmH_2O \cdot L^{-1} \cdot s^{-1}$, respectively. It is obvious that VA has the units of E_{rs} and FA the units of R_{rs}. Substituting for P_{aw} in equation 2 with equation 3 and solving for P_{mus}:

$$P_{mus} = V' \times (R_{rs}\text{-}FA) + V \times (E_{rs}\text{-}VA) + PEEPi \tag{4}$$

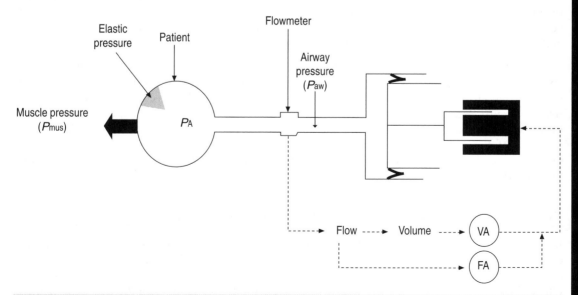

Figure 1. A simplified depiction of the way pressure is generated from instantaneous flow and volume changes. The latter are induced by patient effort. P_{mus}: muscle pressure; P_A: alveolar pressure; P_{aw}: airway pressure; FA: flow assist; VA: volume assist. Reproduced from [21] with permission from the publisher.

It follows that with PAV the inspiratory muscles cope, after triggering, with an afterload that is reduced by an amount equal to VA (for E_{rs}) and FA (for R_{rs}). Assist level can be expressed, instead of an absolute value, as a percentage fraction of R_{rs} (K1) and E_{rs} (K2) and equation 4 is modified as follows:

$$P_{mus} = V' \times R_{rs}(1\text{-}K1) + V \times E_{rs}(1\text{-}K2) + PEEPi \qquad (5)$$

Obviously, K1 and K2 should be always set below 100% of the measured R_{rs} and E_{rs} [24]. Furthermore, if K1 and K2 are equal, elastic and resistive loads are reduced by a similar fraction during inspiration. This is mandatory for proper PAV function since the relative contribution of elastic and resistive loads varies considerably during the inspiratory phase. Setting similar values for K1 and K2 pressure provided by the ventilator (P_{aw}) represents the same percentage of total pressure applied to the respiratory system regardless of the relative contribution of elastic and resistive pressures. As a result, equation 5 is modified as follows:

$$P_{mus} = V' \times R_{rs}(1\text{-}K) + V \times E_{rs}(1\text{-}K) + PEEPi \qquad (6)$$

and

$$P_{aw} = K \times (V' \times R_{rs} + V \times E_{rs}) \qquad (7)$$

It follows that, with PAV, the pressure muscles need to develop is reduced by the percentage of assist set by the physician (K) [25]. During inspiration, the P_{aw}/P_{mus} ratio (proportionality= percentage assist/(100-percentage assist)) is constant and determines the patient's contribution (*i.e.* 1-K) to total pressure. When K is set to zero, breathing is unassisted and P_{mus} undertakes the whole work of inspiration. When K is set to 50%, the proportionality is 1.0 and P_{aw} equals P_{mus} throughout inspiration (assuming that P_{mus} required to trigger the ventilator is negligible). At 80% of assist, the proportionality is 4, implying that 80% of total pressure (which is required to overcome the mechanical load) is provided by the ventilator and 20% by the muscles. Thus, contrary to other assisted modes, with PAV the ventilator simply amplifies patient inspiratory effort without imposing any target either for flow, volume or P_{aw} (table 1). What is set by the physician is the relationship between P_{aw} and P_{mus} (proportionality) and as a result the patient is able to retain considerable control over the desired breathing pattern.

Transition to expiration is also driven by P_{mus}. As the latter declines towards the end of neural inspiration, inspiratory flow gradually decreases and, when it reaches a preselected threshold, the ventilator terminates pressure generation. Thus, contrary to PSV and assist volume control (AVC), cycling off is determined by P_{mus}, minimising expiratory asynchrony (table 1).

It is essential for the proper operation of PAV that VA and FA: 1) are set to lower values than E_{rs} and R_{rs}, respectively; and 2) represent a similar fraction of E_{rs} and R_{rs}. Only under these conditions does the patient always contribute to total pressure, while P_{aw} has a constant and predictable relationship to P_{mus}. It follows that measurement of respiratory system mechanics is a key point in PAV. To the extent that in critically ill patients, resistance and elastance may vary considerably as a function of time, their determination should be performed very often (almost continuously). Otherwise, with PAV, over-assist or under-assist may ensue, whereas the constant relationship between P_{aw} and P_{mus} is lost.

Estimation of resistance and elastance during PAV (PAV+)

In conventional assisted modes (either volume or pressure control modes), mechanical inflation ends either before or after the end of neural inspiration, causing the phenomenon of expiratory asynchrony. Conversely, the unique tight link between P_{aw} and P_{mus} when the patient is on PAV (since P_{mus} drives P_{aw}) causes the end of neural inspiration to coincide with the end of mechanical inflation. This greatly minimises the phenomenon of expiratory asynchrony. Thus, with PAV at the end of mechanical inflation, inspiratory P_{mus} is in the declining phase (or it is already zero), while expiratory muscle activity (if it occurs) usually begins late in neural expiration. It follows that, if the airways are occluded for a short time at the end of mechanical inflation, P_{aw} at the end of the occlusion provides the elastic recoil at the occluded volume (*i.e.* V_T). This is not the case with the other modes, since considerable respiratory activity (inspiratory or expiratory) may be present at the end of mechanical inflation due to expiratory asynchrony.

Taking advantage of the aforementioned feature of PAV, the calculation of respiratory system mechanics is performed automatically by the ventilator by applying, at random intervals of four to 10 breaths, a 300-ms pause manoeuvre at the end of selected inspirations (fig. 2) [21, 22]. Airway pressure at the end of the occlusion ($P_{aw,occlusion}$) is measured and E_{rs} and compliance of the respiratory system ($C_{rs}=1/E_{rs}$) are calculated as follows:

$$E_{rs}=(P_{aw,occlusion}-PEEP)/V_T \qquad (8)$$

and

$$C_{rs}=V_T/(P_{aw,occlusion}-PEEP) \qquad (9)$$

where PEEP is positive end-expiratory pressure. Obviously, in the presence of PEEPi (dynamic hyperinflation), the calculated value of E_{rs} overestimates respiratory system elastance (and the calculated C_{rs} underestimates respiratory system compliance).

Assuming that, early in expiration, flow is driven by the elastic recoil pressure (*i.e.* alveolar pressure (P_A)), expiratory R_{rs} is measured during exhalation following a pause manoeuvre. The software identifies three points on the expiratory flow–time curve corresponding to peak flow and 5 ms and 10 ms later (fig. 2). At these points, P_A and total expiratory resistance (R_{tot}) are calculated as follows:

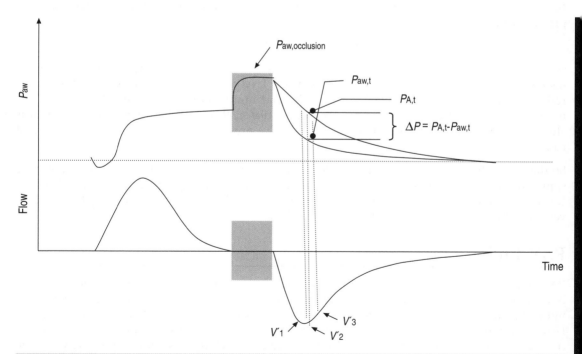

Figure 2. Estimation of resistance and elastance during proportional assist ventilation (updated version; PAV+). The shaded area represents the period of occlusion, which is followed by expiration. The arrows indicate the three points of resistance estimation: peak flow (V'_1) and 5 ms (V'_2) and 10 ms (V'_3) after peak flow. At these points, the ventilator measures instantaneous airway pressure ($P_{aw,t}$), tidal volume exhaled (ΔV) and flow (V'). Elastance of the respiratory system (E_{rs}) is already measured during the occlusion manoeuvre. Alveolar pressure at each point ($P_{A,t}$) is given by the equation $P_{A,t}=P_{aw,occlusion}-\Delta V \times E_{rs}$, where $P_{aw,occlusion}$ is the airway pressure at the end of the occlusion. Thus, from the difference of $P_{A,t}$ minus $P_{aw,t}$ divided by V', R_{tot} (total resistance) is calculated at each point. ΔP: change in pressure.

$$PA = Paw,occlusion - \Delta V \times Ers \tag{10}$$

$$Rtot = (PA - Paw)/V' \tag{11}$$

where ΔV is the exhaled volume up to the point of interest and V' and Paw are the corresponding expiratory flow and airway pressure, respectively. The values of $Rtot$ at these points are averaged and an estimate of $Rtot$ is obtained. $Rtot$ is considered to be the sum of the flow-dependent resistance of the endotracheal tube ($Rtube$) and that of the respiratory system (Rrs,PAV). $Rtube$ is calculated using the following equation:

$$Rtube = a + bV' \tag{12}$$

where a and b are constants, depending on tube length and diameter, estimated using *in vitro* data. Rrs,PAV is derived by subtraction of $Rtube$ from $Rtot$. We should note, however, that this technique measures expiratory resistance, while PAV uses inspiratory resistance. In patients with a large difference between inspiratory and expiratory resistance (*i.e.* patients with obstructive lung disease), this may cause some problems. In addition, in the presence of dynamic hyperinflation, the calculated value of $Rtot$ underestimates the actual value. Finally, in patients with flow limitation during passive expiration, peak flow may exclusively depend on endotracheal tube resistance. In this case, expiratory resistance measured at peak flow is not a reflection of the patient's resistance but of that of the endotracheal tube. Another technique for measuring inspiratory resistance with PAV (pulse technique) may be more suitable [22]. Currently, only one company uses the pulse technique but there are no data regarding the function of this ventilator (SSV; AWSS, Tokyo, Japan).

With the system of automatic measurement of respiratory system mechanics (PAV+; Puritan-Bennett 840; Tyco), the caregiver sets the percentage of unloading (K) and the ventilator delivers pressure as follows:

$$Paw,t = K(V'I,t \times (Rtube,t + Rrs,PAV) + Vt \times Ers,PAV) \tag{13}$$

where Paw,t is instantaneous airway pressure, $V'I,t$ is instantaneous inspiratory flow, Vt is instantaneous lung volume above end-expiratory level and $Rtube,t$ is the endotracheal tube resistance at $V'I,t$ (flow dependent). Because the maximum value of K is limited to 95% of the measured values of elastance and resistance, the ventilator, theoretically, provides pressure that is always a fraction of the measured elastic and resistive pressure, thus avoiding the occurrence of run-away phenomena.

Studies have shown that respiratory system mechanics, as measured with PAV+, are on average similar to those measured during passive mechanical ventilation using standard techniques [21, 22]. It is of interest to note that the values of Ers and Rrs with PAV+ may be used not only to adjust the ventilator function, but also to follow the patient's status.

PAV limitations

PAV is designed to respond to changes in flow and volume detected within the ventilator circuit. It is assumed that the pattern of these changes during the evolution of inspiration expresses, indirectly, variations in diaphragmatic pressure in response to respiratory drive fluctuations. However, flow and volume constitute only the final part of this drive's journey from the brain stem down to the respiratory muscles. Insults in each step along this path may severely impede assist delivery and ventilation.

Central nervous system diseases (cerebrovascular disorders, tumours, infections, injuries, *etc.*), drugs (excessive sedation) and metabolic or (induced by mechanical ventilation) respiratory alkalosis depress the respiratory centre. Neural (polyneuropathy or Guillain–Barré syndrome), neuromuscular (myasthenia gravis, botulism, muscle relaxing drugs, *etc.*) or muscular disorders (muscular dystrophy, critical illness myopathy, muscle fatigue, acid-base or electrolyte derangements, shock, *etc.*) either prevent or diminish transformation of the respiratory centre's impulses into mechanical output (neuromuscular uncoupling). Furthermore, the magnitude of the force generated by the dominant inspiratory muscle, the diaphragm, depends greatly on its shape. When diaphragmatic fibres are shortened or chest configuration is altered, as happens during hyperinflation, force generation as well as its transformation into negative alveolar pressure is reduced [26].

Since, with PAV, the signals for pressure delivery are the inspiratory flow and volume, the operation of this mode is highly susceptible to dynamic hyperinflation, which affects the triggering function. With volume assist or PSV, the ventilator, once triggered, delivers the preset volume or pressure regardless of patient effort beyond the trigger; the patient may relax their respiratory muscles after triggering, leaving the ventilator to deliver the volume, which, depending on the settings, may be substantial. In PAV, instead, immediately after ventilator triggering, pressure delivery is driven exclusively by the patient. Because the assist will automatically terminate at the end of inspiratory effort, any delay in onset of assist reduces the fraction of neural inspiratory time that is being assisted. Moreover, the level of effort required to trigger the ventilator is not assisted throughout the breath and the magnitude of pressure applied during the remaining neural inspiratory time will be proportional to only a fraction of the patient's effort (fig. 3) [17, 27]. It has been shown in critically ill patients that increasing PEEPi from 0.9 to 3.5 cmH$_2$O decreases the portion of supported inspiratory effort from 86% to 66% [27]. Therefore, a large portion of a patient's breath may be unassisted even though maximal gain (K) is used. Every effort should be made in order to reduce the magnitude of dynamic hyperinflation (*i.e.* by using bronchodilators or corticosteroids) or to counterbalance PEEPi (*i.e.* by adding external PEEP; see later in this chapter). Similarly, delayed triggering, due to high threshold of triggering (flow or pressure), slow ventilator response or significant concave shape to the pressure axis of the Pmus–time relationship, also decreases the portion of assisted inspiratory efforts. It follows that events during the triggering phase considerably affect PAV function. In any case, PAV does not support the portion of respiratory effort required to trigger the ventilator.

Another major disadvantage of the original PAV mode was the complicated procedure of respiratory system mechanics quantification. The problem was largely solved with the automatic

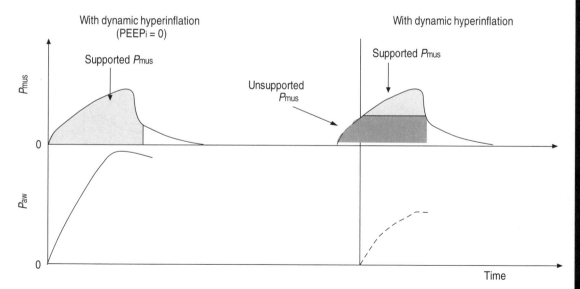

Figure 3. Tracings showing how the presence of intrinsic positive end-expiratory pressure (PEEPi) affects the portion of inspiratory muscle pressure (Pmus) supported. In the left graph, where PEEPi is zero, the total amount of Pmus required to trigger the ventilator is negligible and nearly the total amount of its value is supported. In the right graph, the section of Pmus marked darker grey is consumed entirely to counterbalance PEEPi. The ventilator supports only the remaining part (marked lighter grey). Airway pressure (Paw) provided by the ventilator (dashed line in right graph) is significantly lower than that on the left graph, although the patient's Pmus has not changed.

and continuous noninvasive measurement of mechanics incorporated in PAV+. However, mechanics calculation with PAV+ is far from ideal, especially in patients with expiratory flow limitation and dynamic hyperinflation, and this mode should be used with caution in this patient group.

Due to PAV operation principles, there is the potential for excessive pressure or volume delivery: the "run-away" phenomenon (fig. 4). Run-away occurs when pressure provided by the ventilator is greater than the sum of elastic and resistive pressures at some point during inflation [11, 12, 17, 25]. As a result, the ventilator continues to deliver volume despite the fact that the patient has terminated their inspiratory effort. The volume will continue to increase until an alarm limit (pressure or volume) is activated or the compliance of the respiratory system is decreased because the system approaches total lung capacity due to over-inflation or when expiratory muscles are recruited by the patient attempting to exhale [11, 12, 24, 25]. This phenomenon occurs because VA and/or FA are set to values higher than Ers and Rrs, respectively. Nonlinearity of pressure–volume and pressure–flow relationships may also cause VA or FA to be inappropriately set. For example, if end-expiratory lung volume is near residual volume, where Ers is high and VA is set according to this value, then there is a possibility that during inspiration Ers may decrease because of recruitment, becoming smaller than VA and leading to run-away. Similarly, endotracheal tube resistance does not have a single value but changes depending on flow rates. Therefore, FA that is appropriate for a range of flow rates may not be appropriate with flows outside this range, causing over-assist [24, 25]. Nevertheless, with automatic measurements of respiratory system mechanics (which take into account the nonlinear pressure–flow relationship of the endotracheal tube), run-away occurs rarely and only when the percentage of assist approaches 90% [24]. In our hands, with PAV+, run-away was not observed when the percentage of support was less than 80–85% [22].

Similar to over-assist, air leaks encountered mainly during noninvasive application of PAV dissociate Paw from Pmus, causing run-away [11, 25, 28]. In the presence of leaks, the ventilator misinterprets the flow and volume, abandoning its gas system as a continuous patient effort extending assist delivery into exhalation. Therefore, leak compensation is important in order to

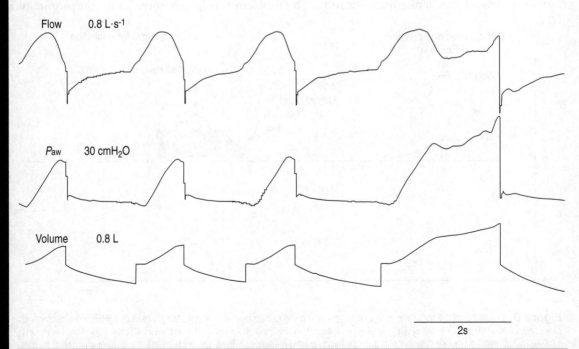

Figure 4. Traces depicting a stretched-out breath (run-away) in a case of over-assist during proportional assist ventilation. Observe the different appearances and magnitudes of flow, airway pressure (Paw) and volume of the stretched-out breath compared with those of previous normal breaths.

apply PAV noninvasively [11, 25, 29]. For the same reasons, the presence of a large bronchopleural fistula is a deterrent for PAV application.

Clinical studies

What distinguishes PAV from conventional assisted modes (PSV and AVC) is the introduction of the concept of patient-driven ventilation: assist delivery follows the patient's effort not only in terms of timing but also in terms of ventilator demand. Several theoretical advantages should be expected from this approach, especially in the fields of optimum patient–ventilator synchrony and respiratory muscles unloading. In the following sections of this chapter, we attempt to address whether the anticipated theoretical benefits are confirmed in practice, quoting evidence from clinical studies published so far. However, it is imperative, for the proper interpretation of clinical data, to separate two distinct eras in the literature, before and after PAV+ introduction.

Studies before PAV+

PAV has been shown to enhance exercise performance and to relieve exercise-induced dyspnoea in normal volunteers [30, 31], in obese adults [32], in stable patients with severe chronic obstructive pulmonary disease (COPD) [33–36] and in patients with pulmonary fibrosis [37]. Significant prolongation of high-intensity exercise in all studies, along with arterial oxygenation improvement in the most recent study [37], have made PAV a suitable adjunct to rehabilitation programmes. Compared with PSV, PAV exhibited a greater improvement in endurance time, dyspnoea and oxygen requirement [34]. Furthermore, inspiratory muscle effort indexes were significantly lower as a result of the linear correlation between changes in oesophageal pressure (Poes) and Paw delivered during PAV, in contrast to PSV [31].

The impact of adding dead space [18, 19], elastic load [15] or increase in the inspired fraction of carbon dioxide [38] in mechanically ventilated patients were used to further explore the performance of PAV under conditions of increased ventilatory requirements. In general, patients preserved the desired minute ventilation, although they managed to do it by adopting different breathing patterns with PAV compared with PSV: a higher respiratory rate was responsible for load compensation during PSV whereas, during PAV, VT was raised following escalation of inspiration effort, without considerable variation in breathing frequency. Moreover, muscle effort and the sense of dyspnoea were greater with PSV [15, 18], with the exception of one study [19], where an increase in resistive load due to higher inspiratory flows might have accounted for the nonsuperiority of PAV over PSV with regard to respiratory muscle unloading.

Apart from experimental respiratory muscle loading, several studies examined how, in daily practice, invasively ventilated patients responded to PAV and compared these responses to those observed during PSV [13, 14, 16, 17, 20, 28, 39, 40]. PAV has been demonstrated to successfully unload inspiratory muscles and improve comfort in patients with acute respiratory failure of various causes [13, 16, 28, 39], allowing, concurrently, greater variability of VT in comparison to PSV, mimicking normal breathing adaptation to alterations in ventilator demand [20, 40]. Nevertheless, it should be mentioned that the efficiency of PAV largely depended on the level of assist selected [20, 39, 40] and, in case of dynamic hyperinflation, on the application of adequate values of external PEEP [13]. With PAV, breathing frequency and VT remained relatively stable over a wide range of assist, being more influenced by ventilator requirements [14, 17]. At high levels of PSV, the lack of feedback between patient and ventilator with respect to VT modulation aggravated dynamic hyperinflation, resulting in the occurrence of missing efforts [14, 17]. In contrast, ineffective triggering was not observed even at the highest levels of PAV [14, 17]. Depending on level of assist, PSV seemed to eliminate arterial carbon dioxide tension (Pa,CO$_2$) to a greater, albeit clinically insignificant, extent compared with PAV, resulting in higher pH values [17, 19, 40]. No further clinically significant differences with respect to haemodynamics and arterial blood gases were observed between the two modes [14, 16, 19].

The improved patient–ventilator synchrony with PAV may affect sleep both in normal subjects and in critically ill patients. Meza et al. [41] compared the effect of PAV and PSV on the development of periodic breathing in 12 healthy participants during sleep. Progressive increase in the assistance level on PSV (average pressure of 5–10 cmH$_2$O) resulted in periodic breathing in all but one participant. In contrast, with PAV at comparable levels of assistance, periodic breathing occurred in only one participant. These results are explained by the tight link between Pmus and Paw observed with PAV but not with PSV. In critically ill patients, Bosma et al. [42] also compared the effects of PAV and PSV on sleep quality. 13 patients suffering weaning failure were assigned to receive PSV and PAV in a randomised crossover manner during two consecutive nights. Bosma et al. [42] demonstrated that, although total sleep time was not different between the two modes, overall sleep quality was significantly better during ventilation with PAV as a result of improvements in both sleep fragmentation and sleep architecture. The difference in sleep quality was attributed to better patient–ventilator synchrony observed with PAV. Indeed, patient–ventilator asynchronies per hour were lower during PAV than PSV and correlated significantly with the number of arousals per hour.

It should be emphasised that, in critically ill patients, an appreciable fluctuation in respiratory system impedance can completely abolish the benefits of PAV if inadequately compensated. Indeed, in many of the aforementioned studies, work of breathing and respiratory drive indexes indicated lack of superiority or even inferiority, at lower levels of assist, for PAV compared with PSV [16, 17, 20, 40]. At least partly, these results might be attributed to the lack of automatic ventilator support adjustment to changing respiratory mechanics, a drawback theoretically eliminated with PAV+.

Studies conducted with PAV+

The first study evaluating PAV+ was conducted by Kondili et al. [27], who assessed, in a small group of critically ill patients, the short-term response of respiratory motor output to added mechanical respiratory load during PSV and during PAV+. Without load, no differences in breathing pattern or magnitude of inspiratory effort were noticed between the two modes. Load addition led to smaller VT values and higher respiratory rates to maintain the desirable minute ventilation, but the percentage of these changes were significantly lower during PAV+. More importantly, while worsening of mechanics raised all indices of inspiratory effort, their values were significantly lower with PAV+ compared with PSV, implying a remarkably higher oxygen cost of breathing with the latter [27]. Although quite different from the study of Grasso et al. [15], these results could be said to be predictable when bearing in mind the different operational characteristics of PAV+ in comparison to the original PAV mode. Load addition amplified the provided pressure, responding both to respiratory mechanics deterioration and to greater patient effort, partly relieving respiratory muscles from the extra workload. Finally, ineffective efforts or run-away breaths were not observed with either mode, despite the notable increase in PEEPi [27].

Of utmost importance, although unaddressed in the literature, was the performance of PAV+ when applied in a long-term fashion, as the dominant mode of assisted mechanical ventilation. Xirouchaki et al. [43] attempted to answer this question in the largest study on PAV published so far. Apart from the size of population studied (208 patients), this study was innovative in that it directly compared the two modes of assisted ventilation, PSV versus PAV+, targeting possible differences in outcomes: failure of assisted ventilation necessitating switch to controlled modes, rates of successful weaning, mortality and patient–ventilator dyssynchrony. Patients, immediately upon fulfilling certain criteria for assisted mechanical ventilation, were randomised either to PSV or PAV+. In the PSV group, the proportion of patients who had to be switched to controlled mechanical ventilation during the 48 hours of the study period was twice the corresponding value in the PAV+ group (11% failure rate in PAV+ versus 22% in PSV; p=0.04) (fig. 5). Additionally, a larger number of patients developed major dyssynchrony in the PSV group (29% in PSV versus 5.6% in PAV+). Liberation from mechanical ventilation, ICU and in-hospital mortality and total amount of sedative, analgesic or vasoactive drugs were similar between the two study groups.

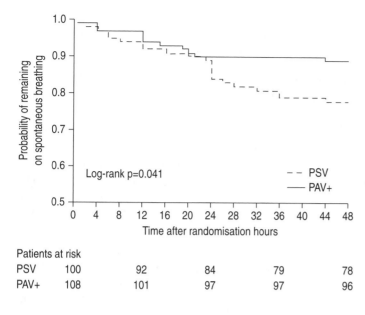

Figure 5. Kaplan–Meier estimates of the probability of remaining on spontaneous breathing in patients randomised to pressure support ventilation (PSV) and proportional assist ventilation (PAV+). Reproduced from [43] with permission from the publisher.

A correlation between neural and mechanical respiratory rate in PAV+ and PSV is shown in figure 6 [43].

By retrospective analysis of data from their previous study, XIROUCHAKI *et al.* [44] revealed that, in the group of patients ventilated with PSV, the mean number of changes in ventilator settings and in the dose of sedatives was significantly higher compared with the group ventilated with PAV+. During PSV, the dominant cause of interventions (more often directed to triggering sensitivity and level of support) was clinical deterioration, as judged by the treating physicians. Conversely, significantly more interventions in the PAV+ group were performed to facilitate weaning [44]. These are interesting results for the daily clinical practice of ICUs, indicating that PAV+ is not only simple in its application but is also time saving.

Apart from improved synchrony between the patient and ventilator, PAV+ may be viewed as a protective mode of mechanical ventilation. With other modes of assisted mechanical ventilation such as PSV or AVC, V_T largely depends on the level of assist, and high assist may be associated with high V_T, a well-known factor for ventilator-induced lung injury. The study of XIROUCHAKI *et al.* [43] showed that, with PAV+ even with high assistance, V_T and end-inspiratory plateau pressure were comparable to those observed during protective controlled mechanical ventilation.

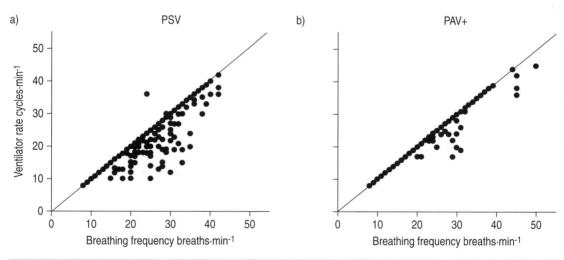

Figure 6. The relationship of patients' breathing frequency and ventilator respiratory rate is shown for a) pressure support ventilation (PSV) and b) proportional assist ventilation (PAV+). Each closed circle represents a measurement during the 48-hour study period. In the PSV group, the patients' respiratory rate differed from the corresponding rate of the ventilator in 13.6% of measurements due to ineffective efforts. Only 2.8% of measurements during PAV+ revealed a difference between patient and ventilator breathing frequency. Reproduced from [43] with permission from the publisher.

Examination of individual end-inspiratory plateau pressures during PAV+ showed that, out of a total of 744 measurements, only on nine (1.2%) occasions and in five (4.6%) patients were plateau pressures above 30 cmH$_2$O (fig. 7). 94% of the end-inspiratory plateau pressures were below 26 cmH$_2$O, a value associated with lung protection [43]. These results can be explained by the operation of reflex feedback (vagally controlled reflexes or Hering–Breuer reflex). These neural reflexes inhibit inspiratory muscle activity if lung distension exceeds a certain threshold that is well below total lung capacity. Contrary to other assisted modes, PAV+ does not interfere with the operation of these reflexes, since, with this mode, inhibition of inspiratory muscle activity results in an automatic termination of pressure delivery.

More recently, another head-to-head comparison between PSV and PAV+ in the field of patient–ventilator interaction was conducted in a small group of difficult-to-wean patients [45]. The results were in line with the existing literature: with PSV, patients suffered a higher proportion of major dyssynchrony and expiratory triggering delay, and spent less time synchronised with neural inspiration pressure delivery [45].

In a different approach, ALEXOPOULOU et al. [46] tested whether, in patients exhibiting harmonious interaction with the ventilator, the large number of end-inspiratory occlusions during PAV+ operation adversely affected sleep quality. PSV and PAV+, each at two levels of assist, were examined in both sedated and nonsedated patients. PAV+ and PSV equally affected sleep efficiency and architecture. Moreover, in patients prone to unstable breathing, high levels of PAV+ promoted, in the same manner as high levels of PSV, the occurrence of periodic breathing [46]. In agreement with the latter, periodic breathing developed at high levels of PAV+ in all but one out of 11 brain damage patients sedated with propofol [47]. In addition to these observations, data from further studies might shed light on the extremely interesting field of sleep in mechanically ventilated patients. As yet, available evidence is inadequate to clarify the exact role of PAV+ in this area.

PAV as a noninvasive mode of mechanical ventilation

The performance of PAV in the field of noninvasive mechanical ventilation has been tested by several investigators [33–36, 48–53]. In rehabilitation programmes in COPD outpatients, PAV used noninvasively has been shown to increase endurance time and relieve exercise-induced dyspnoea [33–36]. Compared with unassisted breathing, PAV through a nasal or full face mask is

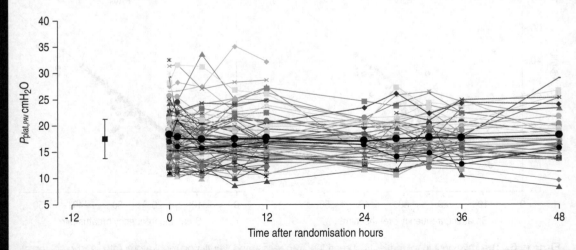

Figure 7. Closed black circles connected by a solid black line represent mean values of airway pressures measured during a 300-ms pause manoeuvre ($P_{\text{plat,PAV}}$). Different colours represent different patients. For comparison the mean ± SD static end-inspiratory airway pressure, obtained up to 8 hours before randomisation, during controlled mechanical ventilation is shown (closed black square). Reproduced from [43] with permission from the publisher.

well tolerated, improves ventilation and gas exchange and alleviates dyspnoea by effectively unloading the inspiratory muscle workload in patients with chronic respiratory insufficiency of various origins [48, 49]. In the same group of patients (stable patients with chronic respiratory failure), PSV and PAV exhibit similar performance in relation to patient tolerance, ventilation and blood gas tension improvement and diaphragmatic activity decrease [50, 51].

In the acute care setting, only two studies have randomised patients admitted with acute respiratory insufficiency to either PAV or PSV with the aim of testing possible differences in outcomes [52, 53]. Both the study of GAY et al. [52] and the larger one of FERNANDEZ-VIVAS et al. [53] failed to prove superiority of one modality over the other with respect to intubation, mortality rates or gas exchange. Dyspnoea scores were initially identical but, at the end of the latter study, a significant deviation in favour of PAV was observed [53]. Refusal rate and complications in the form of nasal bridge ulcerations or conjunctivitis were significantly less often observed during PAV [52, 53]. Furthermore, PAV was combined with higher comfort rates and better tolerance compared with PSV [31, 50, 51]. In patients with acute cardiogenic pulmonary oedema, PAV and continuous positive airway pressure were identical regarding failure and intubation rates or total ventilator time [54]. However, these results should be interpreted with caution due to the lower than planned recruitment, the relatively high failure rate of noninvasive ventilation in this study and the uncertainties concerning elastance and resistance estimation. Of note, there was no evidence for increased risk of myocardial infarction with PAV [54].

A common finding in studies evaluating the noninvasive application of PAV has been the lower mean airway pressures developed in comparison with PSV. This could be clinically important if one considers that, when instituting noninvasive ventilation, high airway pressures have been associated with reduction of cardiac output and oxygen delivery, skin ulcers, barotrauma and leaks [55–57]. Finally, run-away occurred in a small minority of patients ventilated with PAV, especially in those with COPD [52].

It can be concluded that, according to the existing literature, PAV can be utilised as an alternative mode of noninvasive ventilation. Its use is feasible, well tolerated and efficient. However, in the studies already published, it has not prevailed over PSV, while it requires a satisfactory leak compensation algorithm, otherwise deleterious malfunction might occur. Finally the nonautomatic measurement of respiratory system mechanics (PAV+ has been designed for intubated patients) limits the use of PAV for noninvasive ventilatory support.

Applying PAV+ in daily ICU practice

As mentioned earlier in this chapter, PAV without automatic measurements of the respiratory system mechanics is, although feasible, difficult to apply, at least for extensive periods, in critically ill patients. Therefore, in this section, a comprehensive description of how to use PAV+ in intubated critically ill patients is attempted.

There are specific patient characteristics that predict a favourable outcome or, conversely, a high probability of failure. As with other assisted modes, any patient able to bear part of their ventilator requirements is considered eligible for PAV+ application. Nevertheless, its use should be particularly examined in difficult-to-wean patients suffering from acute lung injury (ALI)/acute respiratory distress syndrome (ARDS). These patients often develop distress and require sedation escalation due to either patient–ventilator dyssynchrony or sudden increase in their ventilator demands. By enhancing patient–ventilator interaction and adjusting the assist provided to instantaneous ventilator requirements, PAV+ might decrease sedation and precipitate liberation from mechanical ventilation. Additionally, respiratory system mechanics measurement might give clues regarding the causes of the patient's clinical deterioration (tachypnoea, use of accessory muscles or diaphoresis) or gas exchange deterioration, allowing the appropriate measures to be taken. There is also clinical evidence indicating that PAV+ may minimise the risk of lung overdistension, since this mode does not interfere with the operation of lung protective innate reflexes (*i.e.* Hering–Breuer). However, caution should be exerted in patients with strong signals of nonrespiratory origin (*e.g.* acidosis or brain dysfunction) that drive ventilation.

It should particularly be re-emphasised that PAV+ application might prove problematic in patients with severe airflow obstruction, especially when combined with either a weak drive or muscle weakness. As described in detail earlier in this chapter, extra load imposed by PEEPi absorbs a large part of muscle force leaving neural inspiration totally or partly unassisted. For reasons already analysed, calculated elastance might be overestimated in the presence of remarkable PEEPi, leading to errors in resistance measurement (resistance is calculated utilising elastance value). Moreover, in the presence of expiratory flow limitation during passive expiration, expiratory resistance is highly unreliable. Finally, PAV+ may not be suitable for patients with a large bronchopleural leak, although theoretically the underestimation of E_{rs} by an amount corresponding to the leak may partly offset the error in pressure delivery.

Figure 8 provides an algorithm developed by M. Younes (University of Manitoba, Winnipeg, MB, and University of Calgery, Calgery, AB, Canada; personal communication) and D. Georgopoulos to guide the procedure for placing a patient on PAV+. Using this algorithm, critically ill patients can be ventilated easily, even during the acute phase of their illness. The following key points further facilitate the procedure.

1) Ensure that correct ideal body weight, endotracheal tube size and maximum airway pressure (40 cmH$_2$O) are entered correctly. Setting airway pressure limit is of paramount importance, since it will protect the lungs from overdistension if run-away breaths occur. Nevertheless, the shape of

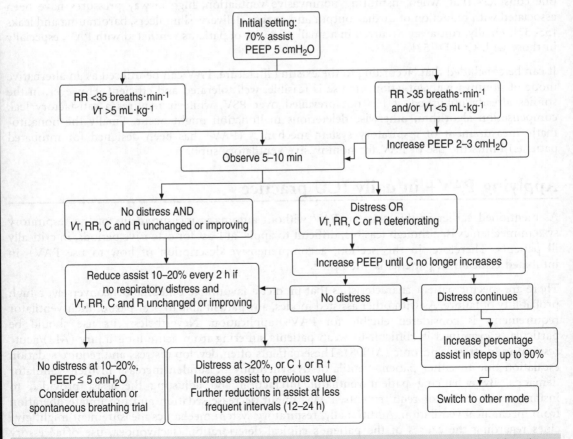

Figure 8. A stepwise approach for proportional assist ventilation implementation in critically ill adult patients. PEEP: positive end-expiratory pressure; RR: respiratory rate; V_T: tidal volume; C: respiratory system compliance; R: respiratory system resistance; ↑: increased; ↓: decreased.

the pressure–volume curve (compliance decreases with increasing lung volume) effectively precludes significant overdistension.

2) With respect to percentage of support, a rational approach is to start with a level sufficiently high to support the patient but well away from the area where run-away phenomena are likely to occur. That is why an initial gain of 70% is proposed in the suggested algorithm.

3) Initial PEEP and inspiratory oxygen fraction (F_{I,O_2}) are set using common criteria. In our unit, as with other modes, the initial value of PEEP is set to $\geqslant 5$ cmH$_2$O. Also, subsequent hypoxaemia is managed as usual, by adjusting PEEP and F_{I,O_2}. The response of compliance (measured automatically and semi-continuously by the ventilator software) may be used to titrate PEEP; PEEP is increased until compliance no longer increases, signifying the end of recruitment (see also key point 8).

4) Immediate response following a change to PAV+ may vary considerably depending on whether the patient was over-assisted and whether there was nonsynchrony on the previous mode. Response may range from "no change" to "very shallow breathing" (an indication of the presence of a significant number of ineffective efforts on previous modes) to "central apnoea" (an indication of over-assist on previous modes). Wait a minute or so to see what the pattern will actually become before deciding on next steps.

5) V_T may be quite variable on PAV+. This is normal, partly reflecting the normal breath variability and partly events on previous modes (mainly over-assist). V_T may be quite low (i.e. 3–4 mL·kg^{-1}) and this is not uncommon. To the extent that respiratory rate does not increase concurrently and there are no other signs of distress, low V_T is not an indication to change assist level.

6) A high respiratory rate (even up to 50 breaths·min^{-1}) need not by itself indicate distress. Other signs of distress should be present (e.g. sustained change in heart rate or blood pressure, accessory muscles use, sweating, etc.). Many patients have high rates even when they are very well supported and this is masked in other modes by nonsynchrony (i.e. ineffective efforts). Ineffective efforts are particularly common with tachypnoea and when the V_T is relatively high (because of high assist) and mechanical inflation extends well into neural expiration (delayed opening expiratory asynchrony). With PAV+ the likelihood of ineffective efforts is reduced significantly because mechanical inflation time is terminated close to the end of neural inspiration (i.e. expiratory asynchrony is minimised), and V_T in most cases remains relatively small even at high assist. The latter is due to the fact that, with PAV+, contrary to other conventional modes of support, the patient retains considerable control of V_T, independent of the level of assist.

7) P_{a,CO_2} may rise after switching to PAV+. Most commonly this is due to over-ventilation before PAV+. In these patients, central apnoeas upon switching to PAV+ may be observed. Be concerned only if the pH decreases below normal (i.e. <7.37). Acidaemia without distress indicates depressed respiratory drive. These patients are not candidates for PAV+ until the cause of depressed drive is corrected.

8) Distress at 70% of assist is uncommon and is usually due to delayed triggering because of severe dynamic hyperinflation and weak muscles (i.e. patients with obstructive lung disease). Alternatively, it may be due to very low compliance at low lung volume (i.e. patients with obesity, abdominal pathology, ALI/ARDS, etc.) and usually these patients exhibit hypoxaemia. Either condition may be improved by increasing PEEP. The increase in PEEP may be guided by response of compliance; increase PEEP until compliance no longer increases. This manoeuvre is commonly effective at the presence of flow limitation during passive expiration (patients with dynamic hyperinflation). In these patients, increasing PEEP does not affect end-expiratory lung volume while it does improve the triggering function. In patients with low compliance at low lung volumes, PEEP escalation increases end-expiratory lung volume and bypasses the respiratory system region with low compliance. However, other factors, such as cardiac output, end-inspiratory plateau pressure and arterial blood pressure, need to be considered in determining how high PEEP can be increased.

9) Very few patients continue to have distress at 70% of assist after adjusting PEEP. In these patients, increase percentage of assist in steps of 5% up to 90%. Wait 15–20 breaths between steps

and observe for stretched out breaths (delayed cycling off or run-away). If stretched out breaths appear, decrease the assist to the previous level.

10) There is a minority of patients in whom, at maximum assist (85–90%) and after properly adjusting PEEP, distress remains. Usually these are patients in whom a large portion of inspiratory effort is not supported because of excessive triggering delay (key point 8) and they cannot be improved by increasing PEEP and percentage of assist. Until the incorporation of better triggering methods, PAV+ cannot adequately support this group of patients.

11) In some patients with clinical signs of severe obstructive lung disease and expiratory flow limitation during passive expiration (*i.e.* expiratory flow spike), the calculated value of expiratory resistance is very low. In these patients, the low expiratory resistance is a reflection of endotracheal tube resistance and not of respiratory system resistance. PAV+ may not sufficiently support these patients even at high assist.

12) Obviously, patients who deteriorate with decreasing assist are not candidates for fast weaning. Percentage of assist and/or PEEP should be reduced slowly (over several hours or days), depending on the individual patient.

New developments

Although it may originally have been perceived as brilliant, the mechanism under which PAV+ works is far from ideal. For example, further developments are needed in the area of triggering. Essentially, PAV did not evolve triggering systems compared with previous assisted modes, thus carrying all their inherent limitations while its performance is even worse in the presence of dynamic hyperinflation. The flow–waveform method of triggering is more sensitive than flow- or pressure-triggered methods but the improvement is only modest [24, 58]. Conversely, it does not work when expiratory flow is very low as is the case with severe airflow limitation [24, 58]. Beyond triggering, flow and airway are located well down the line of neuroventilatory coupling.

Recently, a new technology has been introduced that aims to monitor and improve patient–ventilator interaction (PVI monitor; YRT, Winnipeg, MB, Canada) [59]. With PVI monitor, a signal representing an estimate of the patient's total respiratory muscle pressure ($P_{mus,PVI}$) is calculated *via* the equation of motion, utilising estimated values of resistance and elastance of the respiratory system, obtained noninvasively. The waveform of $P_{mus,PVI}$ is continuously displayed online on a breath-by-breath basis and can be used to trigger the ventilator. It has been shown that this triggering method may substantially shorten the triggering delay (by approximately 70%), even in patients with dynamic hyperinflation [60]. Theoretically, this system should increase the efficiency of PAV+ to support critically ill patients with dynamic hyperinflation. Similarly, measuring inspiratory resistance (instead of expiratory) should further increase the ability of this mode to support patients with obstructive lung disease.

The use of electrical activity of the diaphragm (EA_{di}) signal (neurally adjusted ventilator assist (NAVA)) represents another effort for further improvement of patient–ventilator synchrony [61]. With this mode, pressure delivery from the beginning until the end of mechanical inspiration targets changes in the EA_{di}, which are captured through an array of nine electrodes incorporated in a nasogastric tube [61, 62]. Because EA_{di} is born before the mechanical induction of PEEPi, its signal should be neither delayed nor dampened by its presence [62, 63]. However, a head-to-head comparison between PAV and NAVA has not been made.

Future perspectives: is integration feasible?

Increased life expectancy and accentuated access to healthcare services have (and will continue to) dramatically increased the requirements for ICU beds and the population of patients who are mechanically ventilated. The latter absorbs a significant amount of human and money resources.

In this context, there is more than urgent demand for innovations enhancing the quality of provided care while concurrently saving money and time. The future ventilator could be envisioned as a completely autonomous machine, functioning from the moment of its inception in response to a variety of information transmitted from the patient: blood gases, respiratory mechanics and behavioural responses. PAV+ forms the ideal base for the construction of this "intelligent" ventilator: through the semi-continuous measurement of respiratory mechanics, the calculation of Pmus during inspiration is feasible. Following the inspiratory Pmus signal not only for terminating but also for triggering mechanical assist, any time lapse between mechanical and neural phases of breathing would be eliminated. Consequently, automatic assist titration according to inspiratory Pmus amplitude and shape would involve the whole duration and intensity of patient effort even in the presence of severe dynamic hyperinflation, completely closing the loop between patient and ventilator. In addition, PEEP and F_{I,O_2} could be adjusted based on the principles described in this chapter. Of course, sophisticated alarm systems would be necessary to protect against run-away, high pressures or respiratory drive depression, along with the adoption of better techniques to measure inspiratory resistance (e.g. the pulse technique) upgrading PAV+ performance in patients with airflow obstruction. Furthermore, even with the aid of Pmus, mechanical support should ideally be preserved within the boundaries of patient comfort on the one hand and prevention of excessive muscle relaxation on the other.

Conclusions

In recent years, progress in the field of mechanical ventilation has greatly updated the quality of patient management. Without any doubt, PAV+ has brought us one step closer to the so-called "ideal mechanical assistance". Training in its use, careful monitoring of the patient's response and, above all, deep understanding of the complex mechanisms dictating respiratory physiology, will inevitably help towards the future resolution of the few but real problems regarding its use.

Statement of interest

D. Georgopoulos received €3,000 in 2008 and €1,500 in 2009 for speaking at conferences sponsored by Tyco, and €20,000 research grant for conducting clinical trials from Nellcor Puritan Bennett in the years 2007–2009. None of the flu studies conducted by D. Georgopoulos was sponsored by industry.

References

1. Kress JP, Pohlman AS, O'Connor MF, et al. Daily interruption of sedative infusions in critically ill patients undergoing mechanical ventilation. N Engl J Med 2000; 342: 1471–1477.
2. Schweickert WD, Gehlbach BK, Pohlman AS, et al. Daily interruption of sedative infusions and complications of critical illness in mechanically ventilated patients. Crit Care Med 2004; 32: 1272–1276.
3. Levine S, Nguyen T, Taylor N, et al. Rapid disuse atrophy of diaphragm fibers in mechanically ventilated humans. N Engl J Med 2008; 358: 1327–1335.
4. Vassilakopoulos T, Petrof BJ. Ventilator-induced diaphragmatic dysfunction. Am J Respir Crit Care Med 2004; 169: 336–341.
5. Larsson L, Li X, Edstrom L, et al. Acute quadriplegia and loss of muscle myosin in patients treated with nondepolarizing neuromuscular blocking agents and corticosteroids: mechanisms at the cellular and molecular levels. Crit Care Med 2000; 28: 34–45.
6. Garnacho-Montero J, Madrazo-Osuna J, Garcia-Garmendia JL, et al. Critical illness polyneuropathy: risk factors and clinical consequences. A cohort study in septic patients. Intensive Care Med 2001; 27: 1288–1296.
7. Putensen C, Zech S, Wrigge H, et al. Long-term effects of spontaneous breathing during ventilatory support in patients with acute lung injury. Am J Respir Crit Care Med 2001; 164: 43–49.
8. MacIntyre NR. Respiratory function during pressure support ventilation. Chest 1986; 89: 677–683.
9. Tobin MJ, Jubran A, Laghi F. Patient–ventilator interaction. Am J Respir Crit Care Med 2001; 163: 1059–1063.
10. Kondili E, Prinianakis G, Georgopoulos D. Patient–ventilator interaction. Br J Anaesth 2003; 91: 106–119.
11. Younes M. Proportional assist ventilation, a new approach to ventilatory support. Theory. Am Rev Respir Dis 1992; 145: 114–120.

12. Younes M, Puddy A, Roberts D, *et al.* Proportional assist ventilation. Results of an initial clinical trial. *Am Rev Respir Dis* 1992; 145: 121–129.
13. Appendini L, Purro A, Gudjonsdotiir M, *et al.* Physiologic response of ventilator-dependent patients with chronic obstructive pulmonary disease to proportional assist ventilation and continuous positive airway pressure. *Am J Respir Crit Care Med* 1999; 159: 1510–1517.
14. Giannouli E, Webster K, Roberts D, *et al.* Response of ventilator-dependent patients to different levels of pressure support and proportional assist. *Am J Respir Crit Care Med* 1999; 159: 1716–1725.
15. Grasso S, Puntillo F, Mascia L, *et al.* Compensation for increase in respiratory workload during mechanical ventilation. Pressure support *versus* proportional assist ventilation. *Am J Respir Crit Care Med* 2000; 161: 819–826.
16. Kondili E, Xirouchaki N, Vaporidi K, *et al.* Short-term cardiorespiratory effects of proportional assist and pressure support ventilation in patients with acute lung injury/acute respiratory distress syndrome. *Anesthesiology* 2006; 105: 703–708.
17. Passam F, Hoing S, Prinianakis G, *et al.* Effect of different levels of pressure support and proportional assist ventilation on breathing pattern, work of breathing and gas exchange in mechanically ventilated hypercapnic COPD patients with acute respiratory failure. *Respiration* 2003; 70: 355–361.
18. Ranieri VM, Giuliani R, Mascia L, *et al.* Patient–ventilator interaction during acute hypercapnia: pressure support *versus* proportional assist ventilation. *J Appl Physiol* 1996; 81: 426–436.
19. Varelmann D, Wrigge H, Zinserling J, *et al.* Proportional assist *versus* pressure support ventilation in patients with acute respiratory failure: cardiorespiratory responses to artificially increased ventilatory demand. *Crit Care Med* 2005; 33: 1968–1975.
20. Wrigge H, Golisch W, Zinserling J, *et al.* Proportional assist *versus* pressure support ventilation: effects on breathing pattern and respiratory work of patients with chronic obstructive pulmonary disease. *Intensive Care Med* 1999; 25: 790–798.
21. Younes M, Webster K, Kun J, *et al.* A method for measuring passive elastance during proportional assist ventilation. *Am J Respir Crit Care Med* 2001; 164: 50–60.
22. Younes M, Kun J, Masiowski B, *et al.* A method for noninvasive determination of inspiratory resistance during proportional assist ventilation. *Am J Respir Crit Care Med* 2001; 163: 829–839.
23. Georgopoulos D, Roussos C. Control of breathing in mechanically ventilated patients. *Eur Respir J* 1996; 9: 2151–2160.
24. Georgopoulos D, Plataki M, Prinianakis G, *et al.* Current status of proportional assist ventilation. *Int J Intensive Care Med* 2007; 14: 74–80.
25. Younes M. Proportional assist ventilation. *In:* Tobin MJ, ed. Principles and Practice of Mechanical Ventilation. New York, Mc Graw Hill, 2006; pp. 335–364.
26. Beck J, Sinderby C, Lindström L, *et al.* Effects of lung volume on diaphragm EMG signal strength during voluntary contractions. *J Appl Physiol* 1998; 85: 1123–1134.
27. Kondili E, Prinianakis G, Alexopoulou C, *et al.* Respiratory load compensation during mechanical ventilation: proportional assist ventilation with load-adjustable gain factors *versus* pressure support. *Intensive Care Med* 2006; 32: 692–699.
28. Ranieri VM, Grasso S, Mascia L, *et al.* Effects of proportional assist ventilation on inspiratory muscle effort in patients with chronic obstructive pulmonary disease and acute respiratory failure. *Anesthesiology* 1997; 86: 79–91.
29. Wysocki M, Richard JC, Meshaka P. Non-invasive proportional assist ventilation compared with non-invasive pressure support ventilation in hypercapnic acute respiratory failure. *Crit Care Med* 2002; 30: 323–329.
30. Kleinsasser A, Von Goedecke A, Hoermann C, *et al.* Proportional assist ventilation reduces the work of breathing during exercise at moderate altitude. *High Alt Med Biol* 2004; 5: 420–428.
31. Wysocki M, Meshaka P, Richard JC, *et al.* Proportional assist ventilation compared with pressure-support ventilation during exercise in volunteers with external thoracic restriction. *Crit Care Med* 2004; 32: 409–414.
32. Dreher M, Kabitz HJ, Burgardt V, *et al.* Proportional assist ventilation improves exercise capacity in patients with obesity. *Respiration* 2010; 80: 106–111.
33. Dolmage TE, Goldstein RS. Proportional assist ventilation and exercise tolerance in subjects with COPD. *Chest* 1997; 111: 948–954.
34. Bianchi L, Foglio K, Pagani M, *et al.* Effects of proportional assist ventilation on exercise tolerance in COPD patients with chronic hypercapnia. *Eur Respir J* 1998; 11: 422–427.
35. Hernandez P, Maltais F, Gursahaney A, *et al.* Proportional assist ventilation may improve exercise performance in severe chronic obstructive pulmonary disease. *J Cardiopulm Rehabil* 2001; 21: 135–142.
36. Hawkins P, Johnson LC, Nikoletou D, *et al.* Proportional assist ventilation as an aid to exercise training in severe chronic obstructive pulmonary disease. *Thorax* 2002; 57: 853–859.
37. Moderno EV, Yamaguti WP, Schettino GP, *et al.* Effects of proportional assisted ventilation on exercise performance in idiopathic pulmonary fibrosis patients. *Respir Med* 2010; 104: 134–141.
38. Mitrouska J, Xirouchaki N, Patakas D, *et al.* Effects of chemical feedback on respiratory motor and ventilatory output during different modes of assisted mechanical ventilation. *Eur Respir J* 1999; 13: 873–882.
39. Navalesi P, Hernandez P, Wongsa A, *et al.* Proportional assist ventilation in acute respiratory failure: effects on breathing pattern and inspiratory effort. *Am J Respir Crit Care Med* 1996; 154: 1330–1338.
40. Delaere S, Roeseler J, D'hoore W, *et al.* Respiratory muscle workload in intubated, spontaneously breathing patients without COPD: pressure support *versus* proportional assist ventilation. *Intensive Care Med* 2003; 29: 949–954.

41. Meza S, Mendez M, Ostrowski M, *et al.* Susceptibility to periodic breathing with assisted ventilation during sleep in normal subjects. *J Appl Physiol* 1998; 85: 1929–1940.

42. Bosma K, Ferreyra G, Ambrogio C, *et al.* Patient–ventilator interaction and sleep in mechanically ventilated patients: pressure support *versus* proportional assist ventilation. *Crit Care Med* 2007; 35: 1048–1054.

43. Xirouchaki N, Kondili E, Vaporidi K, *et al.* Proportional assist ventilation with load-adjustable gain factors in critically ill patients: comparison with pressure support. *Intensive Care Med* 2008; 34: 2026–2034.

44. Xirouchaki N, Kondili E, Klimathianaki M, *et al.* Is proportional assist ventilation with load-adjustable gain factors a user-friendly mode? *Intensive Care Med* 2009; 35: 1599–1603.

45. Costa R, Spinazzola G, Cipriani F, *et al.* A physiologic comparison of proportional assist ventilation with load-adjustable gain factors (PAV+) *versus* pressure support ventilation (PSV). *Intensive Care Med* 2011; 37: 1494–1500.

46. Alexopoulou C, Kondili E, Vakouti E, *et al.* Sleep during proportional-assist ventilation with load-adjustable gain factors in critically ill patients. *Intensive Care Med* 2007; 33: 1139–1147.

47. Klimathianaki M, Kondili E, Alexopoulou C, *et al.* Effect of propofol on breathing stability in adult ICU patients with brain damage. *Respir Physiol Neurobiology* 2010; 232–238.

48. Polese G, Vitacca M, Bianchi L, *et al.* Nasal proportional assist ventilation unloads the inspiratory muscles of stable patients with hypercapnia due to COPD. *Eur Respir J* 2000; 16: 491–498.

49. Ambrosino N, Vitacca M, Polese G, *et al.* Short-term effects of nasal proportional assist ventilation in patients with chronic hypercapnic respiratory insufficiency. *Eur Respir J* 1997; 10: 2829–2834.

50. Serra A, Polese G, Braggion C, *et al.* Non-invasive proportional assist and pressure support ventilation in patients with cystic fibrosis and chronic respiratory failure. *Thorax* 2002; 57: 50–54.

51. Porta R, Appendini L, Vitacca M, *et al.* Mask proportional assist *versus* pressure support ventilation in patients in clinically stable condition with chronic ventilator failure. *Chest* 2002; 122: 479–488.

52. Gay PC, Hess DR, Hill NS. Noninvasive proportional assist ventilation for acute respiratory insufficiency. Comparison with pressure support ventilation. *Am J Respir Crit Care Med* 2001; 164: 1606–1611.

53. Fernandez-Vivas M, Caturla-Such J, Gonzalez de la Rosa J, *et al.* Noninvasive pressure support *versus* proportional assist ventilation in acute respiratory failure. *Intensive Care Med* 2003; 29: 1126–1133.

54. Rusterholtz T, Bollaert PE, Feissel M, *et al.* Continuous positive airway pressure *versus* proportional assist ventilation for noninvasive ventilation in acute cardiogenic pulmonary edema. *Intensive Care Med* 2008; 34: 840–846.

55. Patrick W, Webster K, Ludwig L, *et al.* Noninvasive positive-pressure ventilation in acute respiratory distress without prior chronic respiratory failure. *Am J Respir Crit Care Med* 1996; 153: 1005–1011.

56. Diaz O, Iglesia R, Ferrer M, *et al.* Effects of noninvasive ventilation on pulmonary gas exchange and hemodynamics during acute hypercapnic exacerbations of chronic obstructive pulmonary disease. *Am J Respir Crit Care Med* 1997; 156: 1840–1845.

57. Haworth C, Dodd ME, Atkins M, *et al.* Pneumothorax in adults with cystic fibrosis depend on nasal intermittent positive pressure ventilation (NIPPV): a management dilemma. *Thorax* 2000; 55: 620–623.

58. Prinianakis G, Kondili E, Georgopoulos D. Effects of flow waveform method of triggering and cycling on patient–ventilator interaction during pressure support. *Intensive Care Med* 2003; 29: 1950–1959.

59. Younes M, Brochard L, Grasso S, *et al.* A method for monitoring and improving patient–ventilator interaction. *Intensive Care Med* 2007; 33: 1337–1346.

60. Kondili E, Alexopoulou C, Xirouchaki N, *et al.* Estimation of inspiratory muscle pressure in critically ill patients. *Intensive Care Med* 2010; 36: 648–655.

61. Sinderby C, Navalesi P, Beck J, *et al.* Neural control of mechanical ventilation in respiratory failure. *Nat Med* 1999; 5: 1433–1436.

62. Sinderby C, Beck J. Proportional assist ventilation and neurally adjusted ventilatory assist: better approaches to patient ventilator synchrony? *Clin Chest Med* 2008; 29: 329–342.

63. Sinderby C, Spahija J, Beck J, *et al.* Diaphragm activation during exercise in chronic obstructive pulmonary disease. *Am J Respir Crit Care Med* 2001; 163: 1637–1641.

Chapter 8

Neurally adjusted ventilatory assist

P. Navalesi,+,#, D. Colombo¶, G. Cammarota¶ and R. Vaschetto¶*

Summary

Neurally adjusted ventilatory assist (NAVA) is a form of ventilator support in which the electrical activity of the diaphragm (EAdi) drives the ventilator. The signal, obtained from the crural portion of the diaphragm *via* a nasogastric or orogastric feeding tube, is transformed into a waveform that is utilised to regulate the inspiratory assistance. The ventilator applies pressure to the airway throughout inspiration in proportion to EAdi, which is multiplied by an adjustable gain constant (NAVA level). With NAVA, both the timing and the magnitude of ventilator delivered assistance are controlled by the EAdi. In contrast with the conventional pneumatically-driven modes, NAVA has been shown to improve patient–ventilator interaction and yield a remarkable reduction in any asynchronies. Furthermore, with NAVA the patient retains control of her/his breathing pattern, which is more variable in nature; this variability might determine improved oxygenation in patients with acute lung–volume reduction. Because tidal volume is not remarkably increased when augmenting the NAVA level, this novel mode has the potential to maintain protective ventilation in spontaneously breathing patients.

Keywords: Ineffective efforts, neurally adjusted ventilatory assist, patient–ventilator interaction

*Università del Piemonte Orientale "A. Avogadro",
#Anestesia e Rianimazione, Ospedale Sant'Andrea, Vercelli, and
¶Anestesia e Rianimazione, Azienda Ospedaliero-Universitaria "Maggiore della Carità", Novara, Italy.

Correspondence: P. Navalesi, Dipartimento di Medicina Traslazionale, Università del Piemonte Orientale "A. Avogadro", Via Solaroli 17, 28100 Novara, Italy. Email paolo.navalesi@med.unipmn.it

Eur Respir Mon 2012; 55: 116–123.
Printed in UK – all rights reserved
Copyright ERS 2012
European Respiratory Monograph
ISSN: 1025-448x
DOI: 10.1183/1025448x.10002011

Neurally adjusted ventilatory assist (NAVA) became commercially available only a few years ago; however, it was first described more than 10 years ago in a seminal paper outlining the general principles and the potentials of this novel technique [1]. Using data from three experimental records taken from intensive care unit (ICU) patients, the article showed how driving the ventilator through the electrical activity of the diaphragm (EAdi), as opposed to the conventional pneumatic signals (*i.e.* flow, volume, and airway pressure), improved patient–ventilator synchrony [1]. In addition, the response of one healthy subject to NAVA in the course of a single breath and during various breathing manoeuvers was presented, showing that there are continuous proportional adjustments of airway pressure to changes in EAdi, regardless of breathing pattern and end-expiratory lung volume [1]. With NAVA, both the timing and the magnitude of the ventilator-delivered assistance are controlled by the EAdi, which is considered the best available signal to estimate the neural drive to breathe [1–3]. Because with NAVA the airway pressure instantaneously reflects the patient's respiratory drive, patient–ventilator interaction is accordingly improved and patient–ventilator asynchrony eliminated in most cases. Moreover, being based on diaphragm activity, rather than on flow and/or volume, the support delivered by the ventilator in the NAVA mode is unaffected by respiratory system mechanics, presence of intrinsic positive end-expiratory pressure (PEEP) and airleaks.

Randomised trials, which prove a beneficial effect of NAVA on outcome variables, such as duration of mechanical ventilation, rate of tracheotomy, and ICU and hospital length of stay, are lacking; however, several studies performed on animal models, healthy subjects and, more recently, ICU patients, confirm the physiological benefits of NAVA when compared with conventional modes that utilise pneumatic signals.

Technical aspects

Principles of functioning

EAdi is obtained from the crural portion of the diaphragm *via* a nasogastric or orogastric tube with an array of nine electrodes mounted at its proximal end (fig. 1). Because EAdi is acquired through the oesophagus, the risk of cross-talk from postural and expiratory muscles and the negative effects consequent to the subcutaneous layers are avoided; furthermore, changes in lung volume and chest wall configuration do not affect the quality of the signal acquired [3–5]. To reduce the influence of external noise, the measurement of muscle electrical activity is performed by bipolar differential recordings, where the signal difference between two single electrodes is measured (fig. 1). Eight differential electromyographic (EMG) signals are acquired, processed by a double subtraction technique, and displayed as four tracings on the dedicated ventilator screen named EAdi catheter positioning (fig. 2).

The signal is relayed back to the ventilator *via* a cable and module connection. A dedicated piece of software amplifies, band-pass filters and digitises the signal, removes any electrical contamination from the heart and the oesophagus, filters out the environmental noise and replaces the segments of signal presenting residual disturbances with the previously accepted values [1, 6]. At the end of this process, the raw tracings taken from the closet to the diaphragm electrode pairs are transformed into a waveform, (fig. 2 bottom trace) whose x-axis is time and y-axis is μV, and simultaneously utilised to regulate the ventilator-delivered inspiratory assistance and displayed on the ventilator screen for monitoring purposes.

In principle, peak EAdi (EAdi,peak) corresponds to the maximum activation of the muscle during inspiration, while the minimum EAdi (EAdi,min) represents the tonic activity of the diaphragm, although extremely short expiratory time and high peak values could affect this value (fig. 3).

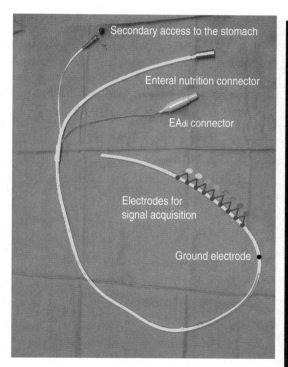

Figure 1. The neurally adjusted ventilatory assist (NAVA) catheter is a feeding tube with nine mounted electrodes and eight for signal acquisition, plus one ground electrode. The signal is fed to the ventilator through a dedicated connector (refer to text for further explanation). EAdi: electrical activity of the diaphragm.

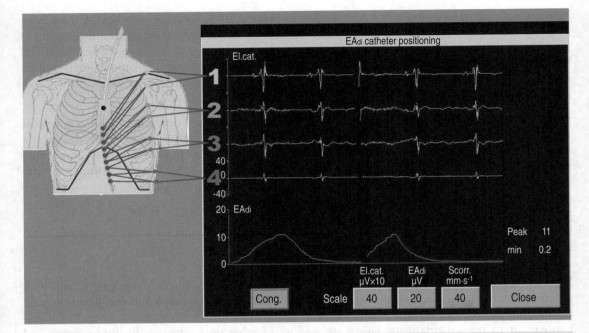

Figure 2. Four raw electromyographic (EMG) tracings, obtained from eight differential electrodes, are displayed on the dedicated ventilator screen labelled as electrical activity of the diaphragm (EAdi) catheter positioning. In the bottom part of the screen, the EMG signal from the closest pair of electrodes to the diaphragm, is transformed into a waveform whose x-axis is time and y-axis is µV (refer to text for further explanation).

With NAVA, the ventilator applies pressure to the airway opening throughout inspiration in proportion to the EAdi signal that is multiplied by an adjustable gain constant, expressed in $cmH_2O/\mu V$, referred to as the NAVA level. During inspiration airway pressure (Paw) is, therefore, instantaneously coupled to EAdi according to the following equation:

$$Paw\ (cmH_2O) = EAdi \cdot \mu V^{-1} \cdot NAVA\ level\ cmH_2O \cdot \mu V^{-1}$$

where the EAdi value multiplied by the NAVA level is $EAdi,peak$ minus $EAdi,min$.

The support delivered is constantly under the patient's control and matches their demand, provided that the respiratory centres, phrenic nerves and the neuromuscular junctions are intact, and the drive to breathe is not suppressed [3].

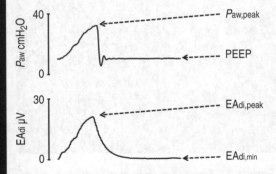

Figure 3. Airway pressure (Paw) and the electrical activity of the diaphragm (EAdi) tracings are shown from the top to the bottom. Paw is instantaneously coupled to EAdi throughout inspiration (refer to text for further explanation). PEEP: positive end-expiratory pressure.

EAdi catheter positioning

The NAVA catheter is a modified nasogastric or orogastric tube that can be used as a normal feeding tube for enteral nutrition and is available in various sizes from newborn to adult. An array of nine electrodes (plus one for the ground signal) is situated at the distal end of the catheter (fig. 1), which has to be placed nearby the crural portion of the diaphragm. Correct positioning is obtained in most cases following the instructions depicted in table 1.

BARWING *et al.* [7] found that EAdi catheter placement, based only on xiphoid-ear-nose distance, allowed adequate positioning in 18 out of 25 patients. The additional tools provided on the

Table 1. Sequence of key actions for electrical activity of the diaphragm (EAdi) catheter positioning

1) Measure the xiphoid-ear-nose distance by means of the graduated scale on the catheter and mark it (nasal insertion only)
2) Put the catheter in saline water
3) Insert the catheter 5–10 cm beyond the measure obtained at the point 1
4) Confirm the position of the catheter tip in stomach appreciating the borborygmi obtained with a syringe insufflation of 50–60 cm^3 of air
5) Connect the catheter to the dedicated cable
6) Select on the ventilator "EAdi catheter positioning" from the menu "Neural access"
7) Observe on the ventilator screen the four tracings, each coming from a couple of paired electrodes, which displays the ECG signal (white colour). Raw electromyogram signal is simultaneously displayed in some of the tracings (blue colour) (fig. 2)
8) Considering that the lowest of the four tracings displaying the raw signals on the ventilator refers to the distal couple on the catheter, pull back the catheter until:
   8.1) The P wave is evident in the upper tracing and progressively diminishes, disappearing or becoming smaller in the lower tracings
   8.2) The QRS complex progressively reduces its voltage from the highest to the lowest tracing
   8.3) The distance between the mark obtained with the aforementioned xiphoid-ear-nose measurement and the tip of the nose is ± 2 cm
   8.4) The raw (blue) EAdi signal (nasal insertion only) is visible in the second and third tracings (fig. 2)

ventilator screen were efficient and necessary to guarantee correct positioning of the EAdi catheter in all patients enrolled in their study [7]. In a more recent study, the same group demonstrated that although PEEP, body position and intra-abdominal pressure may affect EAdi catheter position, the quality of the signal was not compromised and the correct positioning was attained when utilising the dedicated tool for catheter positioning [8]. Green *et al.* [9] confirmed, in a series of 20 mechanical ventilated paediatric patients, the correct positioning of the catheter occurred when following the criteria described in table 1. The authors concluded that this approach is equivalent to standard practice for confirming gastric catheter placement and that radiographic verification may not be necessary [9].

Based on common sense, more than on specific contraindications, we suggest avoiding catheter positioning in the case of recent gastro-oesophageal surgery, recent gastro-oesophageal bleeding, oesophageal varices, recent facial trauma of maxillo-facial surgery, and severe coagulation disorders.

Setting NAVA level

How to choose the optimal NAVA level is still an open question. Colombo *et al.* [10] utilised, in the clinical setting, a ventilator function named "NAVA preview", through which, while applying other forms of ventilator support, the virtual tracing of P_{aw} was obtained by multiplying the actual EAdi by the NAVA level set on the machine. This virtual tracing (white) is overlapped on the ventilator screen on the actual P_{aw} tracing (yellow). By increasing or decreasing the NAVA level, peak P_{aw} ($P_{aw,peak}$) varies accordingly. In this manner, the NAVA level can be set to match the actual and virtual $P_{aw,peak}$ [10]. This approach is simple and overall quite straightforward; however, it does present several limitations. First, it is worth noting that this comparative approach was proposed for the purpose of matching the assistance provided using NAVA with that already applied in a pressure support ventilation (PSV) system found in a clinical setting [10]. Secondly, matching $P_{aw,peak}$ does not guarantee that the level of assistance is similar between NAVA and PSV, as the amount of support actually delivered may be substantially affected by the intra-breath P_{aw} profile. Thirdly, the wide breath-by-breath variability, commonly occurring in NAVA, may make it difficult to assess the matching P_{aw} value [10, 11]. Finally, the NAVA preview function does not consider potential variations in EAdi caused by switching from PSV to NAVA.

Following on from the work by Colombo *et al.* [10], and despite the aforementioned limitations, several investigators have utilised this method to set the NAVA level [11–15]. Alternatively, an optimal NAVA level can be found by following a titration method, this has been described by BRANDER *et al.* [16]. In addition to the tracings that are available on the ventilator screen, *i.e.* flow, volume, Paw and EAdi, the authors measured the oesophageal pressure (Poes) [16]. The optimal NAVA level was identified in 15 ICU patients, who were receiving mechanical ventilation for hypoxaemic acute respiratory failure (ARF), by considering the changes from a steep to a less steep increase in Paw and tidal volume (VT), in response to a stepwise increase in NAVA level from low to high values [16]. The authors reported that at the optimal NAVA level, in comparison with the lowest NAVA level, Poes time product (PTPoes) and EAdi values were reduced by 47% and 18% of the lowest NAVA level, respectively [16]. At the highest NAVA level, PTPoes and EAdi values were reduced by 74% and 36% of the lowest NAVA level, respectively. Based on this observation the authors concluded that the breakpoint on the Paw,peak profile identifies the adequate NAVA level [16]. Considering the difficulty of introducing such a complex technique in the clinical setting, a subsequent study was undertaken by the same group. The authors implemented a mathematical algorithm, based on a polynomial fitting model, for automatically detecting the Paw,peak breakpoint at an increasing NAVA level [17]. They found that this algorithm avoided observer-related bias and inter-individual variability [17].

Another approach for setting the NAVA level in patients being weaned off a ventilator was suggested by ROZÉ *et al.* [18]. In 15 patients, who failed a spontaneous breathing trial, the authors set the NAVA level in order to maintain EAdi, peak at approximately 60% of the value recorded when the spontaneous breathing trial failed, and found this approach feasible and well tolerated [18].

Paucity of studies, limited number of patients included in the studies, and potential confounding factors, such as the different underlying respiratory disorders, type of interface, and level of sedation, make it currently impossible to provide clear-cut indications for establishing an optimal NAVA level in a clinical setting.

NAVA in ICU

Adult ICU patients

COLOMBO *et al.* [10] compared NAVA with PSV in 14 ICU patients with ARF with varied aetiology. PSV was first set to obtain a VT of 6–8 mL·kg^{-1} with an active inspiratory effort, assessed as previously described [19]. NAVA was then set to match Paw,peak using specialised software on the ventilator. The level of assistance was decreased and increased by 50% for both modes. The six assist levels were applied in a random order. There was no difference in gas exchange, regardless of the mode and assist levels [10]. The differences between PSV and NAVA in breathing pattern, ventilator assistance, and respiratory drive and timing were small overall at both the target and lower assist levels [10]. However, at the higher assist level VT was greater, breathing frequency was reduced, and EAdi smaller in the PSV system when compared with NAVA. There was a mismatch between neural and flow-based timing using PSV, but not with NAVA [10]. The rate of asynchronous events (*i.e.* ineffective efforts) exceeded 10% in five (36%) and no (0%) patients with PSV and NAVA, respectively [10]. Breathing pattern variability was always higher in NAVA when compared with PSV. In contrast, EAdi variability was similar at the lowest level of assistance between the two modes, and showed a significant increase when augmenting the support level in PSV, but not NAVA [10].

Similar results were obtained a few years later in 14 nonsedated invasively ventilated patients, 12 of whom had chronic obstructive pulmonary disease (COPD) [12]. Two levels of PSV, *i.e.* lowest tolerable and +7 cmH$_2$O, were matched using Paw,peak with two NAVA levels. Arterial blood gases were no different; the pattern of breathing was similar at the low levels of assistance, while at the higher support level VT was significantly greater and respiratory rate reduced in PSV, as opposed to NAVA [12]. On–off triggering performance was improved with NAVA when compared with PSV, regardless of the assistance level. Ineffective efforts never occurred with NAVA, while at the higher level of assistance, they were observed in six patients during PSV.

In 22 intubated COPD patients, PIQUILLOUD et al. [15] confirmed that NAVA, when compared with PSV, reduced trigger delay, inspiratory time in excess, and patient–ventilator asynchronies. Although the number of patients with an asynchrony index exceeding 10% were 50% less with NAVA than with PSV, the incidence of double triggering was higher in NAVA than with PSV. In a crossover study, COISEL et al. [11] investigated 12 post-surgical patients undergoing 24 hours of PSV and NAVA in random order and found higher arterial oxygen tension/inspiratory oxygen fraction ($P_{a,O_2}/F_{I,O_2}$) with NAVA when compared with PSV and attributed this improvement to the higher breathing pattern variability [11]. TERZI et al. [14] found in acute respiratory distress syndrome (ARDS) patients that NAVA, contrary to PSV, was associated with stable V_T and a negligible occurrence of asynchrony when increasing the assistance level.

KARAGIANNIDIS et al. [20] described a series of six patients ventilated with NAVA, while undergoing extracorporeal membrane oxygenation (ECMO). V_T ranged from 2 to 5 mL·kg^{-1} of the predicted body weight on ECMO, and increased up to 8 mL·kg^{-1} when ECMO was inactivated. When the ECMO gas flow was decreased, the ventilator response rapidly occurred and patients were able to regulate arterial carbon dioxide tension (P_{a,CO_2}) to maintain pH at physiologic values [20].

PASSATH et al. [13] evaluated the impact of different PEEP levels on respiratory muscle load and function in 20 intubated patients ventilated with NAVA. Once the adequate NAVA level was identified, based on the P_{aw} and V_T response to systematic increases in the NAVA level, the PEEP level was set at 20 cmH_2O, which was then decreased stepwise by 1 cmH_2O [13]. By reducing PEEP levels the authors observed that EAdi increased by 34%; the value of P_{aw} above PEEP also increased from 8.5 cmH_2O (range 6.7–11.4 cmH_2O) to 12.2 cmH_2O (range 8.8–16.7 cmH_2O), whereas the V_T and respiratory rate remained unchanged [13].

TUCHSCHERER et al. [21] found that EAdi was preserved enough to titrate and implement NAVA in most of the patients with critical illness-associated polyneuromyopathy. In a randomised cross-over study on 14 conscious, nonsedated mechanically ventilated adults, DELISLE et al. [22] compared the effects of NAVA and PSV on sleep. The authors found that the rapid eye movement (REM) phase of sleep during NAVA was increased (16.5%; range 13–29%) with respect to PSV (4.5%; range 3–11%); on the contrary, the sleep fragmentation index (arousals per hour mean $\pm$ SD) was 40$\pm$20 and 16$\pm$9 with PSV and NAVA, respectively [22].

CAMMAROTA et al. [23] recently compared NAVA with PSV in delivering noninvasive ventilation by helmet in 10 patients with post-extubation hypoxaemic ARF. PSV, NAVA and PSV again were applied, in sequence, to all patients. Gas exchange, breathing pattern and neural effort were similar with the two modes. Compared with PSV, NAVA reduced the inspiratory trigger delay and increased the time during which the diaphragm and the ventilator were acting in phase [23]. The asynchrony index exceeded 10% in 70% and 80% of patients in the first and second PSV trial, respectively, while no patient reached that threshold with NAVA (p<0.001 NAVA versus first and second PSV trial) [23].

Paediatric ICU patients

BECK et al. [24] compared invasive and noninvasive NAVA with PSV or PSV+guaranteed volume, in seven low birth weight infants and found ineffective efforts during conventional ventilation, but not with NAVA. The synchrony with NAVA was maintained while ventilating the patients with the leaky interface [24]. More recently, CLEMENT et al. [25] compared NAVA with volume support in infants with bronchiolitis (aged 1.6$\pm$1.0 months) in a crossover designed study and found that the inspiratory trigger function and ventilator response were improved with NAVA, as opposed to volume support. ALANDER et al. [26] evaluated in 18 paediatric patients, aged from 30 weeks to 16 years, the effect of different triggers on patient–ventilator interaction and reported that NAVA improved patient–ventilator synchrony, without affecting arterial blood gases (ABGs) and V_T.

Recently, COLOMBO et al. [27] presented preliminary data on eight consecutive premature infants ventilated with both NAVA and pressure regulated volume control (PRVC) for 12 hours. Contrary to PRVC, when NAVA was used no asynchrony occurred [27]. Moreover, patient–ventilator interaction and oxygenation was found to have improved with NAVA, as opposed to PRVC [27].

Conclusions

The concept of driving the ventilator through an EAdi is extremely exciting. In the last few years several physiological studies have shown the benefits of NAVA, when compared with the conventional pneumatically driven modes (primarily PSV). NAVA was proven to improve patient–ventilator interaction and eliminate, or at least reduce to a remarkable extent, any asynchronies. It was confirmed that under NAVA the patient retained control of their breathing pattern, which is naturally more variable. This variability might determine an improved oxygenation in patients with acute lung volume reduction. Because V_T is not remarkably increased when augmenting the NAVA level, this novel mode might represent a means to maintain protective ventilation in a spontaneously breathing patient. Whether these physiological advantages translate into an improved outcome remains to be proven.

Statement of interest

P. Navalesi has received a fee for speaking from Maquet Critical Care. Maquet Critical Care provided material for research purposes.

References

1. Sinderby C, Navalesi P, Beck J, et al. Neural control of mechanical ventilation in respiratory failure. Nat Med 1999; 5: 1433–1436.
2. Lourenço RV, Cherniack NS, Malm JR, et al. Nervous output from the respiratory center during obstructed breathing. J Appl Physiol 1966; 21: 527–533.
3. Navalesi P, Costa R. New modes of mechanical ventilation: proportional assist ventilation, neurally adjusted ventilatory assist, and fractal ventilation. Curr Opin Crit Care 2003; 9: 51–58.
4. Beck J, Sinderby C, Lindström L, et al. Effects of lung volume on diaphragm EMG signal strength during voluntary contractions. J Appl Physiol 1998; 85: 1123–1134.
5. Beck J, Sinderby C, Weinberg J, et al. Effects of muscle-to-electrode distance on the human diaphragm electromyogram. J Appl Physiol 1995; 79: 975–985.
6. Sinderby C, Beck J, Spahija J, et al. Inspiratory muscle unloading by neurally adjusted ventilatory assist during maximal inspiratory efforts in healthy subjects. Chest 2007; 131: 711–717.
7. Barwing J, Ambold M, Linden N, et al. Evaluation of the catheter positioning for neurally adjusted ventilatory assist. Intensive Care Med 2009; 35: 1809–1814.
8. Barwing J, Pedroni C, Quintel M, et al. Influence of body position, PEEP and intra-abdominal pressure on the catheter positioning for neurally adjusted ventilatory assist. Intensive Care Med 2011; 37: 2041–2045.
9. Green ML, Walsh BK, Wolf GK, et al. Electrocardiographic guidance for the placement of gastric feeding tubes: a pediatric case series. Respir Care 2011; 56: 467–471.
10. Colombo D, Cammarota G, Bergamaschi V, et al. Physiologic response to varying levels of pressure support and neurally adjusted ventilatory assist in patients with acute respiratory failure. Intensive Care Med 2008; 34: 2010–2018.
11. Coisel Y, Chanques G, Jung B, et al. Neurally adjusted ventilatory assist in critically ill postoperative patients: a crossover randomized study. Anesthesiology 2010; 113: 925–935.
12. Spahija J, de Marchie M, Albert M, et al. Patient-ventilator interaction during pressure support ventilation and neurally adjusted ventilatory assist. Crit Care Med 2010; 38: 518–526.
13. Passath C, Takala J, Tuchscherer D, et al. Physiologic response to changing positive end-expiratory pressure during neurally adjusted ventilatory assist in sedated, critically ill adults. Chest 2010; 138: 578–587.
14. Terzi N, Pelieu I, Guittet L, et al. Neurally adjusted ventilatory assist in patients recovering spontaneous breathing after acute respiratory distress syndrome: physiological evaluation. Crit Care Med 2010; 38: 1830–1837.
15. Piquilloud L, Vignaux L, Bialais E, et al. Neurally adjusted ventilatory assist improves patient-ventilator interaction. Intensive Care Med 2011; 37: 263–271.
16. Brander L, Leong-Poi H, Beck J, et al. Titration and implementation of neurally adjusted ventilatory assist in critically ill patients. Chest 2009; 135: 695–703.
17. Ververidis D, Van Gils M, Passath C, et al. Identification of adequate neurally adjusted ventilatory assist (NAVA) during systematic increases in the NAVA level. IEEE Trans Biomed Eng 2011; 58: 2598–2606.

18. Rozé H, Lafrikh A, Perrier V, *et al.* Daily titration of neurally adjusted ventilatory assist using the diaphragm electrical activity. *Intensive Care Med* 2011; 37: 1087–1094.

19. Foti G, Cereda M, Banfi G, *et al.* End-inspiratory airway occlusion: a method to assess the pressure developed by inspiratory muscles in patients with acute lung injury undergoing pressure support. *Am J Resp Crit Care Med* 1997; 156: 1210–1216.

20. Karagiannidis C, Lubnow M, Philipp A, *et al.* Autoregulation of ventilation with neurally adjusted ventilatory assist on extracorporeal lung support. *Intensive Care Med* 2010; 36: 2038–2044.

21. Tuchscherer D, Z'Graggen WJ, Passath C, *et al.* Neurally adjusted ventilatory assist in patients with critical illness-associated polyneuromyopathy. *Intensive Care Med* 2011; 37: 1951–1961.

22. Delisle S, Ouellet P, Bellemare P, *et al.* Sleep quality in mechanically ventilated patients: comparison between NAVA and PSV modes. *Ann Intensive Care* 2011; 1: 42.

23. Cammarota G, Olivieri C, Costa R, *et al.* Noninvasive ventilation through a helmet in postextubation hypoxemic patients: physiologic comparison between neurally adjusted ventilatory assist and pressure support ventilation. *Intensive Care Med* 2011; 37: 1943–1950.

24. Beck J, Reilly M, Grasselli G, *et al.* Patient-ventilator interaction during neurally adjusted ventilatory assist in low birth weight infants. *Pediatr Res* 2009; 65: 663–668.

25. Clement KC, Thurman TL, Holt SJ, *et al.* Neurally triggered breaths reduce trigger delay and improve ventilator response times in ventilated infants with bronchiolitis. *Intensive Care Med* 2011; 37: 1826–1832.

26. Alander M, Peltoniemi O, Pokka T, *et al.* Comparison of pressure-, flow-, and NAVA-triggering in pediatric and neonatal ventilatory care. *Pediatr Pulmonol* 2012; 47: 76–83.

27. Colombo D, Alemani M, Gavelli F, *et al.* Long term physiologic effects of neurally adjusted ventilatory assist (NAVA) *versus* pressure regulated volume control (PRVC) in premature infants. *Intensive Care Medicine* 2011; 37: Suppl. 1, S188.

Chapter 9

Helium as a therapeutic gas: an old idea needing some new thought

J. Carr, B. Jung, G. Chanques and S. Jaber

Summary

First described in the 1930s', there is a good theoretical rationale for using helium as an adjuvant treatment in the respiratory care of patients with severe airway obstruction. Pure helium has been replaced in clinical practice by "helium–oxygen" mixtures that are safer to use. Helium has no pharmacological effect. The physical properties of this light, single-element gas allow mechanical and physiological effects on the respiratory system that can be used in asthma and chronic obstructive pulmonary disease patients. Helium–oxygen can be used in different conditions (*e.g.* spontaneous ventilation, noninvasive ventilation (NIV) or mechanical ventilation) and with different aims (to increase drug delivery in bronchodilator aerosols, to decrease work of breathing, and to decrease ventilation pressures and air trapping during mechanical ventilation). The clinical success of helium treatment probably depends on technical conditions and devices. In the absence of adapted medical devices it is often used only as a last resort in critical patients. With more information, adapted equipment and experienced intensive care unit teams, more patients could potentially benefit from this very old therapeutic gas.

Keywords: Airway flow, airway obstruction, driving gas, heliox, helium, ventilation

*Intensive Care Unit, Anaesthesia and Critical Care Department B, Saint Eloi Teaching Hospital, Equipe soutenue par la Région et l'Institut National de la Santé et de la Recherche Médicale 25, Université Montpellier 1, Centre Hospitalier Universitaire Montpellier, Montpellier, France.

Correspondence: S. Jaber, Intensive Care Unit, Anaesthesia and Critical Care Department B, University Montpellier 1; 80 avenue Augustin Fliche, 34295 Montpellier, Cedex 5, France.
Email s-jaber@chu-montpellier.fr

Eur Respir Mon 2012; 55: 124–132.
Printed in UK – all rights reserved
Copyright ERS 2012
European Respiratory Monograph
ISSN: 1025-448x
DOI: 10.1183/1025448x.10002111

Helium is a mono-atomic gas that is chemically inert because its filled valence orbitals mean that it is less able to interact with other compounds [1]. Unlike xenon, another noble gas, it has no anaesthetic properties and is generally considered by clinicians to be medically inert. Its usual medical applications are linked to the physical properties of helium gas with clinically negligible cellular effects. Helium–oxygen mixtures have no pharmacological effects and the only therapeutic benefits are related to its physical properties. This is why helium–oxygen should only be considered as a symptomatic treatment and why it can be used as a "bridge therapy" or for "gaining time" while waiting for the effects of the aetiological treatment (*i.e.* antibiotherapy, bronchodilator, steroids, *etc.*).

Helium is used in respiratory care for its physical properties of lesser density and higher viscosity than air with clinically relevant reduction of resistance to gas flow in the airways. It is this last approach that was first described more than 70 years ago [2, 3] and is still of clinical relevance despite persistent technical and practical difficulties. Another well-described application of helium–oxygen is deep sea scuba diving with the same physical rationale of reducing the viscosity of breathing gas in conditions of extreme pressure, thus pushing the limits of depth accessible to human divers. Among the many described potential applications, optimisation of aerosol drug particle delivery, acute respiratory distress in asthma and chronic obstructive pulmonary disease (COPD) appear especially promising. Nevertheless, practical difficulties and lack of controlled randomised clinical trials mean that the place of helium in respiratory care remains controversial. As a result, using helium as a therapeutic gas has never been validated by clinical recommendations [4].

Physical properties and physiological effects of helium

Effects on airway resistance

Helium has a molecular weight of 4 $g \cdot mol^{-1}$ and the lowest melting and boiling points of all elements. It has a much lower density compared with oxygen and nitrogen and higher viscosity as shown in table 1. In the airways, a less dense and more viscous gas, such as a helium–oxygen mixture (heliox), decreases airway resistance in zones of turbulent flow and favours laminar gas flow [5]. This can be demonstrated using Reynolds number which predicts the nature of gas flow. Reynolds number is proportional to the density of the gas and flow rate and inversely proportional to the radius of the tube the gas flows through and to its viscosity [6]. Nevertheless, the density of inhaled gas mixture increases and its viscosity decreases with the proportion of oxygen necessary to ensure patient oxygenation. Thus, the benefit of helium–oxygen mixtures may well be decreased in severe hypoxaemic patients.

Helium also has higher thermal conductivity and may increase heat loss. In clinical practice in adults, this effect is negligible but it may become significant in infants. Helium has low solubility in fat. Thus, unlike xenon, it has no anaesthetic properties, with anaesthetic potency being correlated to water–fat partition coefficient [5].

Application in respiratory care

The physical and mechanical properties of helium on gas flow in the airway of distressed patients can be used in several ways. Helium–oxygen will flow faster than air mixed with oxygen through a smaller opening or airway both in the case of upper or lower airway obstruction and also through medical devices such as nebulisers with a more laminar flow [6].

Spontaneously ventilating patients by reducing airway resistance and work of breathing it may relieve, at least partially, dyspnoea and prevent respiratory exhaustion and acidosis until standard bronchodilator and corticosteroid treatments have time to take effect. This was first described in upper airway obstruction (laryngitis and croup) and may still be used as bridge therapy until either medical or surgical (tracheotomy) resolution of the obstruction [7].

Lower airway obstructive diseases, asthma or acquired COPD are now the best described indications of helium–oxygen in adult and paediatric patients [8] to reduce work of breathing and improve gas exchanges [9, 10].

In intubated patients, lower airway resistance will help reduce the pressure required to adequately ventilate a patient with severe obstruction

Table 1. Density and viscosity of helium and helium–oxygen mixture compared to air and oxygen

	Density $g \cdot m^{-3}$	Viscosity µP
Air (80% N/20% O_2)	1.293	188.5
Oxygen	1.429	211.4
Helium	0.179	201.8
Helium–oxygen (80% He/20% O_2)	0.429	203.6

associated with conventional therapy [11]. Reducing total pressure for a given volume will prevent ventilator-related lung injury, and better minute volume ventilation for a given inspiratory pressure will help control respiratory acidosis in hypercapnic asthma or COPD patients.

Recognised clinical indications

No formal recommendations have been formulated for the use of helium gas in clinical routine but, nevertheless, the theoretical rationale in case of airway obstruction is solid and some indications have been fairly well described in small trials and in case reports, both in adult and paediatric patients.

Severe acute asthma resistant to standard therapy

Severe acute asthma was one of the first indications suggested for helium–oxygen and has been described in several case reports [12–15]. Some small clinical trials combining helium–oxygen with standard therapy showed reversal of acidosis and no adverse effects.

Although it is a generally accepted concept that the objective of severe acute asthma treatment in emergency room and intensive care units (ICUs) is to avoid intubation at all cost, the role of helium–oxygen in reducing work of breathing and increasing aerosol potency remains controversial. It is often described as a last resort when faced with an unstable patient but may have a role as "bridge therapy" to enable bronchodilators and corticosteroids to reach maximum effect without resorting to mechanical ventilation. Difficulty in defining the role of helium in the treatment of severe acute asthma before tracheal intubation may be due to practical difficulties, which will be described later along with limited clinical data from large randomised trials [9, 10, 16].

Once an unstable asthma patient has been intubated, helium–oxygen may also be suggested to reduce airway resistance, ventilation pressure and air trapping with the same theoretical substratum as before. As it is a rare and often critical situation, the literature is limited to case reports of helium as rescue therapy, combined with standard therapy and ventilation or associated with sevoflurane continuous sedation (AnaConDa®; Sedana Medical, Uppsala, Sweden) [17] or with nitrogen protoxide [18]. Efficacy of helium–oxygen in severe hypoxaemic patients will be limited by a necessarily higher inspiratory oxygen fraction (F_{I,O_2}) leading to greater density of the gas mixture because of a lesser proportion of helium.

To date, there is no convincing data in favour of systematic administration of helium–oxygen for severe acute asthma, as confirmed by recent meta-analysis. Interestingly, no data are available regarding the combined use of helium–oxygen and noninvasive ventilation (NIV) in severe acute asthma.

Helium–oxygen instead of air or oxygen as the driving gas improves bronchodilator aerosol delivery to the smaller airways. Drug particles will be carried deeper into the distal airways by improved flow speed and more laminar flow through the most obstructed airways. This indication has recently been studied in children with moderate-to-severe asthma in a randomised controlled clinical trial [8], with favourable clinical results. Nevertheless, results of randomised trials are disparate [19, 20] and do not allow conclusion in favour of a certain clinical benefit [9].

Acute respiratory distress in COPD

Another clinical setting for the potential benefit of the physical properties of helium is COPD, with the same rationale for reducing work of breathing when associated with standard therapy. As well as bridge therapy and aerosol therapy in spontaneous ventilation, and rescue therapy in the most severe intubated patients, using helium has also been described in association with noninvasive positive-pressure ventilation and for weaning of prolonged artificial ventilation.

Artificial ventilation with helium–oxygen

Helium–oxygen will improve airway flow both during inspiration and expiration. In acute COPD patients with severe thoracic hyperinflation more laminar flow and less resistance should reduce air trapping through improved expiratory flow, thus reducing work of breathing in spontaneous ventilation and intrinsic positive-end expiratory pressure in ventilated patients without any undesirable haemodynamic side-effects. Several recent randomised trials and reviews have addressed the issue of helium–oxygen for exacerbated COPD making it one of the better studied and described indications. Nevertheless, it still cannot be recommended as standard of care, as existing data shows small trends favouring helium but no significant difference of outcome or even intubation rate [6, 9].

NIV with helium–oxygen

NIV is routinely used to treat exacerbated COPD, particularly in the case of hypercarbia and respiratory acidosis. The rationale is that it improves alveolar ventilation and carbon dioxide elimination correcting acidosis and also reduces work of breathing allowing many patients to avoid tracheal intubation. Breathing helium–oxygen mixtures, by reducing airway resistance and hyperinflation, could be expected to further help achieve these two goals. This hypothesis has been positively tested in physiological studies. Clinical trials have shown better carbon dioxide elimination and reduced dyspnoea in exacerbated COPD treated with NIV [21, 22]. Unfortunately, randomised controlled trials, including one recent multicentre trial of 204 patients with known or suspected COPD have failed to show a significant difference in NIV failure (need for intubation after initial attempt at NIV treatment) or clinical outcome using 65% helium and 35% oxygen [23]. Recently, stable, severe obstructive chronic respiratory patients receiving a combination of NIV with helium–oxygen during exercise training were studied, highlighting another possible future application outside of the ICU [24].

In the future, it will be important to consider the results of an international, ongoing, adequately powered, randomised clinical trial to better define the impact of helium–oxygen on outcome, not only in combination with NIV, but also during the NIV free periods of spontaneous breathing (NCT01155310; www.ClinicalTrials.gov).

Helium–oxygen to assist prolonged weaning

Reduced work of breathing and air trapping during mechanical ventilation weaning with helium–oxygen have also been described in cases of difficult prolonged weaning of ventilation [25, 26] and after extubation associated with NIV [27].

Upper airway obstruction

One of the very first indications for helium–oxygen breathing described in medical literature is upper airway obstruction in children, such as croup. Croup is usually triggered by viral infection with upper airway inflammation leading to a reduced diameter, which may cause acute respiratory distress. Helium–oxygen is still regularly described as bridge therapy until corticosteroid treatment becomes effective. Recent literature reviews and Cochrane database searches have failed to conclude in favour of a clinical benefit of helium–oxygen, possibly because of lack of well-powered trials [28, 29].

It has since been suggested in post-extubation laryngeal oedema with respiratory distress to avoid re-intubation. Lesser density could result in a more laminar flow through a constricted larynx. Once again, this would be a "bridge" until the effect of corticosteroid treatment is achieved [7, 27].

New perspectives

Experimental *in vitro* and *in vivo* data has shown other potential properties of helium. In animal models of cardiac ischaemia–reperfusion, halogenated fluorocarbons (commonly used anaesthetic gases such as desflurane and sevoflurane) have shown cardio-protective effects after preconditioning [5]. Experimental data suggests similar protective effects of helium for preconditioning before an ischaemia–reperfusion procedure on both cardiac and on neurological tissue. Helium is the first non-anaesthetic gas to induce organ protection (early preconditioning) that could be used safely in patients experiencing ischaemic periods but not undergoing anaesthesia. It has been suggested that the mechanism involved in organ protection is activation of multiple pathways in which reactive oxygen species, protein kinase C and various mitochondrial channels play a crucial role.

Helium has also been discussed to reduce cancer cell proliferation during laparoscopic surgery and a systemic anti-inflammatory effect has been described in healthy human volunteers [5].

Technical and practical aspects of using helium in respiratory care

The persistent controversy surrounding the use of helium–oxygen mixtures to treat critically ill patients is probably linked to lack of conclusive literature and lack of experience of many clinicians regarding this gas. Although almost no serious adverse events have recently been described, technical difficulties and risks may be predominant in many respiratory and intensive care specialists' misgivings about using helium in routine practice [4]. Some notions of the presentations and effects of helium on medical equipment are necessary for those who choose to try it as a rescue technique or more frequently.

Presentation

Helium is provided in 50-L tanks containing a mix of helium–oxygen in varying proportions. The maximum helium content is 80% (20% O_2) providing minimum security of never administering a hypoxic gas mixture when air is replaced with helium–oxygen. Tanks containing a greater percentage of oxygen are available (70% He/30% O_2). Although a mixture of helium and oxygen will always be less dense than a mixture of oxygen and nitrogen (air) [30], it is generally accepted that a maximum of 40% oxygen is acceptable before the physical characteristics of the helium–oxygen mixture (density and viscosity) are too similar to that of air to be clinically relevant in respiratory care. As an indication, a helium–oxygen tank (78%/22%) of 50 L at 200 bar (10,000 L) costs approximately US$275.00.

Transition from compressed gas in the tank to a medical device and breathing system is obtained with a regulator. An air regulator can be screwed to the tank and then connected to the desired medical device (*e.g.* flow meter). Although standard air or oxygen regulators are often used, regulators for use with either pure helium or helium–oxygen mixtures are commercially available [31]. Performance of nonspecific medical devices with helium is a source of concern for many clinicians.

Helium–oxygen as a driving gas for aerosols

One of the most frequent and less controversial indications of helium–oxygen is use as a nebuliser driving gas for β_2-agonists. This has been demonstrated *in vitro* [32] and several trials have described practical requirements to ensure clinical benefit. Aerosol particle delivery to distal airways is increased by up to 50% regardless of which nebulisation technique is used; however, most authors insist that a higher gas flow is necessary. At the usual inspired fractions of helium (70–80%) it is recommended to set the flow rate at 15 L·min^{-1} as opposed to 6 L·min^{-1} for 100% oxygen. Large volume nebulisers may also be useful to meet the minute ventilation requirements of patients. Ideally, specific helium–oxygen nebulisers would probably best exploit the physical properties of helium–oxygen mixtures but very few hospitals are equipped, *i.e.* recommended to use helium.

When setting a flow rate it is necessary to consider the helium fraction of the driver gas. As helium–oxygen flows faster through a flow meter proportionally to helium fraction (inversely proportionally to density), the real flow rate will be greater than the set flow rate [31]. It is possible to determine helium–oxygen flow rate through a meter calibrated for oxygen using a correction factor. Clinicians must at least be aware that helium–oxygen flow rate with an air or oxygen meter will be underestimated.

Helium diffuses and "escapes" easily into room air making actual delivery of a sufficient concentration and flow to the patients' airway with standard breathing mask and nebulisers uncertain. The nebuliser-mask system should ideally be helium tight which implies less leakage [33, 34]. In the non-intubated patient this is difficult to achieve.

Helium–oxygen use with standard ventilators

Despite the advantages of a closed system, several technical problems have limited the indications of helium for artificial ventilation of intubated patients. The same physical properties helium is used for significantly disrupt the functioning of most ventilators, in particular flow meters, inspiratory and expiratory valves and, eventually, gas mixing [11]. In addition, a given ventilator may behave differently in the presence of different concentrations of helium and thus of F_{I,O_2}.

Inaccurate volume delivery in volume control mode

High thermal conductivity makes the use of hot-wire flow meters impossible and screen flow meters may underestimate flow due to lower resistances. In particular, most bench tests found either erratic tidal volume delivery or, in the best case, constant cycles but delivery of tidal volume differed from set tidal volume [35]. In this case it is possible to use a conversion factor, determined *in vitro* for each ventilator [36]. In ventilators with leak compensation, expiratory flow meter malfunction will be wrongly interpreted as leak leading to increased delivered tidal volume [11]. If possible this function should be disabled.

No monitoring of tidal and minute volume in pressure–control modes

Although inspiratory pressure will not be affected by helium ventilation [37], absence of flow meter calibrated for helium will mean erratic and unreliable tidal volume monitoring. In spontaneous breathing modes, the effect of helium on triggering has never been tested *in vitro* to our knowledge.

Inconsistent F_{I,O_2} and measurement

Typically, a tank of helium–oxygen mix (80%/20% or 70%/30%) is attached to the air inlet, and the oxygen inlet to the oxygen. The total oxygen fraction of the respiratory gas may be approximate and/or inconsistent. An oxygen module not intended for use with helium will be unable to accurately measure the F_{I,O_2} the patient is receiving [11]. In clinical conditions, carful saturation and blood gas monitoring must be obtained as minimum security but unreliable F_{I,O_2} remains worrying. In this case, adding a density independent gas monitor close to the patients seems to be a safe option.

Humidification systems

There is no data in recent literature regarding performance and choice of humidification systems for helium–oxygen breathing mixtures.

Ventilators adapted for use with helium–oxygen

Although the behaviour of some standard ventilators may be predictable in the presence of helium with the help of mathematical correction, using them in clinical practice with precise respiratory parameters to achieve a good standard of respiratory care remains complicated [36]. To our knowledge, to date there is only one validated ventilator calibrated for helium available on the market which is the Avea^{TM} (Viasys, Palm Springs, CA, USA).

Potential risks and side-effects

Helium itself has shown no undesirable effects when used on human beings, despite fairly limited clinical trials. Most potential accidents appear linked to previously discussed technical difficulties and particularly to the absence of adequate monitoring. The main pitfalls of therapeutic use of helium–oxygen mixtures are summarised in table 2.

Anoxia and hypoxia

Erratic functioning of medical devices not designed for use with helium may lead to inadequate ventilation parameters and undetected problems.

The risk of accidentally ventilating a patient with a hypoxic gas mixture will be prevented by never using a respirator with pure helium but with helium–oxygen mixtures. In the few bench tests of ventilators used with helium, results differ with some finding that delivered F_{I,O_2} deviated from set F_{I,O_2} in all tested ventilators [37]. Clinicians using standard ventilators not calibrated for helium should assume that the set F_{I,O_2} is unreliable. At best, F_{I,O_2} should be then measured by an independent gas monitor on the inspiratory branch. If this is not available the patients' saturation and blood gases must be the object of extra attention.

Hypoventilation

Erratic ventilator performance may lead to undetected insufficient minute ventilation as the set and measured parameters are unreliable. Flow meters and valves may malfunction leading to some standard ventilators stopping cycling altogether.

Volume-induced lung injury

Variation of tidal volume during helium ventilation may be either towards increased or decreased volumes. In particular, leak compensation will lead to excessively large tidal volumes and must be inactivated in the presence of helium [31].

Insufficient bronchodilator treatment

Well used helium–oxygen can increase the delivery of active drug particles to distal airways through a nebuliser. Clinicians must be attentive to sufficient gas flow (15 L·min^{-1}) to drive bronchodilator aerosols with helium–oxygen, taking into account inaccuracy of flow meters designed for air or oxygen when used with helium.

Hypothermia

Not a risk in adult patients, hypothermia has been described during hood or tent administration of helium–oxygen to pre-term infants where the whole body surface is in contact with the breathing gas

Table 2. Pitfalls with helium in adult respiratory care

Indication	Problem	Preventative action
Nebuliser/face mask	Insufficient drug delivery	Increase flow rate
		Specific helium–oxygen nebuliser
	Excessive room air leak	Large volume nebuliser
		Air-tight mask
		Specific helium–oxygen nebuliser
Noninvasive ventilation	Excessive room air leak	Air-tight mask or hood
	Erratic ventilator function	Careful monitoring
		Helium-adapted ventilator
Invasive ventilation	Incorrect tidal volume	Careful monitoring
		Disable leak compensation
		Helium-adapted ventilator
	Incorrect inspiratory oxygen fraction	Density independent gas monitor
		Helium-adapted ventilator

[31]. High thermal conductivity means adequate warming and humidification are important. When helium is used in NIV, the patients' face may feel cool if the breathing gases are insufficiently warmed.

Transporting an unstable patient

Very few evaluations of helium in a pre-hospital setting have been published. Although its effects on breathing mechanics seem interesting, out of hospital use is probably limited by tank size as well as monitoring problems. For aerosol therapy no extra risks are apparent.

No transport ventilators have been tested in the presence of helium. The possibility of hypoventilation, volume-linked lung trauma and hypoxaemia must be considered before transporting a ventilated patient using helium–oxygen. Potential benefit of reduced airway pressure for ventilation must be weighed up against the risk of "blindly" ventilating an unstable patient with almost no monitoring of ventilation parameters.

Conclusions

There is a good theoretical rationale for using helium as an adjuvant treatment in the respiratory care of patients with severe airway obstruction, as was first described in 1930. Pure helium has been replaced in clinical practice by "helium–oxygen" mixtures that are safer to use. Helium has no pharmacological effect. The physical properties of this light single element gas allow mechanical and physiological effects on the respiratory system that can be used in asthma and COPD patients. Upper airway obstruction, although the first known indication of helium in respiratory medicine, is poorly described in modern medical literature and cannot be currently recommended. Within the described indications, helium–oxygen can be used in different conditions (spontaneous ventilation, NIV or mechanical ventilation) and with different aims (to increase drug delivery in bronchodilator aerosols, decrease work of breathing in spontaneous ventilation or NIV and decrease ventilation pressures and air trapping during mechanical ventilation).

Clinical success of helium treatment probably depends on technical conditions and devices. Aerosol therapy remains relatively easy with nonspecific equipment, given a few adaptations, and carries few risks of accident. However, mechanical ventilation can be more difficult and not without risks. The clinicians' experience of using helium and the knowledge of underlying mechanisms in case of homemade adaptations of medical devices. Flow meters, nebulisers and ventilators calibrated for helium are not usually available. In case of occasional use careful monitoring is essential.

The place of helium in respiratory care remains unclear. In the absence of adapted medical devices it is often only used as a last resort in critical patients. With more information, adapted equipment and experienced ICU teams more patients could potentially benefit from this very old therapeutic gas.

Statement of interest

None declared.

References

1. Thomson E. Helium. *Science* 1927; 65: 299–300.
2. Barach AL, Eckman M. The effects of inhalation of helium mixed with oxygen on the mechanics of respiration. *J Clin Invest* 1936; 15: 47–61.
3. Doll R. Helium in the treatment of asthma. *Thorax* 1946; 1: 30–38.
4. Hurford WE, Cheifetz IM. Respiratory controversies in the critical care setting. Should heliox be used for mechanically ventilated patients? *Respir Care* 2007; 52: 582–591.
5. Oei GT, Weber NC, Hollmann MW, *et al*. Cellular effects of helium in different organs. *Anesthesiology* 2010; 112: 1503–1510.
6. Gainnier M, Forel JM. Clinical review: use of helium-oxygen in critically ill patients. *Crit Care* 2006; 10: 241.

7. Wittekamp BH, van Mook WN, Tjan DH, *et al.* Clinical review: post-extubation laryngeal edema and extubation failure in critically ill adult patients. *Crit Care* 2009; 13: 233.

8. Kim IK, Saville AL, Sikes KL, *et al.* Heliox-driven albuterol nebulization for asthma exacerbations: an overview. *Respir Care* 2006; 51: 613–618.

9. Colebourn CL, Barber V, Young JD. Use of helium-oxygen mixture in adult patients presenting with exacerbations of asthma and chronic obstructive pulmonary disease: a systematic review. *Anaesthesia* 2007; 62: 34–42.

10. Rodrigo G, Pollack C, Rodrigo C, *et al.* Heliox for nonintubated acute asthma patients. *Cochrane Database Syst Rev* 2006; 4: CD002884.

11. Venkataraman ST. Heliox during mechanical ventilation. *Respir Care* 2006; 51: 632–639.

12. Kass JE, Castriotta RJ. Heliox therapy in acute severe asthma. *Chest* 1995; 107: 757–760.

13. Manthous CA, Hall JB, Caputo MA, *et al.* Heliox improves pulsus paradoxus and peak expiratory flow in nonintubated patients with severe asthma. *Am J Respir Crit Care Med* 1995; 151: 310–314.

14. Tobias JD, Garrett JS. Therapeutic options for severe, refractory status asthmaticus: inhalational anaesthetic agents, extracorporeal membrane oxygenation and helium/oxygen ventilation. *Paediatr Anaesth* 1997; 7: 47–57.

15. Bathke P, Gallagher T. Respiratory problems in accident and emergency – the role of helium-oxygen mixtures. *Anaesthesia* 2009; 64: 576.

16. Rodrigo GJ, Rodrigo C, Pollack CV, *et al.* Use of helium-oxygen mixtures in the treatment of acute asthma: a systematic review. *Chest* 2003; 123: 891–896.

17. Nadaud J, Landy C, Steiner T, *et al.* Association helium-sevoflurane: une therapeutique de sauvetage dans l'asthme aigu grave [Helium-sevoflurane association: a rescue treatment in case of acute severe asthma]. *Ann Fr Anesth Reanim* 2009; 28: 82–85.

18. Phatak RS, Pairaudeau CF, Smith CJ, *et al.* Heliox with inhaled nitric oxide: a novel strategy for severe localized interstitial pulmonary emphysema in preterm neonatal ventilation. *Respir Care* 2008; 53: 1731–1738.

19. Dorfman TA, Shipley ER, Burton JH, *et al.* Inhaled heliox does not benefit ED patients with moderate to severe asthma. *Am J Emerg Med* 2000; 18: 495–497.

20. Rose JS, Panacek EA, Miller P. Prospective randomized trial of heliox-driven continuous nebulizers in the treatment of asthma in the emergency department. *J Emerg Med* 2002; 22: 133–137.

21. Jaber S, Fodil R, Carlucci A, *et al.* Noninvasive ventilation with helium-oxygen in acute exacerbations of chronic obstructive pulmonary disease. *Am J Respir Crit Care Med* 2000; 161: 1191–1200.

22. Jolliet P, Tassaux D, Thouret JM, *et al.* Beneficial effects of helium:oxygen *versus* air:oxygen noninvasive pressure support in patients with decompensated chronic obstructive pulmonary disease. *Crit Care Med* 1999; 27: 2422–2429.

23. Maggiore SM, Richard JC, Abroug F, *et al.* A multicenter, randomized trial of noninvasive ventilation with helium-oxygen mixture in exacerbations of chronic obstructive lung disease. *Crit Care Med* 2010; 38: 145–151.

24. Allan PF, Thomas KV, Ward MR, *et al.* Feasibility study of noninvasive ventilation with helium-oxygen gas flow for chronic obstructive pulmonary disease during exercise. *Respir Care* 2009; 54: 1175–1182.

25. Diehl JL, Mercat A, Guerot E, *et al.* Helium/oxygen mixture reduces the work of breathing at the end of the weaning process in patients with severe chronic obstructive pulmonary disease. *Crit Care Med* 2003; 31: 1415–1420.

26. Flynn G, Mandersloot G, Healy M, *et al.* Helium-oxygen reduces the production of carbon dioxide during weaning from mechanical ventilation. *Respir Res* 2010; 11: 117.

27. Jaber S, Carlucci A, Boussarsar M, *et al.* Helium-oxygen in the postextubation period decreases inspiratory effort. *Am J Respir Crit Care Med* 2001; 164: 633–637.

28. Vorwerk C, Coats TJ. Use of helium-oxygen mixtures in the treatment of croup: a systematic review. *Emerg Med J* 2008; 25: 547–550.

29. Vorwerk C, Coats T. Heliox for croup in children. *Cochrane Database Syst Rev* 2010; 2: CD006822.

30. Hess DR, Fink JB, Venkataraman ST, *et al.* The history and physics of heliox. *Respir Care* 2006; 51: 608–612.

31. Fink JB. Opportunities and risks of using heliox in your clinical practice. *Respir Care* 2006; 51: 651–660.

32. Martin AR, Ang A, Katz IM, *et al.* An *in vitro* assessment of aerosol delivery through patient breathing circuits used with medical air or a helium-oxygen mixture. *J Aerosol Med Pulm Drug Deliv* 2011; 24: 225–234.

33. Roche-Campo F, Vignaux L, Galia F, *et al.* Delivery of helium-oxygen mixture during spontaneous breathing: evaluation of three high-concentration face masks. *Intensive Care Med* 2010; 37: 1787–1792.

34. Standley TD, Smith HL, Brennan LJ, *et al.* Room air dilution of heliox given by facemask. *Intensive Care Med* 2008; 34: 1469–1476.

35. Brown MK, Willms DC. A laboratory evaluation of 2 mechanical ventilators in the presence of helium-oxygen mixtures. *Respir Care* 2005; 50: 354–360.

36. Tassaux D, Jolliet P, Thouret JM, *et al.* Calibration of seven ICU ventilators for mechanical ventilation with helium-oxygen mixtures. *Am J Respir Crit Care Med* 1999; 160: 22–32.

37. Oppenheim-Eden A, Cohen Y, Weissman C, *et al.* The effect of helium on ventilator performance: study of five ventilators and a bedside Pitot tube spirometer. *Chest* 2001; 120: 582–588.

Chapter 10

Extracorporeal membrane oxygenation

A. Zanella*, V. Scaravilli*, G. Grasselli#, N. Patroniti*,# and A. Pesenti*,#

Summary

For the last three decades, extracorporeal lung assist (ECLA) has been employed as a life-saving therapy in few highly-specialised centres. A deeper understanding of acute respiratory distress syndrome (ARDS) pathophysiology, improved technology and the positive results of recent trials have led to a reassessment of ECLA in the clinical setting. The referral and transfer of sicker patients to specialised extracorporeal membrane oxygenation (ECMO) centres has been shown to improve clinical outcome. The CESAR (conventional ventilator support *versus* extracorporeal membrane oxygenation for severe adult respiratory failure) trial was the first positive randomised controlled trial to investigate ECMO use in adult patients with ARDS. In 2009, many healthcare systems worldwide successfully faced the influenza A (H1N1) pandemic, instituting networks of specialised intensive care units (ICUs), for transfer of the sickest patients and management with ECMO. There is also an increasing interest in new and less invasive extracorporeal techniques, primarily aimed at carbon dioxide removal, which may be more widely applied in combination with a strictly protective ventilatory strategy.

Keywords: Acute respiratory distress syndrome, extracorporeal carbon dioxide removal, extracorporeal membrane oxygenation

*Dept of Experimental Medicine, University of Milan-Bicocca, and #Dept of Perioperative Medicine and Intensive Care, San Gerardo Hospital, Monza, Italy.

Correspondence: A. Pesenti, University of Milan-Bicocca, Via Cadore 48, Monza, Italy. Email antonio.pesenti@unimib.it

Eur Respir Mon 2012; 55: 133–141.
Printed in UK – all rights reserved
Copyright ERS 2012
European Respiratory Monograph
ISSN: 1025-448x
DOI: 10.1183/1025448x.10002311

Until recently, the use of extracorporeal membrane oxygenation (ECMO) in patients with acute respiratory failure (ARF) has been the prerogative of a few highly specialised centres due to technical difficulties, side-effects and a lack of strong scientific evidence. In recent years, the results of important clinical trials and the diffuse application of ECMO in patients with influenza A (H1N1)-associated ARF have given new impetus to a more widespread use of ECMO in ARF patients. Moreover, important technological and conceptual improvements have led to the development of new and less invasive extracorporeal techniques, with potential application in earlier phases of the disease.

Definitions

Extracorporeal life support (ECLS) is a generic term used to describe the application of prolonged artificial cardiac and/or respiratory support. Extracorporeal lung assist (ECLA) is a specific subset of ECLS, optimised for pulmonary function replacement. ECLA includes several techniques, based on different pathophysiological principles and with specific clinical indications (table 1): extracorporeal carbon dioxide removal ($ECCO_2R$) [1], ECMO [2], interventional lung assist (ILA) [3] and arteriovenous carbon dioxide removal ($AVCO_2R$) [4] (fig. 1). In this chapter, we will discuss the latest innovations in these techniques but will not describe the extracorporeal techniques used for cardiac support and neonatal applications.

Update on clinical applications

The interest in ECMO has increased worldwide as a result of two meaningful events: the results of the CESAR (conventional ventilator support *versus* extracorporeal membrane oxygenation for severe adult respiratory failure) trial [5] and the H1N1 pandemic [6].

The CESAR trial

A solid argument for the institution of an organised network of centres capable of ECMO support arises from the results of the CESAR trial [5]. It was the first positive randomised controlled trial (RCT) on the use of ECMO in patients with acute respiratory distress syndrome (ARDS). Two previous RCTs failed to demonstrate any advantage of ECMO over a conventional treatment strategy. The first study, by ZAPOL *et al.* [2] in 1979, was probably performed too early; ECMO was employed as a salvage procedure for the most severely hypoxaemic patients, with the aim of preserving normal blood gases while maintaining roughly unchanged, and potentially harmful, ventilatory patterns. Less than 10% of the patients survived in both arms of the study. Such results can be explained by the patient selection criteria, the use of rudimentary ECMO technology and by the fact that in 1979, the pathophysiology of ARDS was not completely understood and the concept of ventilator-induced lung injury (VILI) was as yet unknown. In addition, the second RCT [7] was performed using old technology; further, it was a single-centre trial comparing ECMO to an alternative and unconventional mode of ventilation (inverse-ratio ventilation). Patients in the ECMO group suffered from important coagulation problems that caused an elevated number of uncontrolled bleeding episodes and prompted emergency discontinuation of the bypass.

Table 1. Characteristics of different extracorporeal life support systems

	VA-ECMO	AV-ECMO	VV-ECMO	ECCO$_2$R	Low-flow ECCO$_2$R
Indications	Severe respiratory and heart failure	Severe respiratory failure	Severe respiratory failure	Severe respiratory failure	Respiratory failure
Need for blood pump	Yes	No	Yes	Yes	Yes
Blood flow L·min^{-1}	3–5	1.5#	>2.5	1–2	0.5
Cardiac support	Yes	No	No	No	No
Oxygenation	Total	Low	Total	Low	No
Carbon dioxide removal	Total	Total–partial	Total	Total–partial	Partial
Incannulation	VA	AV	VV	VV	Venous (double-lumen catheter)

VA: veno-arterial; AV: arteriovenous; VV: veno-venous; ECMO: extracorporeal membrane oxygenation; ECCO$_2$R: extracorporeal carbon dioxide removal. #: dependant on cardiac output.

The recently published CESAR study was a large and complex multicentre trial carried out by G.J. Peek and co-workers [5]. The study enrolled 180 patients from 68 UK centres, involved thousands of clinicians, and required years of planning and execution. Patients with severe but potentially reversible ARF (Murray score of at least 3 or uncompensated hypercapnia with a pH of less than 7.20) were randomised to either consideration for ECMO (which was only performed in a single ECMO-specialised centre in Leicester, UK, to which all the patients in this arm were transferred) or to conventional management (as performed at the referral

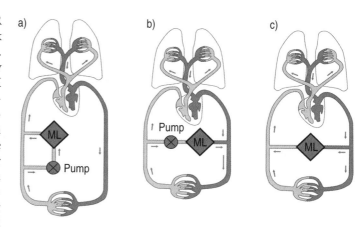

Figure 1. Schematic of possible extracorporeal membrane oxygenation (ECMO) circuitry: a) veno-venous ECMO; b) veno-arterial ECMO; c) arteriovenous ECMO. ML: membrane lung; pump: blood pump.

tertiary care hospitals). The majority of the patients in the ECMO group were treated with a veno-venous bypass *via* percutaneous cannulation. The drainage cannula was positioned in the jugular or femoral vein, while the reinfusion drain was positioned in the femoral vein. ECMO support was maximal, with extracorporeal blood flow higher than 5 L·min^{-1}; this allowed a gradual but substantial reduction of mechanical ventilation, with peak inspiratory pressure as low as 20 cmH$_2$O, a positive end-expiratory pressure (PEEP) of 10 cmH$_2$O, a respiratory rate of 10 breaths per minute and an inspiratory oxygen fraction (F_{I,O_2}) of approximately 30%. Coagulation was managed with heparin infusion to achieve an activated clotting time of between 160 and 220 seconds. The bypass was employed for 9 days on average. Investigators performed an intention-to-treat survival analysis, an evaluation of disability at 6 months and a cost analysis. The results showed a significantly improved outcome without disability at 6 months (63% *versus* 47%) in patients randomised to ECMO, with a number needed to treat (NNT) of six patients. Mortality was also lower in the ECMO group than in the conventional management group, but the study was not powered to assess this outcome and the difference was not significant. The major causes of death were respiratory failure in the control group and multiorgan failure in the ECMO group; in addition, five patients in the ECMO group died of complications related to the transport. Overall, the incidence of ECMO-related complications was low. The cost-effectiveness analysis showed a more than double cost for ECMO patients, but the lifetime-predicted cost utility was within the range considered to be cost-effective.

Two major weaknesses of this trial have been highlighted [8–13]. First, there was no specific management protocol in the conventional treatment arm of the study; the referral centres were only recommended to follow a low-volume, low-pressure ventilation strategy with a plateau pressure lower than 30 cmH$_2$O. Secondly, as the trial was an intention-to-treat study, only 68 of the 90 patients randomised to ECMO were actually treated with ECMO. For these reasons, the CESAR trial [5] could not answer the claim: "is ECMO a valuable alternative to conventional treatment in patients with severe ARF?" Nevertheless, this trial strongly pointed out that patients with severe refractory ARDS should be referred to a specialised centre capable of ECMO, as part of an integrated, strictly protective ventilatory strategy.

ECMO in H1N1

During 2009, many healthcare systems worldwide successfully faced the H1N1 pandemic, instituting networks of specialised intensive care units (ICUs) in which the sickest patients could be transferred and managed with ECMO, if necessary [14–18]. ECMO support was regionalised and patients were centralised to a few ECMO centres. Regionalisation of the ECMO service led to concentration of know-how and resources in highly specialised centres; this was associated with a reduction of complications and improvement in clinical outcome but, unavoidably, exposed the patients to the risk of transport.

A clinical example of this policy is the Italian Extracorporeal Membrane Oxygenation Network (ECMOnet) [19], instituted by the Italian Ministry of Health to fight H1N1 pandemic spread in the course of the period December 2009 to March 2010. Fourteen ICUs were selected according to their expertise in ECMO, experience in caring for ARDS patients and geographical distribution. Five of these ICUs guaranteed all inter-hospital transport. A call centre service was created to organise and redirect all requests from any hospital in Italy. Moreover, training courses were administered to all the ECMO teams. Eligibility criteria were promulgated by the Ministry of Health, who provided the following indications for ECMO: oxygenation index >30 (computed as F_{I,O_2} × mean airway pressure × 100/ arterial oxygen tension (Pa,O_2)); $Pa,O_2/F_{I,O_2}$ <70 with PEEP $\geqslant$15 cmH$_2$O (in patient already admitted to one of the ECMOnet centres); $Pa,O_2/F_{I,O_2}$ <100 with PEEP >10 cmH$_2$O (in patients still to be transferred); pH <7.25 for at least 2 hours; and haemodynamic instability.

Of the 685 H1N1 patients admitted to Italian ICUs during the winter of 2009, 153 were referred to an ECMOnet centre. Seventy-one patients were transferred by ambulance [20], helicopter [8] or aircraft [2] from a referring hospital to an ECMO centre. Sixty patients were treated with ECMO, 59 of them with a veno-venous circuit. In 28 cases, ECMO was instituted by the ECMOnet team at the local hospital and the patients were transferred while already on ECMO. No major complications were reported during transportation. The incidence of ECMO-related complications was low, with bleeding being the most important; only one death could have been directly ascribed to ECMO treatment (cerebral haemorrhage).

It is obviously impossible to predict whether the application of ECMO actually challenged the patients' clinical outcome; however, this experience shows that centralisation of most severe ARDS patients to a limited number of tertiary hospitals capable of ECMO is feasible and safe.

Recently, in a cohort study, NOAH et al. [21] compared the hospital mortality (intention-to-treat principle) of a group of patients with H1N1-related ARDS transferred for ECMO to one of the four adult ECMO centres in the UK, with matched patients who were not referred for ECMO. 80 ECMO-referred patients and 80 controls from a pool of 1,756 patients were matched using three different matching techniques (individual matching, 59 patients; propensity score matching, 75 patients; and GenMatch matching, 75 patients). Among the 80 ECMO-referred patients, 69 (86.3%) received ECMO and 22 (27.5%) died prior to discharge from the hospital. Hospital mortality for matched control patients was approximately twice that of ECMO-referred patients; this result was consistent across the three alternative matching methods. The authors concluded that for patients with H1N1-related ARDS, referral and transfer to an ECMO centre was associated with lower hospital mortality compared with matched non-ECMO-referred patients.

Evolution of technologies, techniques and knowledge

The results of the CESAR trial [5] and the work by NOAH et al. [21] are consistent with previous insights on ARDS pathophysiology (VILI concept) [22]. The most severe ARDS patients have extremely diseased lungs; hence, acceptable gas exchanges cannot be obtained with conventional mechanical ventilation without leading to structural lesions of the lung that are open to ventilation, even when a "protective" ventilatory strategy is applied.

It is reasonable to state that mechanical ventilation does not substitute lung function but simply does the respiratory muscles' job, while ECMO could be a substitute of lung function; in other words, mechanical ventilation may effectively rest the respiratory muscles but not the lung as in the way that ECMO would.

KOLOBOW and co-workers [1, 23] and GATTINONI et al. [24] introduced the concept of separately assisting the two gas exchange functions of the lung: oxygenation and carbon dioxide removal.

Oxygenation may require high levels of airway pressure or a veno-venous bypass with extracorporeal blood flow higher than 3–4 L·min^{-1}. Carbon dioxide removal may be achieved through tidal ventilation of the lungs at the expense of inducing VILI, or by use of a veno-venous bypass (ECCO$_2$R) with extracorporeal blood flow of 1–2 L·min^{-1}. Lower extracorporeal blood flows may be suitable for ECCO$_2$R of just a portion of the total carbon dioxide production of a patient.

ECCO$_2$R

Following in the path of Kolobow and Gattinoni, several new devices and technical approaches have been recently implemented to accomplish ECCO$_2$R in a way that is less invasive and has fewer side-effects [1, 23, 24].

In a recent publication, TERRAGNI et al. [25] employed a new ECCO$_2$R technique consisting of a modied continuous veno-venous haemofiltration system equipped with a membrane lung (Decap®; Hemodec, Salerno, Italy). It was used to enhance lung protection while limiting respiratory acidosis in ARDS patients in whom even a "protective" ventilation with a low tidal volume (6 mL·kg^{-1} of predicted body weight) resulted in elevated and dangerous plateau pressures. The same device was used safely and effectively in different clinical scenarios [26–29].

Thanks to new technologies, it now seems possible to treat ARDS patients with an ECCO$_2$R support associated with a really protective mechanical ventilation, or even without any form of mechanical ventilation but with some degree of continuous positive airway pressure (CPAP) and adequate FI,O_2. A new strategy could be foreseen in which selected awake, nonintubated patients would receive ECCO$_2$R and noninvasive CPAP while being treated for ARF. Such a goal may be achieved by employing a minimally invasive technology, capable of removing a substantial amount of carbon dioxide from a low extracorporeal blood flow (less than 0.5–1 L·min^{-1}). This approach may reduce the onset of VILI, ventilator-associated pneumonia, and decrease the need for sedation while allowing the patient to preserve verbal communication.

A new extracorporeal veno-venous carbon dioxide removal device (Hemolung; Alung Technologies, Pittsburg, PA, USA) is being tested on animals [30, 31] and human patients. Unlike conventional passive oxygenators, which require a pump to generate the extracorporeal blood flow, this gas exchanger drives blood flow by means of rotational motion, while increasing gas exchange efficiency.

Other new and interesting technologies, tested in animal models but not yet available for clinical application, are the intravascular systems such as the intravascular oxygenator and the Hattler catheter [32–34]. These systems are directly placed in the vena cava where they exert the gas exchange. Their efficacy is enhanced by an intravascular microaxial blood pump or by a pulsating balloon that conveys the blood flow toward the gas exchange fibres.

As most of the carbon dioxide carried in the blood is in the form of bicarbonate ions, while only physically dissolved carbon dioxide (10% of the total blood carbon dioxide content) can cross the artificial lung membranes, at least 1–2 L·min^{-1} of extracorporeal blood flow are required to remove a clinically significant amount of carbon dioxide. With the target of lowering the extracorporeal blood flow while performing an efficient ECCO$_2$R, our group recently tested two different strategies of enhanced ECCO$_2$R in an animal model, based on bicarbonate ultrafiltration and its substitution by sodium hydroxide [35] or on conversion of the bicarbonate ions into physically dissolved carbon dioxide by means of blood acidification [36]. Both techniques need further development before reaching possible clinical application.

The pumpless arteriovenous ILA

The first report on arteriovenous ECMO dates back to the 1980s [37]. Since then, the technology has evolved and the pumpless arteriovenous extracorporeal respiratory support technique, also called ILA, now has several different clinical indications, such as severe asthma, transportation of patients affected by severe ARDS, trauma, thoracic surgery, bridge to lung transplantation and as a means of achieving a protective mechanical ventilation [38–47]. Like other ECCO$_2$R strategies, the ILA technique has been recently reviewed by MIELCK and QUINTEL [48]. The system employs a simplified extracorporeal circuit with a high-performance membrane lung, which offers an exceptionally low resistance to blood flow and high gas transfer efficiency. The bypass usually connects the femoral artery to the femoral vein; hence, it is an arterio-venous shunt and does not need an extracorporeal pump to generate the blood flow. Consequently, the blood flow cannot be regulated and is governed by the mean systemic arterial pressure and the size of the arterial catheter. The cannulas are commonly inserted percutaneously using Seldinger's technique. The maximum extracorporeal blood flow that is usually achievable is 2.5 L·min^{-1}, which is certainly sufficient to obtain an appropriate carbon dioxide removal but cannot guarantee an adequate oxygenation support.

In a recent report on 90 patients, the use of ILA allowed for a reduction in the need for mechanical ventilation and ameliorated blood oxygenation [49]. The major complication reported in 22% of the patients was ischaemia of the leg distal to the site of arterial cannulation.

This technology has been employed more recently, with some technical improvements, in patients with severe H1N1-related ARF [49]. In such patients, the pumpless bypass was able to reduce carbon dioxide levels, improve pH and offer a more protective mechanical ventilation; no major complications related to the use the ILA were recorded.

During ILA support, it is mandatory to monitor limb perfusion, measuring foot temperature and pulse oximetry. For ischaemia, the prompt removal of the device can at least partially prevent permanent damage to the lower limb.

Materials

In the second half of the last century, the extracorporeal gas exchange devices that were available provided direct exposure of the blood to oxygen; this limited the usage of these devices to a few hours, due to important complications such as haemolysis, haemorrhage and thrombocytopenia. Following this, new oxygenators were introduced featuring a specialised membrane to separate blood from gases. Such membrane lungs, originally made from a spiral coil of silicon rubber as designed by KOLOBOW and BOWMAN [50], have been employed in the clinical setting for many years, especially for neonatal indications.

To increment the gas transfer properties while reducing resistance to blood flow, microporous membranes were then developed; however, their polypropylene fibres could not prevent plasma leakage [51], which limited their usage to short-term applications. This problem was recently well addressed by the introduction of microporous polymethylpentene (PMP) membranes, which offer an extremely elevated performance for several days without any plasma leakage [52–54].

Since the contact between the blood and the artificial surfaces triggers a systemic inflammatory response and activates the coagulation cascade, systemic anticoagulation remains necessary for long-term ECLA application. Thus, major bleeding remains a dreadful complication of ECLA: patients enrolled in the two aforementioned pivotal RCTs required an extremely elevated level of transfusion support (on average, more than 3.5 L blood·day^{-1}).

Today, the introduction of "biocompatible" or "heparinised" surfaces has significantly reduced anticoagulant requirements, thereby lowering the incidence of major uncontrollable bleeding episodes; nevertheless, the real clinical advantage of this very promising technology still needs to be assessed in focused clinical investigations.

A promising strategy for management of this problem may be loco-regional anticoagulation. Unfortunately, citrate loco-regional anticoagulation (which is employed with positive result during dialysis and haemofiltration) is difficult to apply in the ECMO settings, as the extracorporeal blood flows are much higher and the amount of citrate needed to obtain an effective anticoagulation exceeds the body's metabolising capacity, with the risk of dangerous citrate accumulation [55].

Finally, another important technological improvement is represented by the evolution of driving pumps for extracorporeal blood flow. The substitution of the original sub-occlusive roller pumps with less-traumatic centrifugal pumps has led to a significant reduction in the mechanical stress applied to the blood flowing through the extracorporeal circuit, with a consequent lower risk of haemolytic complications [56].

Cannulation

Today, vascular access for veno-venous ECMO in adult patients is generally obtained *via* percutaneous cannulation of two large-calibre veins, usually the internal jugular and/or femoral veins. This approach, compared with the previously used surgical cut-down, ensures reduced bleeding problems. As both cannulae are positioned within the venous system, a fraction of the extracorporeally oxygenated and decarboxylated blood may be drained once again into the extracorporeal circuit; this phenomenon is known as recirculation [57]. Recirculation obviously limits gas exchange efficiency, particularly oxygenation. Moreover, cannulation of two vessels may limit the patient's movement and nursing care. To address these issues, and following the experiences in neonates [58], several double-lumen cannulae have been designed and recently approved for adult veno-venous ECMO [59]. A double-lumen cannula has several potential advantages: 1) it avoids double-vessel cannulation; 2) it augments patient comfort; and 3) it facilitates patient movement. Fluoroscopic [60] or trans-oesophageal echographic [20, 61] guidance is needed during insertion, and perforation of the right atrium is a possible catastrophic complication. More clinical experience is needed for these devices to be recommended.

Conclusions

For the last two decades, ECLA has been considered a life-saving measure for the treatment of patients in desperate clinical conditions. Nonetheless, in light of the recent findings on ARDS pathophysiology and thanks to continuous technological improvements, clinicians might reconsider the place of extracorporeal lung support to be a mainstay in ARDS treatment.

Statement of interest

The department of A. Pesenti has received: funds for research and reimbursement for attending a symposium from Hemodec; reimbursement for attending a symposium and fees for speaking from Maquet; and consultancy agreement fees from Bellco.

References

1. Kolobow T, Gattinoni L, Tomlinson TA, *et al*. Control of breathing using an extracorporeal membrane lung. *Anesthesiology* 1977; 46: 138–141.
2. Zapol WM, Snider MT, Hill JD, *et al*. Extracorporeal membrane oxygenation in severe acute respiratory failure. A randomized prospective study. *JAMA* 1979; 242: 2193–2196.
3. Bein T, Weber F, Philipp A, *et al*. A new pumpless extracorporeal interventional lung assist in critical hypoxemia/hypercapnia. *Crit Care Med* 2006; 34: 1372–1377.
4. Conrad SA, Green R, Scott LK. Near-fatal pediatric asthma managed with pumpless arteriovenous carbon dioxide removal. *Crit Care Med* 2007; 35: 2624–2629.
5. Peek GJ, Mugford M, Tiruvoipati R, *et al*. Efficacy and economic assessment of conventional ventilatory support *versus* extracorporeal membrane oxygenation for severe adult respiratory failure (CESAR): a multicentre randomised controlled trial. *Lancet* 2009; 374: 1351–1363.
6. Bautista E, Chotpitayasunondh T, Gao Z, *et al*. Clinical aspects of pandemic 2009 influenza A (H1N1) virus infection. *N Engl J Med* 2010; 362: 1708–1719.
7. Morris AH, Wallace CJ, Menlove RL, *et al*. Randomized clinical trial of pressure-controlled inverse ratio ventilation and extracorporeal CO$_2$ removal for adult respiratory distress syndrome. *Am J Respir Crit Care Med* 1994; 149: 295–305.
8. Wallace DJ, Milbrandt EB, Boujoukos A. Ave, CESAR, morituri te salutant! [Hail, CESAR, those who are about to die salute you!]. *Crit Care* 2010; 14: 308.
9. Zwischenberger JB, Lynch JE. Will CESAR answer the adult ECMO debate? *Lancet* 2009; 374: 1307–1308.
10. Hubmayr RD, Farmer JC. Should we "rescue" patients with 2009 influenza A (H1N1) and lung injury from conventional mechanical ventilation? *Chest* 2010; 137: 745–747.

11. Park PK, Dalton HJ, Bartlett RH. Point: Efficacy of extracorporeal membrane oxygenation in 2009 influenza A(H1N1): sufficient evidence? *Chest* 2010; 138: 776–778.

12. Morris AH, Hirshberg E, Miller RR 3rd, *et al.* Counterpoint: Efficacy of extracorporeal membrane oxygenation in 2009 influenza A(H1N1): sufficient evidence? *Chest* 2010; 138: 778–781.

13. Dalton HJ, MacLaren G. Extracorporeal membrane oxygenation in pandemic flu: insufficient evidence or worth the effort? *Crit Care Med* 2010; 38: 1484–1485.

14. Davies A, Jones D, Bailey M, *et al.* Extracorporeal membrane oxygenation for 2009 influenza A (H1N1) acute respiratory distress syndrome. *JAMA* 2009; 302: 1888–1895.

15. Freed DH, Henzler D, White CW, *et al.* Extracorporeal lung support for patients who had severe respiratory failure secondary to influenza A (H1N1) 2009 infection in Canada. *Can J Anaesth* 2010; 57: 240–247.

16. Norfolk SG, Hollingsworth CL, Wolfe CR, *et al.* Rescue therapy in adult and pediatric patients with pH1N1 influenza infection: a tertiary center intensive care unit experience from April to October 2009. *Crit Care Med* 2010; 38: 2103–2107.

17. Schellongowski P, Ullrich R, Hieber C, *et al.* A surge of flu-associated adult respiratory distress syndrome in an Austrian tertiary care hospital during the 2009/2010 influenza A H1N1v pandemic. *Wiener klinische Wochenschrift* 2011; 123: 209–214.

18. Roch A, Lepaul-Ercole R, Grisoli D, *et al.* Extracorporeal membrane oxygenation for severe influenza A (H1N1) acute respiratory distress syndrome: a prospective observational comparative study. *Intensive Care Med* 2010; 36: 1899–1905.

19. Patroniti N, Zangrillo A, Pappalardo F, *et al.* The Italian ECMO network experience during the 2009 influenza A(H1N1) pandemic: preparation for severe respiratory emergency outbreaks. *Intensive Care Med* 2011; 37: 1447–1457.

20. Trimlett RH, Cordingley JJ, Griffiths MJ, *et al.* A modified technique for insertion of dual lumen bicaval cannulae for venovenous extracorporeal membrane oxygenation. *Intensive Care Med* 2011; 37: 1036–1037.

21. Noah MA, Peek GJ, Finney SJ, *et al.* Referral to an extracorporeal membrane oxygenation center and mortality among patients with severe 2009 influenza A(H1N1). *JAMA* 2011; 306: 1659–1668.

22. Tremblay LN, Slutsky AS. Ventilator-induced lung injury: from the bench to the bedside. *Intensive Care Med* 2006; 32: 24–33.

23. Kolobow T, Gattinoni L, Tomlinson T, *et al.* An alternative to breathing. *J Thorac Cardiovasc Surg* 1978; 75: 261–266.

24. Gattinoni L, Kolobow T, Tomlinson T, *et al.* Low-frequency positive pressure ventilation with extracorporeal carbon dioxide removal (LFPPV-ECCO2R): an experimental study. *Anesth Analg* 1978; 57: 470–477.

25. Terragni PP, Del Sorbo L, Mascia L, *et al.* Tidal volume lower than 6 ml·kg^{-1} enhances lung protection: role of extracorporeal carbon dioxide removal. *Anesthesiology* 2009; 111: 826–835.

26. Ruberto F, Pugliese F, D'Alio A, *et al.* Extracorporeal removal CO$_2$ using a venovenous, low-flow system (Decapsmart) in a lung transplanted patient: a case report. *Transplant Proc* 2009; 41: 1412–1414.

27. Ricci D, Boffini M, Del Sorbo L, *et al.* The use of CO$_2$ removal devices in patients awaiting lung transplantation: an initial experience. *Transplant Proc* 2010; 42: 1255–1258.

28. Moscatelli A, Ottonello G, Nahum L, *et al.* Noninvasive ventilation and low-flow veno-venous extracorporeal carbon dioxide removal as a bridge to lung transplantation in a child with refractory hypercapnic respiratory failure due to bronchiolitis obliterans. *Pediatr Crit Care Med* 2010; 11: e8–e12.

29. Iacovazzi M, Oreste N, Sardelli P, *et al.* Extracorporeal carbon dioxyde removal for additional pulmonary resection after pneumonectomy. *Minerva Anestesiol* 2011; [Epub ahead of print PMID 21602748].

30. Svitek RG, Frankowski BJ, Federspiel WJ. Evaluation of a pumping assist lung that uses a rotating fiber bundle. *ASAIO J* 2005; 51: 773–780.

31. Batchinsky AI, Jordan BS, Regn D, *et al.* Respiratory dialysis: reduction in dependence on mechanical ventilation by venovenous extracorporeal CO$_2$ removal. *Crit Care Med* 2011; 39: 1382–1387.

32. Zwischenberger JB, Tao W, Bidani A. Intravascular membrane oxygenator and carbon dioxide removal devices: a review of performance and improvements. *ASAIO J* 1999; 45: 41–46.

33. Cattaneo G, Strauβ A, Reul H. Compact intra- and extracorporeal oxygenator developments. *Perfusion* 2004; 19: 251–255.

34. Hattler BG, Lund LW, Golob J, *et al.* A respiratory gas exchange catheter: *in vitro* and *in vivo* tests in large animals. *J Thorac Cardiovasc Surg* 2002; 124: 520–530.

35. Cressoni M, Zanella A, Epp M, *et al.* Decreasing pulmonary ventilation through bicarbonate ultrafiltration: an experimental study. *Crit Care Med* 2009; 37: 2612–2618.

36. Zanella A, Patroniti N, Isgrò S, *et al.* Blood acidification enhances carbon dioxide removal of membrane lung: an experimental study. *Intensive Care Med* 2009; 35: 1484–1487.

37. Kasama A, Katada M, Koyama T, *et al.* [A simple method of extracorporeal membrane oxygenation (ECMO)-1. The effects of blood flow through the ECMO, using arterio-venous shunt on the oxygenation of arterial blood]. *Masui* 1987; 36: 1608–1615.

38. Mallick A, Elliot S, McKinlay J, *et al.* Extracorporeal carbon dioxide removal using the Novalung in a patient with intracranial bleeding. *Anaesthesia* 2007; 62: 72–74.

39. Kjaergaard B, Christensen T, Neumann PB, *et al.* Aero-medical evacuation with interventional lung assist in lung failure patients. *Resuscitation* 2007; 72: 280–285.

40. Renner A, Neukam K, Rosner T, *et al.* Pumpless extracorporeal lung assist as supportive therapy in a patient with diffuse alveolar hemorrhage. *Int J Artif Organs* 2008; 31: 279–281.

41. Twigg S, Gibbon GJ, Perris T. The use of extracorporeal carbon dioxide removal in the management of life-threatening bronchospasm due to influenza infection. *Anaesth Intensive Care* 2008; 36: 579–581.
42. Elliot SC, Paramasivam K, Oram J, *et al.* Pumpless extracorporeal carbon dioxide removal for life-threatening asthma. *Crit Care Med* 2007; 35: 945–948.
43. Zimmermann M, Philipp A, Schmid F-X, *et al.* From Baghdad to Germany: use of a new pumpless extracorporeal lung assist system in two severely injured US soldiers. *ASAIO J* 2007; 53: e4–e6.
44. McKinlay J, Chapman G, Elliot S, *et al.* Pre-emptive Novalung-assisted carbon dioxide removal in a patient with chest, head and abdominal injury. *Anaesthesia* 2008; 63: 767–770.
45. Iglesias M, Jungebluth P, Petit C, *et al.* Extracorporeal lung membrane provides better lung protection than conventional treatment for severe postpneumonectomy noncardiogenic acute respiratory distress syndrome. *J Thorac Cardiovasc Surg* 2008; 135: 1362–1371.
46. Fischer S, Hoeper MM, Bein T, *et al.* Interventional lung assist: a new concept of protective ventilation in bridge to lung transplantation. *ASAIO J* 2008; 54: 3–10.
47. Fischer S, Simon AR, Welte T, *et al.* Bridge to lung transplantation with the novel pumpless interventional lung assist device NovaLung. *J Thorac Cardiovasc Surg* 2006; 131: 719–723.
48. Mielck F, Quintel M. Extracorporeal membrane oxygenation. *Curr Opin Crit Care* 2005; 11: 87–93.
49. Johnson P, Fröhlich S, Westbrook A. Use of extracorporeal membrane lung assist device (Novalung) in H1N1 patients. *J Card Surg* 2011; 26: 449–452.
50. Kolobow T, Bowman RL. Construction and evaluation of an alveolar membrane artificial heart-lung. *Trans Am Soc Artif Intern Organs* 1963; 9: 238–243.
51. Ko WJ, Hsu HH, Tsai PR. Prolonged extracorporeal membrane oxygenation support for acute respiratory distress syndrome. *J Formos Med Assoc* 2006; 105: 422–426.
52. Shimono T, Shomura Y, Hioki I, *et al.* Silicone-coated polypropylene hollow-fiber oxygenator: experimental evaluation and preliminary clinical use. *Ann Thorac Surg* 1997; 63: 1730–1736.
53. Toomasian JM, Schreiner RJ, Meyer DE, *et al.* A polymethylpentene fiber gas exchanger for long-term extracorporeal life support. *ASAIO J* 2005; 51: 390–397.
54. Agati S, Ciccarello G, Fachile N, *et al.* DIDECMO: a new polymethylpentene oxygenator for pediatric extracorporeal membrane oxygenation. *ASAIO J* 2006; 52: 509–512.
55. Cardenas VJ, Miller L, Lynch JE, *et al.* Percutaneous benovenous CO_2 removal with regional anticoagulation in an Ovine model. *ASAIO J* 2006; 52: 467–470.
56. Yamagishi T, Kunimoto F, Isa Y, *et al.* Clinical results of extracorporeal membrane oxygenation (ECMO) support for acute respiratory failure: a comparison of a centrifugal pump ECMO with a roller pump ECMO. *Surg Today* 2004; 34: 209–213.
57. Lindstrom SJ, Mennen MT, Rosenfeldt FL, *et al.* Quantifying recirculation in extracorporeal membrane oxygenation: a new technique validated. *Int J Artif Organs* 2009; 32: 857–863.
58. Otsu T, Merz SI, Hultquist KA, *et al.* Laboratory evaluation of a double lumen catheter for venovenous neonatal ECMO. *ASAIO Trans* 1989; 35: 647–650.
59. Wang D, Zhou X, Liu X, *et al.* Wang-Zwische double lumen cannula-toward a percutaneous and ambulatory paracorporeal artificial lung. *ASAIO J* 2008; 54: 606–611.
60. Javidfar J, Wang D, Zwischenberger JB, *et al.* Insertion of bicaval dual lumen extracorporeal membrane oxygenation catheter with image guidance. *ASAIO J* 2011; 57: 203–205.
61. Dolch ME, Frey L, Buerkle MA, *et al.* Transesophageal echocardiography-guided technique for extracorporeal membrane oxygenation dual-lumen catheter placement. *ASAIO J* 2011; 57: 341–343.

Chapter 11

Extracorporeal lung support to remove carbon dioxide

P. Terragni, A. Birocco and V.M. Ranieri

Summary

Acute respiratory distress syndrome with 30–50% mortality affects approximately 150,000 patients per year and together with chronic obstructive pulmonary disease causes one in every seven deaths in the USA. Conventional mechanical ventilatory assistance, although a life-saving procedure, is itself injurious causing ventilator-induced lung injury.

The use of lung protective strategies poses challenges for patient management, motivating research for improved lung support approaches. A possible valuable strategy consists of letting the lungs rest by means of apnoeic oxygenation diffusion and extracorporeal carbon dioxide elimination.

Starting from the first approaches with oxygenators or haemodialysis to the current new and improved technologies and experiences, the use of extracorporeal gas exchange has become the key management strategy for respiratory failure, making clinicians rethink the treatment algorithm of all severe respiratory failure.

Keywords: Extracorporeal carbon dioxide removal, extracorporeal membrane oxygenation, lung support, protective ventilation, ventilator-induced lung injury

Dipartimento di Discipline Medico Chirurgiche, Università di Torino, Azienda Ospedaliero-Universitaria San Giovanni Battista di Torino, Turin, Italy.

Correspondence: V.M. Ranieri, Dept of Anesthesia and Intensive Care Medicine, University of Turin, S. Giovanni Battista Molinette Hospital, Corso Dogliotti 14, 10126 Turin, Italy.
Email marco.ranieri@unito.it

Eur Respir Mon 2012; 55: 142–152.
Printed in UK – all rights reserved
Copyright ERS 2012
European Respiratory Monograph
ISSN: 1025-448x
DOI: 10.1183/1025448x.10002411

M echanical ventilation is known to be deleterious and inadequate in some cases of severe acute respiratory distress syndrome (ARDS) [1, 2], so one possible strategy to reduce ventilator-induced lung injury (VILI) is to improve extracorporeal carbon dioxide removal ($ECCO_2R$) with or without apnoeic oxygenation. [3, 4].

An alternative form of the extracorporeal support used in cardiac surgery was represented by the empirical observation of carbon dioxide reduction during renal replacement therapy (RRT). In 1972, SHERLOCK *et al.* [5] observed transient mild hypoxaemia in patients treated with haemodialysis as a consequence of alveolar hypoventilation due to carbon dioxide removal by the haemofilter. This concept suggested that respiration could be controlled *via* an artificial kidney or an artificial lung leading the way to further development of these theories [6].

In order to increase the carbon dioxide reduction ratio from extracorporeal circuits, GILLE et al. [7] experimented with acidification of a venous blood model using aqueous polyelectrolyte solution. This concept was based on the rationale that the extracorporeal circulation removes only the dry form of carbon dioxide (dissolved carbon dioxide) while haemodialysis removes the wet form (bicarbonates) as reported by experimental data. GILLE et al. [7] developed the concept that carbon dioxide removal limiting factors are represented by the physiological low speed of dehydration and the consecutive rise in carbon dioxide concentration. This is the reason 25% of cardiac output is required to eliminate metabolic carbon dioxide production. In order to investigate less invasive extracorporeal circuits the authors experimented with solution acidification (achieved through HCl injection) to enhance carbon dioxide removal by forcing the shift to dissolved carbon dioxide equilibrium. The "in vitro" experimental setting gave good results with observed significant carbon dioxide reduction but the suspected iatrogenic injury due to acid infusion in animal models was considered a significant limiting factor.

More recently, CRESSONI et al. [8] and ZANELLA et al. [9] developed ARDS experimental models with ECCO$_2$R implementation. The former demonstrated the technical feasibility of carbon dioxide removal with a blood haemofilter and infusion of sodium hydroxide solution to replace bicarbonate. Blood ultrafiltrate containing half of the metabolic production of carbon dioxide was removed and minute ventilation ($V'E$) was lowered to less than half of its baseline value. The study gave good results in terms of acid-base equilibrium and blood gas management, but because the models were sacrificed it was not possible to discuss survival and potential toxic effects of basic fluid infusion.

ZANELLA et al. [9] proposed that blood acidification in association with extracorporeal support could enhance carbon dioxide removal. In the experimental setting, lactic acid was infused at different rates facilitating the dissociation of bicarbonate ions into dissolved carbon dioxide which was then removed by the artificial lung. The rationale is intriguing because in ARDS patients a substantial fraction of carbon dioxide production by the body can be removed through an extracorporeal membrane lung to allow effective protective ventilation, but limits imposed by the available technology are represented by the need for an extracorporeal blood flow of at least 1.5 L·minute^{-1} with large bore cannulas. The dissolved carbon dioxide can cross the artificial lung membranes and this is less than 10% of the total blood carbon dioxide content. Increasing the carbon dioxide transfer through the membrane lung may lower the demand for extracorporeal blood flow and therefore decrease the complications related to this technique. In their study, the maximum carbon dioxide removal was achieved at the highest acid infusion rate (5 mEq·minute^{-1}) and the resulting pH drop was constantly ~0.5 pH units; furthermore, adding acid to blood not only increased the carbon dioxide removal, but also buffered the respiratory alkalosis resulting in a safer level of pH at the membrane lung outlet.

Extracorporeal life support (ECLS) is a variant of cardiopulmonary bypass. Whereas cardiopulmonary bypass facilitates open-heart surgery for a limited number of hours, ECLS maintains tissue oxygenation for days to weeks in patients with life threatening respiratory or cardiac failure.

Veno-venous extracorporeal membrane oxygenation (ECMO) cannulation is used for isolated respiratory failure (tissue hypoxia secondary to hypoxaemia), whereas veno-arterial cannulation is used for cardiac failure (tissue hypoxia secondary to hypoperfusion) with or without respiratory failure.

In particular, veno-arterial ECMO for cardiopulmonary failure supports life when the native organs cannot. In cases of total support the use is time limited and systemic anticoagulation is mandatory. This extracorporeal device is not a treatment for the underlying disease but it is indicated in high mortality patients requiring physiological stabilisation and reduces the risk of iatrogenic injury. It also allows time for diagnosis, treatment and recovery from the primary disease. Total support is defined as blood flow through the circuit of 60–100 mL·kg^{-1}·minute^{-1} (entire cardiac output) [10]. Bleeding (7–34%) and thrombosis (8–17%) are the most common serious complications. All organ systems can be affected by hypoxia and hypoperfusion before and during extracorporeal life support, but the brain is particularly vulnerable to damage by each of the above mechanisms and so, in addition to haemorrhage, seizures (2–10%) and infarction (1–8%) are common complications.

In 1979, GATTINONI and co-workers [11, 12] began to explore a new way to treat ARDS, based on an approach that was called extracorporeal carbon dioxide removal and apnoeic oxygenation with "pulmonary rest". Based on the assumption that oxygenation and carbon dioxide removal require different physiological mechanisms, the authors introduced the concept of dissociating respiratory functions. In particular, with carbon dioxide complete removal in the blood through an extracorporeal circuit, the need for alveolar ventilation is overcome and the only exchanged gas is the oxygen supplied by the native lung. This is a new concept of apnoeic oxygenation. After promising results from former experiments, low-frequency positive-pressure ventilation (LFPPV) with $ECCO_2R$ was later introduced to prevent the fall in functional residual capacity (FRC) and total lung compliance in order to preserve elastic properties of the native lungs [11]. Thus, considering the feasibility and safety of the procedure, the authors indicated $LFPPV-ECCO_2R$ in cases of severe ARDS in order to prevent barotrauma by avoiding the abnormal distribution of ventilation in nonhomogeneous lung areas, to put the "lung to rest" and to foster healing of the diseased lung while maintaining a selected arterial carbon dioxide tension (Pa,CO_2) and normalising the pH into physiological range [12].

In cases of cardiac support vascular access is veno–arterial and the circuit components are selected to support a blood flow of 3 $L \cdot m^{-2} \cdot minute^{-1}$ (adults 60 $mL \cdot kg^{-1} \cdot minute^{-1}$) with a goal of venous saturation greater than 70% as a measure of adequate systemic perfusion. Considering respiratory support, membrane lung and blood flow should be capable of oxygen delivery and carbon dioxide removal at least equal to the patient's basal metabolism (adults 3 $mL \cdot kg^{-1} \cdot minute^{-1}$), usually equivalent for adults to veno-venous blood flow of 60–80 $mL \cdot kg^{-1} \cdot minute^{-1}$. Carbon dioxide removal always exceeds oxygen delivery when the circuit is planned for full support, so if the circuit is planned for carbon dioxide removal only, access can be veno-arterial, veno-venous or arteriovenous and typical blood flow is approximately 25% of cardiac output, which is sufficient to remove the carbon dioxide produced by metabolism (3–6 $mL \cdot kg^{-1} \cdot minute^{-1}$) [13]. Unfortunately, the $ECCO_2R$ system required all of the components of a standard ECMO circuit. Despite the early success shown by $ECCO_2R$, studies comparing $ECCO_2R$ with mechanical ventilation showed no difference in mortality, although the results of these studies were disappointing for some investigators, others began to look for simpler carbon dioxide removal devices that would offer the benefits of gentle ventilation without all of the ECMO or $ECCO_2R$ risks [14]. But a cornerstone of any extracorporeal circuit is its capability to generate adequate blood flow. Venous blood contains large amounts of carbon dioxide, most carried as bicarbonate ions (approximately 500 $mL \cdot L^{-1}$ of carbon dioxide under normocapnic conditions). Thus, with a blood flow through the extracorporeal circuit of 500 $mL \cdot minute^{-1}$, the tidal volume (VT) could be reduced to zero [15]. With the development of very efficient devices capable of removing a substantial amount of carbon dioxide production (30–100%) with blood flows of 250–500 $mL \cdot minute^{-1}$, we could assume the possibility of avoiding tracheal intubation, nosocomial infections and the need for sedation [16].

Looking for devices less invasive than $ECCO_2R$, two approaches derived from the RRT and from the Interventional Lung Assist (iLA) Novalung (Novalung GmbH, Hechingen, Germany) were developed. PESENTI et al. [17] suggested that $ECCO_2R$, when applied by a system comparable in complexity and invasiveness to continuous RRT, might be preferable to endotracheal intubation (ETI), mechanical ventilation and sedation and, thus, to ECMO. It allows the patient full contact with the environment, normal airway physiology and enlargement of the noninvasive ventilation (NIV) application range. Natural lung ventilation can be decreased in proportion to the amount of carbon dioxide removed by the extracorporeal device. This technique was demonstrated to be safe and feasible and in a different application of a similar device $ECCO_2R$ can be coupled with RRT in order to achieve the desired continuum in organ support [2].

A new approach is also represented by an iLA membrane lung coupled in series with a blood pump through a veno-venous vascular access. This device promises to cover a full range of respiratory support from low-flow $ECCO_2R$ (500–1,000 $mL \cdot minute^{-1}$) to full ECMO support with 4.5 $L \cdot minute^{-1}$.

Clinical trials

Over the years different studies approached the carbon dioxide removal concept: Bartlett's experience in 1993, initially reported by ANDERSON *et al.* [18], demonstrated a 47% survival in adults with severe acute respiratory failure (ARF). In a retrospective review, KOLLA *et al.* [19] described their experience with ECLS in 100 adult patients with severe ARF to define techniques, efficacy and analyse outcome predictors. The duration of ECLS was 11 ± 10 days and overall hospital survival was 54%. The main group of patients presented with hypoxaemic ARF with a ratio of arterial oxygen concentration to the fraction of inspired oxygen ($Pa,O_2/FI,O_2$) of 55.7 ± 15.9 supported with veno-venous percutaneous access; only a small number of patients enrolled presented with hypercapnic ARF or the need for arteriovenous access.

In the first trials in the 1970s, only 10% of ARF patients with ECMO support survived, this rose to 49% in 1986 using new techniques with low-flow and veno–venous vascular access. The report changed the worldwide practice of mechanical ventilation by identifying the beneficial effects of "resting" the lung from high pressure and high-inspired oxygen, and relying on the native lung for oxygenation [3, 4].

In 1993, BRUNET *et al.* [20] used LFPPV-ECCO$_2$R to improve oxygenation in ARDS patients who did not respond favourably to mechanical ventilation, avoiding pulmonary over-inflation and barotrauma; they achieved a mortality rate of 50%.

Despite these hopeful results, in 1994, MORRIS *et al.* [21] presented results from a randomised clinical trial of pressure-controlled inverse-ratio ventilation *versus* ECCO$_2$R in ARDS patients. The trial showed no significant difference in survival (38%) between the two groups. Even though the observed mortality rate was lower than expected, several episodes of severe bleeding were reported due to the complexity of technical equipment and the need for major anticoagulation with consequent haemorrhagic complications.

At the end of the 1990s there was a decrease in enthusiasm for ECLS and a need for technological innovation. New theoretical assumptions about VILI will open the way in the 2000s for protective low V_T ventilation theories in severe ARDS patients and the necessity for new implemented lung support technologies [2].

VILI: new concepts of treatment in mechanical stress

Mechanical ventilation is a supportive and life-saving therapy in patients with ARDS. Despite advances in critical care, mortality remains high. Since the first report by GREENFIELD *et al.* [22] demonstrated that mechanical ventilation with large V_T and pressures alters the surface properties of canine lung extracts, it became obvious in both *in vitro* and *in vivo* studies that although mechanical ventilation is a life-saving tool in patients with ARDS, it can aggravate pre-existing or even cause *de novo* lung injury. For almost two decades, ARDS was considered a homogeneous process associated with relatively uniform lung injury. Quantitative assessment of chest computed tomography (CT) images, however, revealed that the ARDS lung consisted of normally aerated, poorly aerated and non-aerated tissue, and the amount of normally aerated tissue was roughly equivalent to that of a healthy male child aged 5 or 6 years (hence the introduction of the baby lung concept) [23, 24]. The use of low V_T and limited inspiratory plateau pressure (P_{plat}) has been proposed to prevent lung as well as distal organ injury [1]. However, the reduction in V_T may result in alveolar derecruitment, cyclic opening and closing of atelectatic alveoli and distal small airways leading to VILI if inadequate low positive end-expiratory pressure (PEEP) is applied. Mechanical ventilation can be a powerful inflammatory stimulus and VILI has been the object of extensive research.

In acute lung injury (ALI), metabolic activity can be measured by positron-emission tomography (PET) imaging of ^{18}F-fluoro-2-deoxy-D-glucose as an estimate of the intensity of inflammation. If CT scans allow for the measurement of regional aeration and changes induced by mechanical ventilation, PET can detect the presence of metabolically active inflammatory cells, including neutrophils, which have been shown to be primary effectors of VILI. The main finding demonstrated that Pplat was significantly correlated with metabolic activity of the whole lung and the correlation was even stronger for the normally aerated tissue, whereas for poorly aerated tissue it was weaker. Interestingly, the correlation increased steeply above 26 to 27 cmH$_2$O of Pplat [25].

Thus, confirming that Pplat lower than 26 cmH$_2$O is associated with a lower degree of mechanical stress, reducing Pplat below the threshold of 26 cmH$_2$O with the implementation of ECCO$_2$R may enhance lung protection and reduce mortality [1, 2].

Carbon dioxide removal technology

ECCO$_2$R technologies can be classified according to their ability to support total or partial respiratory exchange (table 1).

It is therefore possible to identify two different categories of devices: 1) total extracorporeal support (ECMO) with veno-venous devices (blood flow 2–5 L·minute^{-1}) and veno-arterial devices (blood flows equal to entire cardiac output); and 2) partial extracorporeal support (ECCO$_2$R) with pumpless devices with arteriovenous bypass (blood flow 1–2.5 L·minute^{-1}) and low blood flows (300–500 mL·minute^{-1}) veno-venous devices.

Total support devices: ECMO

Total support devices are able to completely supply the physiological blood gas exchanges normally performed by the native lungs and perfusion. These are invasive and complex systems, which need high blood flows and high diameter and length cannulas to drain venous blood flow from the vena cava and through the artificial lung and reinfuse the blood in the aorta (for arteriovenous bypass) or in the right atrium (for veno-venous bypass) to obtain cardiac and or total lung support. It is also necessary to use high heparin doses and elevated volumes of priming for the device to function correctly.

These devices can be connected to the patient according to a veno-arterial setting, therefore, in parallel with pulmonary circulation and able to support the cardiac functionality, or in a veno–venous setting, sequentially to the pulmonary circulation, which is preferred in cases of respiratory failure alone.

These devices are capable of oxygen delivery (3 mL·kg^{-1}·minute^{-1}) and carbon dioxide removal (carbon dioxide produced by metabolism is 3–6 mL·kg^{-1}·minute^{-1}) equal to the normal metabolism of the patient.

If the circuit is planned for full support with 60–100 mL·kg^{-1}·minute^{-1} blood flow (in cases of cardiac and lung failure) carbon dioxide removal always exceeds oxygen delivery.

The ECMO device can be also utilised for carbon dioxide removal alone, in this case blood flow has to be set at 25% of cardiac output, which is adequate to remove metabolic carbon dioxide. The ability to

Table 1. Classification of carbon dioxide removal technologies

Extracorporeal support	Vascular access	Blood flow L·minute^{-1}	Indications
Total			
ECMO	V–A	5–6	Severe cardio-pulmonary failure
	V–V	2–5	Severe hypoxaemic ARDS
Partial			
ECCO$_2$R	A–V (pumpless)	1–2.5	Severe ARDS
	V–V	0.3–0.5	

ECMO: extracorporeal membrane oxygenation; ECCO$_2$R: extracorporeal carbon dioxide removal; V: venous; A: arterial; ARDS: acute respiratory distress syndrome.

remove carbon dioxide correlates with blood flow level, membrane lung proprieties, sweep gas rate and the patient's basal carbon dioxide production.

During the extracorporeal procedures, complications may arise from malfunction of the device or from patient-related adversities. Technical complications occur in 5% of the treated patients and are represented by pump and cannula malfunction. Regarding patient-related complications, the most frequent is bleeding, which occurs with a frequency of up to 30% [10], haematological changes during extracorporeal support as haemolysis, coagulation problems with clotting in the circuit and trombocytopenia due to heparin use or to blood surface exposure.

Partial support devices: $ECCO_2R$

Partial support devices refer to an extracorporeal support, focused on the removal of blood carbon dioxide, rather than on the improvement of oxygenation. As the use of total extracorporeal support is characterised by a high incidence of complications, in the context of non-refractory oxygenation, the use of partial support should be preferred.

KOLOBOW et al. [6] and GATTINONI et al. [4] exploited the concept that if carbon dioxide is removed by a membrane lung through a low-flow veno-venous bypass, it is possible to reduce the ventilatory support in ARF and severe ARDS, maintaining oxygenation simply with the patient's alveoli diffusion, also called "apnoeic oxygenation", which allows the lung to rest. The entire carbon dioxide production of a resting adult can be removed using blood flows of no more that 1 L·minute^{-1}.

Following this, different technologies have been developed through the years, with the aim of obtaining the best compromise between low blood flows, efficiency and minimal invasiveness.

Pumpless devices with arteriovenous bypass

The pumpless arteriovenous bypass is an artificial shunt with an interposed membrane oxygenator made of polymetylpentene, a polymer that allows optimal gas exchange with minimal plasma leakage. The surface of the lung membrane is approximately 1.3 m^2 with a low internal resistance. The extravascular side of the oxygenator is exposed to high oxygen flows of up to 12 L·minute^{-1}, while the blood flow is secured by the arteriovenous gradient.

After ultrasound assessment of vascular access, the device is connected to the patient through a 13 French (Fr) cannula in the femoral artery: the size of the cannula is individually selected based on vessel diameter to ensure peripheral blood flow with a residual lumen of 30% after insertion. The femoral vein, in order to allow low flow resistance, has to be connected to the artificial lung with a cannula at least two Fr sizes larger than the arterial one [26]. This device is able to remove up to 50% of the total body carbon dioxide production, with a blood flow of around 1–2 L·minute^{-1} (fig. 1).

The pumpless device, depending on the arteriovenous shunt provided by the patient's hemodynamics, can only be used if the left ventricular function is preserved with mean arterial pressure higher than 70 mmHg and without severe peripheral vascular disease.

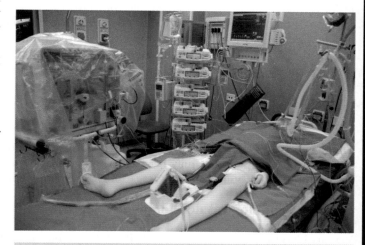

Figure 1. Continuous pumpless arteriovenous carbon dioxide removal technique (Interventional Lung Assist Novalung GmbH, Hechingen, Germany) and renal replacement therapy haemofiltration system.

Originally, up to 25% of patients supported by the device suffered from complications, and in a limited number of cases these complications were serious (lower limb ischaemia and cannula thrombosis) [27], but the improvements in the technology and limitation of cannula size reduced these risks making the pumpless artificial lung a more utilisable extracorporeal device [28]. Moreover, because the same dose of systemic anticoagulation therapy necessary for critically ill immobilised patients is required to utilise the device, it also allows the use of this pumpless lung in patients with a high risk of bleeding [29].

Low flow veno-venous devices

Recent studies proposed new, noninvasive, extracorporeal lung support systems that selectively remove only a portion of carbon dioxide. The new devices are often modifications of RRT circuits that are characterised by veno-venous bypass, low blood flow, small bore catheters or single co-axial catheter and minimal priming volumes. The following technical approaches can be classified into this category.

Devices with a peristaltic pump

This particular lung support is able to reduce P_{a,CO_2} by 20–30% (60 mL·minute^{-1}). Blood is removed through a double-lumen co-axial femoral vein catheter, and moved (maximum of 450 mL·minute^{-1}) through a non-occlusive rotating pump to an artificial membrane lung that filters carbon dioxide with a constant 100% oxygen flow (6–8 L·minute^{-1}). After emerging from the oxygenator, blood passes through a haemofilter from which a peristaltic pump re-circulates the "plasma water" toward the oxygenator. The two filters are in series in order to increase the pressure within the membrane lung (capillary side) to reduce the risk of the development of gas bubbles.

Plasma water recirculation minimises the need for heparin by decreasing haematocrit and increases the efficiency of extraction of carbon dioxide. This lung support technique allows the use of a protective ventilatory strategy with very low V_T as it helps to minimise/prevent respiratory acidosis [2, 30].

Devices with a centrifugal pump

This system is a veno-venous carbon dioxide removal motor-driven device (V_2CO_2R) that is able to remove approximately 40% of carbon dioxide (72 mL·minute^{-1}) with a flow rate of 450 mL·minute^{-1} and allows for maintenance of normocapnia in spite of a 50% reduction in V'_E [31].

The centrifugal pump withdraws venous blood from the superior vena cava and reinfuses it after carbon dioxide removal into the right atrium through the distal opening of the dual-lumen catheter. Inside the oxygenator blood flows centrally into a rotating core and then it is pumped radially through a stationary annular fibre bundle; at the end of the circle, blood without carbon dioxide returns to the patient *via* an outlet port. The core uses a motor-driven rotational motion to increase gas exchange efficiency. This motion increases the amount of carbon dioxide removal relative to the surface area of the fibre bundles, which is just 0.59 m^2. This increase in efficiency allows reduction of blood flows to 300–600 mL·minute^{-1}.

The system is interfaced with the patient through a custom dual-lumen jugular vein 15 Fr catheter similar to a dialysis catheter.

The device is primed with only 300 mL of normal saline containing 5,000 UI of heparin. Further studies are needed as it has only been tested on animal models and with a few cases of end-stage chronic obstructive pulmonary disease (COPD) respiratory failure.

Further technological developments

Venous blood carries approximately 500 mL·L^{-1} carbon dioxide either in a dry (dissolved carbon dioxide) or wet (bicarbonates) form. The dissolved portion is only about 10% of the total amount of carbon dioxide, and it is also the only one that can pass through the oxygenator membrane. This explains the necessity for high blood flows in order to obtain acceptable carbon dioxide removal.

Hypothetically, if the membrane lung could exchange the total amount of venous carbon dioxide, the V_T could be reduced to zero with a blood flow through the extracorporeal circuit of 500 mL·minute^{-1}, and the oxygenation provided by simple alveolar diffusion (apnoeic oxygenation) [15, 32].

To overcome this problem different approaches are possible: the first is to project more and more performing membrane oxygenators and the second way is to increase the carbon dioxide dissolved portion with inlet blood acidification. The second approach was abandoned due to the complexity of the procedure and because the membrane oxygenator method was easier to perform [7, 9].

BRIMIOULLE et al. [33] used systematic acidification in a clinical situation for the treatment of hypercapnia associated with metabolic alkalosis; but the iatrogenic effects of acid infusion meant the technique was abandoned [7].

Recently, blood acidification has been studied in an experiment that aimed to increase the carbon dioxide transfer through the membrane lung, therefore lowering the demand of extracorporeal flows by acidifying the blood entering the membrane lung itself. In a swine model, lactic acid was infused to convert bicarbonate ions into dissolved carbon dioxide, which is then able to pass through the lung membrane. This technique was highly efficient but further laboratory investigations are required to devise strategies applicable for long-term use in a human model [9].

If these efforts to search for a new, more effective and safe extracorporeal procedure are successful, it will allow even more protective ventilation settings, and might also represent a new path for mechanical ventilation, which could become even less invasive, with only the aim of providing enough end-expiratory positive pressure and F_{I,O_2}.

Current applications

Total ECMO support represents the most used extracorporeal gas exchange technique in spite of the high invasiveness, but due to discouraging studies [21] its use was confined only as a rescue therapy for refractory hypoxaemia. Nowadays, the epidemic H1N1 swine flu resulted in a renaissance with an intensive application of this technique [34, 35].

Over the past few years, with the creation of newer and less invasive devices for partial extracorporeal support, the ECCO$_2$R techniques have found new fields of use and development; less iatrogenic injuries and easier device management have allowed broader use.

Present clinical applications of this minimally invasive ECCO$_2$R include prevention of VILI associated with ultra-protective ventilation (with a reduced V_T) during severe ARDS treatment, end-stage COPD respiratory failure and as a bridge to lung transplant.

In ARDS patients, ARDSNet demonstrated that setting V_T to 6 mL·kg^{-1} of predicted body weight and limiting P_{plat} to between 28–30 cmH$_2$O, were the gold standard ventilatory strategies, avoiding physiological and morphological signs of hyperinflation and, consequently, VILI [1, 36].

In a preliminary study, TERRAGNI et al. [2] demonstrated that in ARDS patients a reduction of V_T (at 4 mL·kg^{-1}) correlated with pulmonary damage index and pro-inflammatory cytokine decrease. The hypercapnia and respiratory acidosis resulting from the V'_E reduction were titrated with the implementation of an extracorporeal carbon dioxide removal device needing extremely low flows (300 mL·minute^{-1}) and allowing a 20% decrease in P_{a,CO_2}.

A pioneering application field of the low flow extracorporeal support is the bridge to lung transplantation. The increasing numbers of patient and morbidity and mortality during waiting times has led to an evolution of advanced respiratory support. Patients waiting for a transplant might develop a ventilation-refractory hypercapnia and respiratory acidosis, despite optimal ventilatory support. A standard option for these patients is ECMO, but it can be applied for a very limited period of time because of the high incidence of side-effects and the worsening of transplant outcome [37]. FISCHER et al. [38] presented a series of 168 patients waiting for transplant, in which 30 of them developed a ventilation-refractory hypercapnia and respiratory acidosis. The Hanover group treated these patients with a pumpless device with arteriovenous bypass, which represented an effective and efficient strategy as a bridge to lung transplant. In this pumpless mode the device is able to achieve sufficient carbon dioxide removal, but not oxygenation, due to blood flow limitation, which does not exceed 20% of the cardiac output. Recently, with the development of a new veno-venous pump-driven artificial lung, less invasive than ECMO, but capable of high flows, the same group was able to treat respiratory failure with a predominant hypoxaemia in patients waiting for transplant [39].

Moreover, preliminary data published by the lung transplant group of Turin University (Turin, Italy) described their experience in managing mild hypoxia and severe ventilator-refractory hypercapnia with a low flow extracorporeal device. Data are limited but these techniques may represent a promising approach in a bridge to lung transplantation [40].

Future applications

Extracorporeal gas exchange techniques are not limited to severe ARDS therapies or as a bridge to lung transplant, since low extracorporeal blood flow combined with high efficiency $ECCO_2R$ can be the key to a revolutionary approach in other lung pathologies. Fields of application may be severe COPD, ARDS combined with intracranial bleeding and asthma.

COPD is a syndrome characterised by progressive airflow limitation caused by airways and lung parenchyma chronic inflammation, and by ventilatory failure due to muscle fatigue.

During COPD exacerbations, the expiratory volume flow cannot be increased by active expiration and consequently not all VT can be exhaled. The consequence is an increase in the end-expiratory lung volume (and FRC). This situation may be described as a dynamic hyperinflation, which occurs at rest and worsens during exercise. Hyperinflation causes an increase in the length of inspiratory muscles placing them at a mechanical disadvantage.

Inspiratory muscles have to counterbalance intrinsic PEEP (due to end-expiratory elastic recoil) and the action of the expiratory muscles, in order to maintain an alveolar positive pressure. This situation causes hypercapnia and acidosis because the rise of airway resistance increases the work of breathing, which results in muscular fatigue and respiratory pump failure. Moreover, dynamic hyperinflation, reducing VT and increasing residual ones, causes a reduction in volumes effectively useful for gas exchange, therefore worsening hypercapnia.

Nowadays, COPD exacerbation treatment is represented by NIV or by ETI and mechanical ventilation when NIV failure occurs (*e.g.* worsened respiratory function or mask intolerance) [41].

With this rationale, it is possible to suggest that in patients suffering from COPD exacerbations with NIV failure, it could be possible to avoid ETI with the implementation of extracorporeal partial support in order to correct respiratory acidosis and hypercapnia.

Partial extracorporeal support proved to be effective and safe in protective ventilation management in severe ARDS patients; such an early approach in cases of NIV failure should support respiratory function avoiding ETI.

Preliminary studies and case reports have been recently published researching this topic: for example, using a low flow veno-venous extracorporeal device, equipped with a centrifugal pump and a low resistance gas exchange membrane, it was possible to successfully remove carbon dioxide in a patient suffering from a severe COPD exacerbation, which allowed a reduction in the patient's V'E, recovery of gas exchange and an improvement in the dynamic hyperinflation [42].

Another field of future application is the management of severe ARDS patients with acute intracranial bleeding. The difficult management of this critical patient lies in the ability to provide lung protective ventilation while controlling the resulting hypercapnia (with increase of intracranial pressure). A solution may be the use of ECMO, but in this kind of patient high dosage of anticoagulation therapies are strongly contra-indicated.

In a case report of intracranial bleeding with high levels of carbon dioxide despite an optimal ventilatory management, the use of a partial extracorporeal support device without systemic anticoagulation, was therefore suggested to control hypercapnia [43]. Moreover, a retrospective analysis to evaluate the feasibility of a pumpless device with arteriovenous bypass in a trauma patient suffering from intracranial bleeding was reported. Patients were also affected by ARDS and needed protective ventilation: the use of extracorporeal support minimised hypercapnia and the V_T was therefore safely reduced [29].

Conclusion

Extracorporeal carbon dioxide removal support has evolved to become a key strategy in the management of respiratory failure and helped clinicians to look beyond mechanical ventilation.

Statement of interest

V.M. Ranieri is a member of the advisory board for Hemodec.

References

1. Terragni PP, Rosboch G, Tealdi A, *et al.* Tidal hyperinflation during low tidal volume ventilation in acute respiratory distress syndrome. *Am J Respir Crit Care Med* 2007; 175: 160–166.
2. Terragni PP, Del Sorbo L, Mascia L, *et al.* Tidal volume lower than 6 mL·kg^{-1} enhances lung protection: role of extracorporeal carbon dioxide removal. *Anesthesiology* 2009; 111: 826–835.
3. Gille JP, Bagniewski AM. Ten years of use of extracorporeal membrane oxygenation (ECMO) in the treatment of acute respiratory insufficiency (ARI). *Trans Am Soc Artif Intern Organs* 1976; 22: 102–109.
4. Gattinoni L, Pesenti A, Mascheroni D, *et al.* Low-frequency positive-pressure ventilation with extracorporeal carbon dioxide removal in severe acute respiratory failure. *JAMA* 1986; 256: 881–886.
5. Sherlock JE, Yoon Y, Ledwith JW, *et al.* Respiratory gas exchange during hemodialysis. *Proc Clin Dial Transplant Forum* 1972; 2: 171–174.
6. Kolobow T, Gattinoni L, Tomlinson TA, *et al.* Control of breathing using an extracorporeal membrane lung. *Anesthesiology* 1977; 46: 138–141.
7. Gille JP, Lautier A, Tousseul B. ECCO2R: oxygenator or hemodialyzer? An *in vitro* study. *Int J Artif Organs* 1992; 15: 229–233.
8. Cressoni M, Zanella A, Epp M, *et al.* Decreasing pulmonary ventilation through bicarbonate ultrafiltration: an experimental study. *Crit Care Med* 2009; 37: 2612–2618.
9. Zanella A, Patroniti N, Isgrò S, *et al.* Blood acidification enhances carbon dioxide removal of membrane lung: an experimental study. *Intensive Care Med* 2009; 35: 1484–1487.
10. Bartlett RH, Gattinoni L. Current status of extracorporeal life support (ECMO) for cardiopulmonary failure. *Minerva Anestesiol* 2010; 76: 534–540.
11. Gattinoni L, Pesenti A, Kolobow T, *et al.* A new look at therapy of the adult respiratory distress syndrome: motionless lungs. *Int Anesthesiol Clin* 1983; 21: 97–117.
12. Gattinoni L, Kolobow T, Agostoni A, *et al.* Clinical application of low frequency positive pressure ventilation with extracorporeal carbon dioxide removal (LFPPV-ECcarbon dioxideR) in treatment of adult respiratory distress syndrome (ARDS). *Int J Artif Organs* 1979; 2: 282–283.
13. ELSO Guidelines for Cardiopulmonary Extracorporeal Life Support. Extracorporeal Life Support Organization, Version 1:1. Ann Arbor, 2009. www.elso.med.umich.edu
14. Lynch JE, Hayes D Jr, Zwischenberger JB. Extracorporeal carbon dioxide removal in ARDS. *Crit Care Clin* 2011; 27: 609–625.
15. Bigatello LM, Pesenti A. Ventilator-induced lung injury: less ventilation, less injury. *Anesthesiology* 2009; 111: 699–700.
16. Terragni PP, Birocco A, Faggiano C, *et al.* Extracorporeal carbon dioxide removal. *Contrib Nephrol* 2010; 165: 185–196.
17. Pesenti A, Patroniti N, Fumagalli R. Carbon dioxide dialysis will save the lung. *Crit Care Med* 2010; 38: Suppl. 10, S549–S554.
18. Anderson H III, Steimle C, Shapiro M, *et al.* Extracorporeal life support for adult cardiorespiratory failure. *Surgery* 1993; 114: 161–172.
19. Kolla S, Awad SS, Rich PB, *et al.* Extracorporeal life support for 100 adult patients with severe respiratory failure. *Ann Surg* 1997; 226: 544–564.
20. Brunet F, Mira JP, Belghith M, *et al.* Extracorporeal carbon dioxide removal technique improves oxygenation without causing overinflation. *Am J Respir Crit Care Med* 1994; 149: 1557–1562.

21. Morris AH, Wallace CJ, Menlove RL, *et al.* Randomized clinical trial of pressure-controlled inverse ratio ventilation and extracorporeal carbon dioxide removal for adult respiratory distress syndrome. *Am J Respir Crit Care Med* 1994; 149: 295–305.
22. Greenfield LJ, Ebert PA, Benson DW. Effect of positive pressure ventilation on surface tension properties of lung extracts. *Anesthesiology* 1964; 25: 312–316.
23. Plataki M, Hubmayr RD. The physical basis of ventilator-induced lung injury. *Expert Rev Respir Med* 2010; 4: 373–385.
24. Gattinoni L, Caironi P, Pelosi P, *et al.* What has computed tomography taught us about the acute respiratory distress syndrome? *Am J Respir Crit Care Med* 2001; 164: 1701–1711.
25. Bellani G, Guerra L, Musch G, *et al.* Lung regional metabolic activity and gas volume changes induced by tidal ventilation in patients with acute lung injury. *Am J Respir Crit Care Med* 2011; 183: 1193–1199.
26. Zimmermann M, Bein T, Arlt M, *et al.* Pumpless extracorporeal interventional lung assist in patients with acute respiratory distress syndrome: a prospective pilot study. *Crit Care* 2009; 13: R10.
27. Bein T, Weber F, Philipp A, *et al.* A new pumpless extracorporeal interventional lung assist in critical hypoxemia/hypercapnia. *Crit Care Med* 2006; 34: 1372–1377.
28. Muller T, Lubnow M, Philipp A, *et al.* Extracorporeal pumpless interventional lung assist in clinical practice: determinants of efficacy. *Eur Respir J* 2009; 33: 551–558.
29. Bein T, Scherer MN, Philipp A, *et al.* Pumpless extracorporeal lung assist (pECLA) in patients with acute respiratory distress syndrome and severe brain injury. *J Trauma* 2005; 58: 1294–1297.
30. Terragni PP, Urbino R, Rosboch G, *et al.* Protective ventilation with CO2-removal technique in patients with ARDS. *Intensive Care Med* 2007; 33: Suppl. 2, S235.
31. Batchinsky AI, Jordan BS, Regn D, *et al.* Respiratory dialysis: reduction in dependence on mechanical ventilation by venovenous extracorporeal carbon dioxide removal. *Crit Care Med* 2011; 39: 1382–1387.
32. Kolobow T, Gattinoni L, Tomlinson T, *et al.* An alternative to breathing. *J Thorac Cardiovasc Surg* 1978; 75: 261–266.
33. Brimiouille S, Vincent JL, Berre J, *et al.* Hydrochloric acid infusion for treatment of hypercapnia. *Intensive Care Med* 1983; 9: 196.
34. Extracorporeal membrane oxygenation for 2009 influenza A(H1N1) acute respiratory distress syndrome. *JAMA* 2009; 302: 1888–1895.
35. Domínguez-Cherit G, Lapinsky SE, Macias AE, *et al.* Critically ill patients with 2009 influenza A(H1N1) in Mexico. *JAMA* 2009; 302: 1880–1887.
36. Hager DN, Krishnan JA, Hayden DL, *et al.* Tidal volume reduction in patients with acute lung injury when plateau pressures are not high. *Am J Respir Crit Care Med* 2005; 172: 1241–1245.
37. Fischer S, Struber M, Haverich A. Aktuelles bei der Lungentransplantation. Patienten, Indikationen, Techniken und Ergebnisse [Current status of lung transplantation: patients, indications, techniques and outcome]. *Med Klin (Munich)* 2002; 97: 137–143.
38. Fischer S, Simon AR, Welte T, *et al.* Bridge to lung transplantation with the novel pumpless interventional lung assist device NovaLung. *J Thorac Cardiovasc Surg* 2006; 131: 719–723.
39. Fischer S, Hoeper MM, Tomaszek S, *et al.* Bridge to lung transplantation with the extracorporeal membrane ventilator novalung in the veno-venous mode: the initial Hannover experience. *ASAIO J* 2007; 53: 168–170.
40. Ricci D, Boffini M, Del Sorbo L, *et al.* The use of carbon dioxide removal devices in patients awaiting lung transplantation: an initial experience. *Transplant Proc* 2010; 42: 1255–1258.
41. Sutherland E, Cherniack R. Management of chronic obstructive pulmonary disease. *N Engl J Med* 2004; 350: 2689–2697.
42. Cardenas VJ Jr, Lynch JE, Ates R, *et al.* Venovenous carbon dioxide removal in chronic obstructive pulmonary disease: experience in one patient. *ASAIO J* 2009; 55: 420–422.
43. Mallick A, Elliot S, McKinlay J, *et al.* Extracorporeal carbon dioxide removal using the Novalung in a patient with intracranial bleeding. *Anaesthesia* 2007; 62: 72–74.

Chapter 12

Prevention of VAP: role of the artificial airway, body position and setting the ventilator

G. Li Bassi[*,#,¶], M. Ferrer[*,#,¶], O.T. Ranzani[+], J-D. Marti[*,¶], L. Berra[§], L. Fernandez[*,#,¶] and A. Torres[*,#,¶]

Summary

Ventilator associated pneumonia (VAP) is associated with increased morbidity, mortality and burden for the healthcare system. Oropharyngeal secretions, pooled above the endotracheal tube (ETT) cuff, are the primary source of pathogens in this iatrogenic infection. Improvements in the ETT cuff design to achieve tracheal sealing and maintaining the internal cuff pressure within the recommended range (25–30 cmH$_2$O) have a pivotal role in the prevention of pulmonary aspiration of colonised oropharyngeal secretions and VAP. Additionally, ETTs coated with antimicrobial agents prevent colonisation of their internal lumen and biofilm formation; however, further evidence is necessary to assess the role of biofilm in the pathogenesis of VAP. The semirecumbent position is universally recommended; yet, laboratory studies challenge the benefits of such a position. Finally, during positive pressure ventilation, the ventilatory parameters that influence the inspiratory flow, *i.e.* the duty cycle, have a significant effect on retention of mucus and, potentially, on risks of lung infections. Further clinical evidence is necessary to assess benefits and limitations of ventilatory settings on VAP prevention.

Keywords: Endotracheal tube, mechanical ventilator, mucus, positive end-expiratory pressure, semi-recumbent position, ventilator-associated pneumonia

*Respiratory Intensive Care Unit, Thorax Institute, Hospital Clínic,
#Institut d'Investigacions Biomèdiques August Pi i Sunyer (IDIBAPS),
¶Centro de Investigación Biomédica en Red de Enfermedades Respiratorias (CIBERES), Barcelona, Spain.
+Respiratory Intensive Care Unit, Pulmonary Division, Heart Institute (InCor), Faculdade de Medicina da Universidade de São Paulo, São Paulo, Brazil.
§Dept of Anaesthesia, Critical Care and Pain Medicine, Massachusetts General Hospital, Harvard Medical School, Boston, MA, USA.

Correspondence: A. Torres, Servei de Pneumologia i Al·lèrgia Respiratòria, Hospital Clínic, Calle Villarroel 170, Esc 6/8 Planta 2, 08036 Barcelona, Spain.
Email atorres@clinic.ub.es

Eur Respir Mon 2012; 55: 153–168.
Printed in UK – all rights reserved
Copyright ERS 2012
European Respiratory Monograph
ISSN: 1025-448x
DOI: 10.1183/1025448x.10002511

Ventilator-associated pneumonia (VAP) is an infection that develops in approximately 15–20% of the patients who are mechanically ventilated for at least 48 hours [1]. The development of VAP in critically ill patients is a reason of great concern because of the associated morbidity, mortality and burden for the healthcare system [2–4]. Indeed, patients who develop VAP consistently spend a longer time on the mechanical ventilator in the intensive care unit (ICU) and in the hospital.

Investigators have critically emphasised that the term "VAP" could be a potential misnomer, and hardly define the pathophysiology of the disease [5, 6]. Indeed, it is currently believed that the placement of an endotracheal tube (ETT) into the trachea is the main culprit for the cascade of events that lead to the development of pneumonia. Additionally, since the 1990s gastro-pulmonary aspiration related to the supine body position has been accepted as an additional risk factor in the pathophysiology of the disease [7, 8]. Nevertheless, evidence from recent experimentation is raising awareness on additional features, such as ventilatory settings and mucus retention, seldom considered in the daily clinical practice, which may facilitate respiratory infections in mechanically ventilated patients.

The purpose of this chapter is to elucidate the main pathophysiological mechanisms and preventive strategies for the development of lung infections in intubated and ventilated patients, with particular focus on new insights into the role of the artificial airway, body position and ventilator settings.

Role of the artificial airway

In healthy subjects, the larynx's structures prevent aspiration of pathogens into the airways. Indeed, the adduction of the true and false vocal folds allows full closure of the airways; additionally, the epiglottis moves over the top of the larynx to divert any fluid or solids from reaching the trachea. Following intubation, the tracheal tube completely bypasses these anatomical barriers and creates a direct conduit for pathogens to reach the lower airways. The primary sources of pathogens are retained secretions and biofilm on the ETT internal lumen and the oropharyngeal secretions pooled above the ETT cuff. In particular, the key role of colonised subglottic secretions on VAP pathogenesis is confirmed by the reduction of respiratory infections via the use of dedicated ETTs that allow aspiration of secretions above the cuff [9]. The latest trial by LACHERADE et al. [10] evaluating the efficacy of an ETT comprising aspiration of subglottic secretions, reported a reduction of both early- and late-onset VAP. The investigators included 333 patients randomised to be intubated with either an ETT that allowed drainage of subglottic secretions or a standard ETT and found an incidence of late-onset VAP in 18.6% of patients in the treatment group versus 33.0% of patients in the control group (p=0.01).

Endotracheal tube cuff

The ETT used in the ICU for prolonged mechanically ventilated patients, most commonly comprises a high-volume low-pressure (HVLP) cuff. The outer diameter of the HVLP cuff is vastly larger than the tracheal diameter; hence, upon inflation, the cuff does not stretch and the internal cuff pressure approximates the pressure exerted against the tracheal wall, thus improving safety [11]. The main drawback is that folds are invariably formed along the cuff surface to accommodate its large circumference within the narrower trachea (fig. 1). As already shown some three decades ago [13, 14], oropharyngeal contents are aspirated through these folds and may potentially increase the risk of VAP. Clearly, to understand the factors that may play a role in leakage past the cuff, the reader needs to be acquainted with the underpinning physics that regulate the flow of fluids through these folds. First, leakage rate is determined by the differential pressure between: 1) the head pressure exerted by oropharyngeal secretions above the cuff, and 2) the airways pressure. To date, no studies have quantified the hydrostatic pressure above the cuff, nevertheless, considering an approximately 5 cm distance between the vocal folds and the cuff, a 5-cm secretions column should be present in the subglottic space. The resulting hydrostatic pressure is dependent on the density of oropharyngeal secretions and tracheal orientation, since patients are commonly placed in the semi-recumbent position. Secondly, assuming a homogeneous cylindrical channel, formed by the folded cuff, the

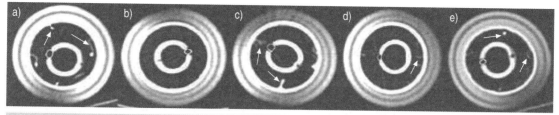

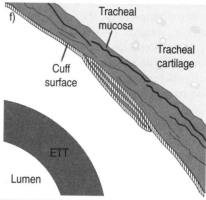

Figure 1. Computed tomography (CT) of high-volume low-pressure (HVLP) cuffs within a 20-mm internal diameter polyvinylchloride tracheal model. The following tubes are shown: a) Mallinckrodt™ Hi-Lo® (Covidien-Nellcor™ and Puritan Bennett™, Boulder, CO, USA); b) Microcuff® HVLP ICU (Kimberly-Clark Health Care, Roswell, GA, USA); c) Portex Profile Soft-Seal® (Smiths Medical-Portex™, St Paul, MN, USA); d) Rüsch® Super Safety Clear Plus (Teleflex Inc., Limerick, PA, USA); and e) Sheridan CF (Hudson RCl®, Durham, NC, USA). CT (spiral CT, Picker PQ 5000; Philips, Best, the Netherlands) was performed after bathing the tube cuffs in contrast medium (Ultravist 300; Schering, Berlin, Germany). All cuffs were inflated to a pressure of 20 cmH2O. The scan level was set at the middle of the cuffs. All cuffs, except the Microcuff® HVLP ICU (b), show additional contrast enhancement within the cuff area due to occurring folds (arrows). Adapted from [12], with permission from the publisher. f) As shown on the right, folds are invariably formed along the surface of HVLP cuffs, to accommodate its large circumference within the narrower trachea. Subglottic secretions may leak through the folds increasing the risk of respiratory infections. ETT: endotracheal tube.

resistance to the seepage of oropharyngeal secretions is theoretically determined by: 1) the viscosity of these fluids, and 2) the fourth power of the channel radius and its length.

HVLP cuffs, as originally designed, were made of polyvinylchloride (PVC). PVC is a low cost, versatile thermoplastic material highly tear- and flame-resistant, chemically inert and with desirable physical and mechanical properties for its efficient fabrication into an ETT cuff. Cuffs made of PVC have an approximate thickness of 50–80 μm [12]. As shown in table 1, several *in vitro* studies have been conducted throughout the years to study sealing effectiveness of cuffs made of different materials or with novel designs. In particular, polyurethane [12], silicone [26], latex [30] and lycra polyurethane [15] cuffs have been recently developed and tested in laboratory and clinical trials. A polyurethane cuff has an approximate thickness of 5–10 μm; hence, upon inflation, smaller folds form, probably because the channels formed by such a thin cuff could be compressed more easily by a rise in cuff pressure. In a bench top study by Dullenkopf *et al.* [12], the sealing efficacy of five different cuffs made of polyurethane and PVC were tested within a 20-mm internal diameter tracheal model. Interestingly, they found that the cuff made of polyurethane, and with the outer diameter best approximating the tracheal internal diameter, was the most effective. Indeed, as shown in figure 1, all large PVC cuffs inflated at 20 cmH2O formed folds. Cuffs made of latex [24, 30], silicone [26, 37] and lycra polyurethane [15] are highly compliant, thus, they behave as low-volume low-pressure cuffs. Upon inflation, these cuffs never form folds, allowing a perfect seal of the trachea. Recent *in vitro* studies on latex [16, 24] and lycra polyurethane [15] cuffs confirmed the high efficacy of these novel cuffs. These prototypes, although currently noncommercialised, offer important insights into future designs to ultimately overcome limitations of HVLP cuffs.

Investigators have also attempted to improve tracheal sealing using cuffs with a tapered shape [21, 30]. The rationale behind the use of a tapered shaped cuff is that folds can be eliminated for a full lower circumference of the trachea/cuff contact zone. Unfortunately, limited clinical and laboratory evidence is available to ultimately confirm the efficacy of this new cuff design. In particular, it seems logical that the outer diameter of a tapered cuff still plays a significant role on the sealing efficacy. As shown in figure 2, the larger the conical cuff, the lesser its sealing capabilities should be.

Among these novel cuffs, only cuffs made of polyurethane and silicone have been tested in humans. LORENTE et al. [36] compared an ETT with a polyurethane cuff and aspiration of subglottic secretions with a standard PVC-cuffed ETT. They found a reduced incidence of VAP of 7.9% using the new ETT compared with 22.1% using the standard (p=0.001). A single-centre study by MILLER et al. [33] tested the use of a polyurethane cuff ETT *versus* a standard PVC cuff ETT, with a before and after design, and found that VAP rates decreased from 5.3 per 1,000 ventilator days before the use of the polyurethane-cuffed ETT to 2.8 per 1,000 ventilator days during the intervention year (p=0.0138). The polyurethane-cuffed ETT has also shown benefits in reducing early post-operative pneumonia in cardiac surgical patients. POELAERT et al. [35] studied 134 cardiothoracic surgery patients and demonstrated that the incidence of early post-operative pneumonia was significantly lower in the polyurethane group than in the PVC group (23% *versus* 42%, p<0.03). Finally, in a clinical trial on patients undergoing anaesthesia or admitted to the ICU, YOUNG et al. [26] demonstrated the high effectiveness of a silicone cuff in reducing pulmonary aspiration.

Internal cuff pressure

Although oropharyngeal secretions leak through the folds of HVLP cuffs, there is consistent evidence that internal cuff pressure partially limits such phenomenon [12, 24, 28]. The cuff pressure is transmitted to the tracheal wall and SEEGOBIN et al. [38] elegantly demonstrated obstruction of tracheal blood flow in humans, when the internal cuff pressure was above 30 cmH$_2$O, with total absence of flow, particularly to the mucosa over the tracheal rings, at a cuff pressure of 50 cmH$_2$O. Thus, in clinical practice, it is recommended that the internal cuff pressure is maintained between 25–30 cmH$_2$O, to prevent macroaspiration and catastrophic complications such as tracheal necrosis, rupture and tracheo-oesophageal fistulae [39–41]. The risk of lung infection, due to aspiration of pathogen-laden oropharyngeal secretions across a deflated cuff, was initially corroborated by RELLO et al. [42]. The authors reported an association between intracuff pressure persistently below 20 cmH$_2$O and development of VAP.

In the daily clinical practice, the manual estimation of the cuff pressure through palpation of the ETT pilot balloon is inaccurate [43–46]. Thus, the intermittent use of a manometer could be a better solution to maintain the cuff pressure within the recommended range, although implementation of this practice is frequently overlooked [47]. A few devices that automatically control the cuff pressure have been evaluated in clinical trials [48, 49]. These studies confirmed that using standard management, the ETT cuff was frequently deflated or hyperinflated; conversely, through continuous control, the cuff pressure was more consistently maintained within the recommended range. NSEIR et al. [50] recently randomised 122 patients to receive continuous control of the cuff through a pneumatic device or standard management and found lower occurrences of microaspiration (18% *versus* 46%, p=0.002), bacterial burden in tracheal aspirates (mean±SD 1.6±2.4 *versus* 3.1±3.7 log$_{10}$ cfu·mL^{-1}, p=0.014) and VAP rate (9.8% *versus* 26.2%, p=0.032; OR (95% CI) 0.30 (0.11–0.84)) in patients with cuff pressure continuously controlled.

Endotracheal tube biofilm

The ETT is commonly made of PVC and pathogens easily adhere to its internal surface (fig. 3). Once attached to a surface, several microbes are capable of forming a complex structure called biofilm. A biofilm comprises sessile bacteria, embedded within a self-produced exopolysaccharide matrix [51]. Biofilms on the internal surface of ETTs can be identified early following tracheal intubation [52, 53]. Sessile bacteria undergo phenotypic differentiation when embedded within the biofilm and gain survival advantages. Indeed, biofilms protect pathogens from antibiotics and the host immune response. During mechanical ventilation, biofilm particles may dislodge into the airways, *i.e.* due to inspiratory airflow [53] or tracheal aspiration [54]. The role of bacterial biofilm on the pathogenesis of VAP is difficult to assess *in vivo*, as causative pathogens could originate from within the biofilm, or equally from subglottic secretions. However, in an interesting study by ADAIR et al. [55], the genotype of bacteria retrieved from the lower airways and the ETT were compared. The authors found matching

Table 1. Significant clinical studies on the sealing efficacy of endotracheal tube (ETT) cuffs

First author [ref.]	Year	Primary aims	Setting	Leaking fluid	Study time
KOLOBOW [15]	2011	To study the sealing efficacy of a novel lycra polyurethane cuff *versus* PVC and polyurethane cuffs	*In vitro*	Methylene blue water	24 hours
ZANELLA [16]	2011	To evaluate the effects of different cuff materials (PVC, polyurethane and guayule latex), shapes (cylindrical and conical) and PEEP on fluid leakage across the cuff	*In vitro*	Methylene blue water	24 hours
OUANES [17]	2011	To evaluate effects of PEEP levels, inspiratory effort intensity and ETT characteristics on fluid leakage past the cuff	*In vitro*	Methylene blue water	1 hour
DAVE [18]	2011	To compare the effects of closed tracheal suction on fluid aspiration across the PVC and polyurethane cuffs varying ventilatory modes	*In vitro*	Clear water	Upon tracheal suctioning
DAVE [19]	2011	To compare the effects of closed tracheal suction on fluid aspiration across cylindrical PVC cuffs	*In vitro*	Clear water	1 hour and upon tracheal suctioning
DAVE [20]	2010	To test the sealing properties of cuffs in a static and dynamic ventilation bench-top model and the effects of cuff lubrication	*In vitro*	Clear water	1 hour
DAVE [21]	2010	To compare the fluid leakage across tapered and cylindrical cuffs	*In vitro*	Clear water	5 minutes and 1 hour
PITTS [22]	2010	To assess effects of cuff design characteristics and mechanical ventilator settings on leakage	*In vitro*	Red-coloured vitamin water®	30 minutes
LUCANGELO [23]	2008	To compare the efficacy of cylindrical PVC and tapered polyurethane cuffs, an *in vitro* and *in vivo* study varying PEEP levels	*In vitro* and *in vivo*	Methylene blue water	1, 5 and 12 hours
ZANELLA [24]	2008	To assess the sealing properties of a novel latex rubber cuff in comparison with commercially available cuffs	*In vitro*	Methylene blue water	2 hours
WINKLMAIER [25]	2006	To evaluate leakage of liquids, *i.e.* water and saliva, past low-pressure cuffs of tracheostomy tubes	*In vitro*	Water artificial saliva	Up to 15 minutes
YOUNG [26]	2006	To assess the sealing efficacy of a low-volume low-pressure cuff with high-volume low-pressure cuffs	*In vitro*	Blue dyed water	≤1 hour
DULLENKOPF [12]	2003	To evaluate the sealing properties of a polyurethane cuff in comparison with commercially available cuffs	*In vitro*	Methylene blue water	≤1 hour
BLUNT [27]	2001	To assess the effects of cuff lubrification on sealing efficacy	*In vitro* and *in vivo*	Blue dyed water	≤15 minutes
ASAI [28]	2001	To study the sealing effectivness of high-volume low-pressure cuffs	*In vitro*	Methylene blue water	5 minutes
YOUNG [29]	1999	To assess the sealing properties of a novel highly compliant high-volume low-pressure cuff in comparison with commercially available high-volume low-pressure cuffs	*In vitro*	Blue dyed water	15 minutes

Table 1. Continued.

First author [ref.]	Year	Primary aims	Setting	Leaking fluid	Study time
YOUNG [30]	1999	To assess fluid leakage through a novel compliant latex cuff in comparison with standard high-volume low-pressure cuffs	In vitro	Blue dyed water	15 minutes
YOUNG [31]	1998	To compare fluid leakage across a novel cuff design versus standard high-volume low-pressure cuffs	In vitro	Water	24 hours
YOUNG [32]	1997	To assess the sealing properties of high-volume low-pressure cuffs during different ventilatory modes and tracheal suctioning	In vitro	Methylene blue water	6 hours
MILLER [33]	2011	To retrospectively assess the incidence of VAP in patients intubated with polyurethane- versus PVC-cuffed ETTs	In vivo	NA	NA
NSEIR [34]	2010	To assess microaspiration of gastric contents and the variations of internal cuff pressure between cuffs made of polyurethane or PVC and with cylindrical and tapered shapes	In vivo	NA	NA
POELAERT [35]	2008	To study incidence of early VAP in cardiac ICU patients intubated with cuffs made of polyurethane or PVC	In vivo	NA	NA
LORENTE [36]	2007	To compare the incidence of VAP between patients intubated with an ETT comprising polyurethane cuff and subglottic drainage versus conventional PVC cuff	In vivo	NA	NA
YOUNG [37]	2000	To evaluate the sealing effectiveness of a silicone cuff	In vivo	Blue dyed water	NA

PVC: polyvinylchloride; PEEP: positive end-expiratory pressure; VAP: ventilator-associated pneumonia; ICU: intensive care unit; NA: not available.

genotypes between microbes of the lower airways and the biofilm in 70% of the samples obtained from patients with VAP. Moreover, the authors confirmed that antibiotic susceptibility was lower in pathogens isolated from within the biofilm.

Thus, coating the ETT with antimicrobial agents such as silver (fig. 4), is a promising strategy to prevent biofilm formation within its internal surface and, hence, to prevent VAP. Several animal studies [52, 56] evaluated the antimicrobial effects of silver-coated ETTs, consistently finding a delay in the ETT colonisation and decreased lung bacterial burden. Interestingly, investigators from the National Institutes of Health (NIH) found that the efficacy of silver-based coatings decreased over time [57] and raised a controversial remark on the use of coated ETT in long-term intubated patients [58]. In line with this argument, only one laboratory study [57] has reported the absence of ETT colonisation and biofilm up to 168 hours of mechanical ventilation via intermittent cleaning of the internal lumen of a coated ETT with the Mucus Shaver [59]. This device was devised to keep the ETT lumen free of mucus and to mechanically remove biofilm formation. A very recent clinical study [60] confirmed the potential of the Mucus Shaver in 24 patients expected to be mechanically ventilated for more than 72 hours. Upon extubation, only one ETT from the Mucus Shaver group was colonised, compared with 83% of the ETTs retrieved from patients in the control group. One large randomised clinical trial, the North American Silver-Coated Endotracheal Tube (NASCENT) trial [61] evaluated 2,003 patients expected to be mechanically ventilated for more than 24 hours and randomised to be intubated with either a silver-coated or a conventional tube. The silver-coated ETT was associated with a lower incidence of microbiologically confirmed VAP (37 (4.8%) out of 766 *versus* 56 (7.5%) out of 743; p=0.03) and a relative risk reduction of 35.9%. A retrospective cohort analysis by AFESSA *et al.* [62] on these patients additionally found a reduction in mortality of patients with VAP intubated with the coated tube (silver ETT *versus* control, five (14%) out of 37 *versus* 20 (36%) out of 56, p=0.03), but mortality was higher in those without VAP (silver ETT *versus* control, 228 (31%) out of 729 *versus* 178 (26%) out of 687, p=0.03). Importantly, in a cost-efficacy analysis by SHORR *et al.* [63], assuming marginal VAP costs of US$16,620 and costs of US$90.00 for coated and US$2.00 for uncoated ETTs, the authors found that savings per case of VAP prevented were US$12,840.

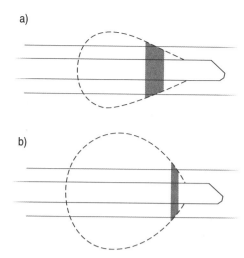

Figure 2. Tapered shaped high-volume low-pressure cuffs allow the elimination of folds for a full lower circumference of the trachea/cuff contact zone. Theoretically, the outer diameter of a tapered cuff still plays a significant role on the sealing efficacy, since the sealing zone develops where the cuff's diameter approximates the tracheal internal diameter. a) Endotracheal tube within a tracheal model. A tapered cuff with an outer diameter approximating the tracheal internal diameter is shown. This design theoretically allows a longer sealing region in comparison with b), in which a very large tapered cuff creates a very short sealing zone.

Body position

In healthy subjects, colonisation of the stomach is prevented by the highly acidic environment. Conversely, mechanically ventilated patients routinely receive drugs for stress ulcer prophylaxis and continuous enteral nutrition, resulting in alkalinisation of gastric contents, and potential colonisation with pathogens. The role of the stomach in the pathogenesis of VAP is a matter of great controversy. Gastric pathogens may potentially translocate into the oropharynx because of the increased gastro-oesophageal reflux, particularly when large-bore gastric feeding tubes are in place [64]. Some investigators emphasised that a gastric pH higher than 4 was associated with bacterial growth [65, 66], and consequently, pulmonary infections [67, 68]. In other studies [69–72] the role of the stomach in VAP pathogenesis was not confirmed.

When patients are positioned with the upper body obliquely oriented, as in the semi-recumbent position, the reflux of gastric contents is reduced and pathogens are potentially compartmentalised within the stomach. We have recently reviewed in detail the most significant evidence supporting the use of the semi-recumbent position in mechanically ventilated patients [73]. Importantly, the semi-recumbent position has been endorsed by the Centers for Disease Control and Prevention (CDC) [74] and several other international medical societies [1, 75], as one of the most effective and feasible strategies to prevent VAP.

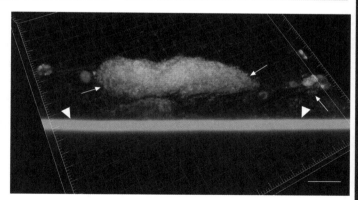

Figure 3. Three-dimensional reconstruction of a bacterial biofilm within the endotracheal tube using confocal laser scanning imaging. The mushroom-shaped multicellular biofilm structure originating from the endotracheal tube (ETT) surface can be observed. The ETT sample was obtained from experimental studies in pigs. The animals were challenged through oropharyngeal instillation of *Pseudomonas aeruginosa* and mechanically ventilated thereafter. Samples were stained with Live/Dead® BacLight kit™ (Invitrogen, Paisley, UK) and imaged using a 25x, 0.95 NA water immersion objective. Arrowheads depict the internal surface of the ETT. The arrows underline biofilm regions where rod-shaped *P. aeruginosa* are clearly visible. Scale bar=20 μm.

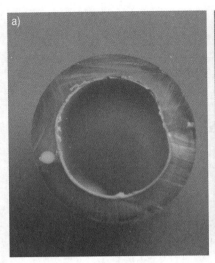
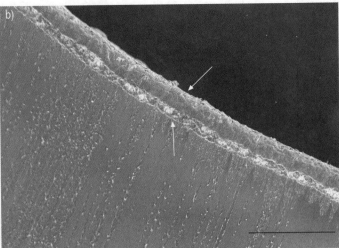

Figure 4. a) Transversal cut of an endotracheal tube (ETT) internally coated with silver-sulfadiazine, chlorhexidine and polyurethane [52]. b) Scanning electron micrograph of the internal surface of a newly coated ETT. The arrows depict the nonhomogeneous coating of silver-sulfadiazine and chlorhexidine, approximately 50 µm, visible on the ETT surface. Scale bar=250 µm.

As mentioned previously, it is important to emphasise that in tracheally intubated patients a tracheal orientation above horizontal potentially increases the hydrostatic pressure exerted by subglottic secretions above the cuff and, as a result, the risk of pulmonary aspiration. In clinical practice, oropharyngeal colonisation is not routinely monitored; hence, it is impossible to identify patients already colonised upon intubation, or who develop pathological oropharyngeal colonisation during the course of tracheal intubation. Theoretically, in these patients, the semi-recumbent position would not provide any additional benefit, and its use may be unsafe, due to the associated risks of pulmonary aspiration.

Several reports from the NIH challenged the role of the semi-recumbent position as a preventive VAP strategy [76, 77]. These studies suggest that gravity plays a key role in the pathogenesis of VAP, and keeping the ETT/trachea obliquely oriented allows leakage across the ETT cuff and translocation of oropharyngeal pathogens into the lungs. In particular, in a study by this group the effects of ETT/trachea orientation on mucus clearance and lung infections were evaluated in 16 sheep [76]. Interestingly, they found that following tracheal intubation mucus was transported by cilia at a mean rate of 2.0 ± 1.9 mm·min^{-1} and 2.1 ± 1.1 mm·min^{-1} in sheep with ETT/trachea oriented above and below horizontal, respectively, confirming that gravity did not affect mucociliary transport. However, when the ETT/trachea axis was above horizontal, mucus retained at the inflated ETT cuff eventually moved backward into the lungs *via* gravitational force. Secretions retained at the proximal trachea were consistently colonised by oropharyngeal pathogens (10^3–10^9 cfu·mL^{-1}); consequently, the gravity-driven flow of mucus toward the lungs led to an intratracheal route of lung colonisation. Indeed, the same pathogens were isolated from both proximal trachea and the lungs. Conversely, with the ETT/trachea axis oriented below horizontal, mucus consistently cleared outward, avoiding bacterial colonisation of airways and lung infections.

To the best of our knowledge, only two clinical trials [78, 79] have attempted to translate these findings into clinical practice. In humans an ETT/trachea orientation below horizontal can be obtained through a semi-lateral Trendelenburg position. In particular, according to a mid-trachea placement of the ETT cuff, the axis from the sternal notch to the mouth should be theoretically maintained horizontal or slightly below horizontal in order to avoid leakage across the ETT cuff. A feasibility study by MAURI *et al.* [78] compared 10 patients placed in a lateral position *versus* 10 patients in the semi-recumbent position. In the lateral position, patients were turned from one side to the other every

2–4 hours for up to 24 hours. Tracheal aspirates were collected at baseline and every 8 hours (in the semi-recumbent group) or every 4 hours (in the lateral-horizontal group). The study showed that the lateral-horizontal position was feasible and did not cause serious adverse events. The presence of pepsin in tracheal aspirates, an index of gastro-pulmonary aspiration, did not increase in the lateral position and was found in seven patients in the semi-recumbent group (33% of all tracheal aspirate samples) and five (38% of all tracheal aspirate samples) in the lateral-horizontal group ($p=0.32$), despite the fact that the lateral-horizontal group was sampled more frequently over a shorter period. Interestingly, the authors found more ventilator-free days and a trend of lower incidence of VAP when the lateral position was applied, but clear conclusions cannot be established given the small sample size. Finally, a study of 60 intubated infants provided further evidence on the role of gravity in the pathogenesis of VAP [79]. Patients were randomised to be positioned either supine horizontal with the ETT held upright in the vertical position or on their side with the ETT maintained horizontal. After 5 days of mechanical ventilation tracheal cultures were positive in 26 (87%) out of 30 and nine (30%) out of 30 of the patients positioned in the supine and lateral position, respectively ($p<0.01$).

Ventilator settings

Ventilatory settings can potentially influence translocation of microbes from the upper to the lower airways, systemic spread of the infection, clearance of pathogens and the overall lung pathogenic burden. Overall, scant investigation in this field limits our ability to accurately define the role of each ventilatory parameter in the pathogenesis of VAP. In fact, experimental and clinical studies have been particularly centred on the potential effects of positive end-expiratory pressure (PEEP). Nevertheless, during positive pressure ventilation, the inspiratory flow is the driving force to translocate pathogens toward the lower airways and may play a significant role in VAP pathogenesis.

Positive end-expiratory pressure

The effects of PEEP on incidence of VAP have recently been evaluated by MANZANO et al. [80] in 131 ICU patients who were nonhypoxaemic and without lung injury. Patients were randomised to receive either 5–8 cmH_2O of PEEP or no PEEP. Microbiologically confirmed VAP occurred in 9.4% of the patients in the PEEP group *versus* 25.4% in the control group ($p=0.017$). PEEP mainly prevented early-onset pneumonia.

PEEP may prevent VAP through several mechanisms. First, PEEP counterbalances hydrostatic pressure exerted by oropharyngeal secretions and consequently, as mentioned previously, seepage of colonised fluids across the folds of the ETT cuff. In *in vitro* studies by OUANES et al. [17] the leakage across four different HVLP cuffs was tested upon volume-control ventilation with a PEEP level of 0, 5, 10, 15 and 20 cmH_2O. As expected, the leakage flow rate was inversely related to the PEEP level ($r^2=0.39$, $p<0.001$). Similarly, in bench-top studies by ZANELLA et al. [16] and PITTS et al. [22], leakage of a 10-cm fluid column across a variety of cuffs made of polyurethane, latex and PVC was assessed. In both studies a consistent prevention of leakage was found only when PEEP was set at 15 cmH_2O. These findings are consistent with the *in vivo* study by LUCANGELO et al. [23], in which 40 patients were randomised to be intubated with either a PVC or polyurethane-cuffed ETT. Under mechanical ventilation, with 5 cmH_2O of PEEP, leakage of dye poured above the cuffs was assessed and remarkably only two out of 20 patients with PVC-cuffed ETT presented dye below the cuff. Conversely, when PEEP was removed dye leaked through all these cuffs within 1 hour; whereas in patients intubated with polyurethane-cuffed ETTs, leakage was delayed for up to 8 hours. However, at 12 hours from removal of PEEP, only 15% of these patients did not present leakage.

Another potential effect of PEEP on prevention of VAP is related to a reduction in the degree of lung atelectasis. In an important report by VAN KAAM et al. [81], newborn piglets were tracheally challenged with Group B streptococci, following pulmonary lavage with saline to induce surfactant deficiency and alveolar collapse. Piglets were then either mechanically ventilated with low levels of tidal volume (V_T) and PEEP or underwent therapeutic and ventilatory interventions to revert atelectasis either: 1) through the use of exogenous surfactant, or 2) by applying a ventilatory strategy with high peak inspiratory pressure and PEEP to stabilise opened lung regions. Interestingly, the authors found a consistent lower lung bacterial proliferation and bloodstream translocation when strategies to reduce atelectasis were applied. These findings are consistent with earlier studies [82, 83]. In particular, SHENNIB et al. [83] first suggested a potential explanation for these discoveries; indeed, they found that alveolar macrophages retrieved from collapsed lung regions of piglets presented a significant depression of their phagocytic activity. Additionally, the use of mechanical ventilation to reopen the atelectatic areas resulted in improvement of macrophage function. Further evidence from *in vitro* and *in vivo* studies is needed to comprehensively elucidate effects of PEEP on local and systemic immune defences and to ultimately translate these findings into clinical practice. As a matter of fact, to date, no clear evidence is available to choose a proper level of PEEP to reduce the risk of infection. In fact, CHARLES et al. [84] found that in rabbits intratracheally challenged by *Enterobacter aerogenes*, 5 cmH$_2$O of PEEP resulted in reduced lung bacterial burden; conversely, when the level of PEEP was increased to 10 cmH$_2$O no beneficial effects in lung bacterial concentration were found; in addition worse extrapulmonary translocation was demonstrated, as shown by higher spleen bacterial burden.

Ventilatory airflow, mucus retention and risk of infections

The lungs of a mechanically ventilated patient are exposed daily to several thousand litres of inhaled air, which potentially transport pathogens from within the ETT lumen and proximal airways. One of the most important defence mechanisms of the respiratory system is mucus, which is a physical barrier and a medium with antimicrobial and immunomodulatory properties [85]. Mucus is continuously cleared through the ciliated cells. Each ciliated cell has approximately 200 cilia on its surface, which move at approximately 8–15 Hz [86]. Mucociliary clearance rates are between 4–20 mm·min^{-1} [87, 88]. Importantly, mechanically ventilated patients frequently develop retention of mucus because of several factors. First, following tracheal intubation mucociliary velocity is approximately 80% slower than normal [89]. SACKNER et al. [90], in particular, demonstrated that inflation of ETT cuff lowers mucociliary velocity by half after only 2 hours. Secondly, when mucus reaches the proximal trachea outward clearance is not possible because of the inflated cuff; therefore, mucus accrues, unless it is aspirated through suctioning or enters the ETT. Thirdly, continuous leakage [12, 23] of bacteria-laden oropharyngeal secretions sustains airways infection and hypersecretion of mucus. Finally, critically ill patients are often incapable of effectively clearing retained mucus secondary to immobilisation, weak cough and muscle weakness. A few arguments support the association between retention of mucus and increased risks for lung infections. Indeed, mucus retained in the peripheral airways potentially causes atelectasis, which, as described previously, ultimately results in an impairment of the cellular immune response. Also, pathogens entangled within the mucus need to be promptly cleared because the microbicidal products contained in mucus exert a time-limited effectiveness. This was clearly demonstrated by COLE et al. [91], who found that bacteria added to nasal mucus acquired resistance to the antimicrobial factors within 24 hours.

When mucus builds up within the airways, airflow exerts an effect on its surface and can eventually influence its movement *via* a two-phase gas–liquid flow. The critical conditions necessary to move mucus through this mechanism were comprehensively evaluated in the late 1980s by KIM and co-workers [92–94]. They developed a glass model of human airways, positioned either vertically or horizontally, with a continuous supply of simulant mucus of differing rheological properties. Thus, the effects of continuous or cyclic airflow patterns were studied, and they found that the main factors regulating mucus transport consisted of: 1) shear stress exerted by the airflow on the liquid layer; 2) the ratio between thickness of the mucus layer and the airway diameter; and 3) the rheological properties of secretions. Importantly, during mechanical ventilation, inspiratory and expiratory airflows exert opposite shear forces on the mucus layer. KIM et al. [94] assessed *in vitro* the effects of tidal inspiratory–expiratory airflows on movement of mucus simulants and found that mucus velocity can be predicted as follows:

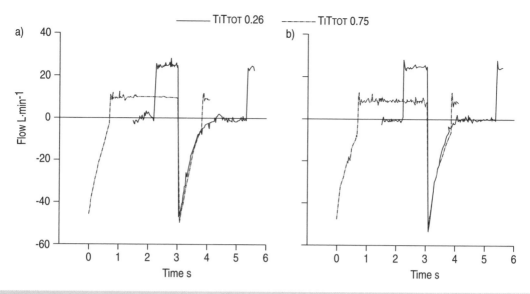

Figure 5. Effects of duty cycle (TI/TTOT) and positive end-expiratory pressure (PEEP) on expiratory–inspiratory flow bias. a) Flow waveforms, TI/TTOT 0.26 and 0.75, with no PEEP. The change of TI/TTOT from 0.26 to 0.75 decreased the inspiratory flow and consequently increased expiratory–inspiratory flow bias. b) Flow waveforms, TI/TTOT 0.26 and 0.75, with 5 cmH$_2$O PEEP. An increase of peak expiratory flow was found when extrinsic PEEP was applied or when intrinsic PEEP developed and when the TI/TTOT was maintained at 0.75. Reproduced from [97] with permission from the publisher.

$$\sim \rho v^2 \times (1\text{-}\mathrm{TI/TTOT}) \times \eta^{-1}$$

where ρ is the gas density, v is the absolute value of the highest airflow velocity throughout the respiratory cycle, which is inversely related to the total cross-sectional area of the airways, TI/TTOT is the duty cycle and η is the mucus viscosity. Interestingly, the authors found that during volume-control mechanical ventilation mucus moved in waves, and the mucus speed was not influenced by the inspiratory flow until its rate reached 90% of the expiratory flow. In a recent *in vitro* study by VOLPE *et al.* [95], using a horizontal tracheal model, the significant effect of peak expiratory flow on mucus transport was corroborated. Additionally, the authors found that: 1) an expiratory–inspiratory flow difference of 17 L·min^{-1} was a threshold to achieve outward mucus clearance, and 2) intrinsic PEEP caused by either elevated minute ventilation or expiratory resistance, respectively, improved and worsened mucus clearance. Theoretically, during mechanical ventilation, the difference between inspiratory and expiratory flow rate can be easily modulated by adjusting parameters that influence the inspiratory flow. Expiration is frequently passive in ventilated patients; thus, the major determinants of expiratory flow rate are lung elastance, lung volume and airway resistances. Only two experimental studies *in vivo* [96, 97] have assessed whether adjustments of ventilatory parameters could influence mucus clearance, specifically addressing the effects of duty cycle and PEEP. BENJAMIN *et al.* [96] studied in six sheep, positioned prone horizontal, transport of artificial mucus instilled into the trachea *via* adjustment of duty cycle to 0.27, 0.65 and 0.75. Applying duty cycles of 0.65 and 0.75, 30 and 49%, respectively, of the instilled simulated mucus was transported outward, whereas with a duty cycle of 0.27, no mucus was recovered. In a recent study by our group [97] we studied eight pigs, positioned in a model of the semi-recumbent position and mechanically ventilated for up to 84 hours. This study arose from the rationale that mechanically ventilated patients are often positioned with the trachea oriented above the horizontal (*i.e.* the semi-recumbent position); as a result, mucus transport *via* the two-phase gas–liquid mechanism mainly depends on a balance between the airflow shear forces on the liquid layer and gravitational force. Animals were ventilated in volume-control, square-wave inspiratory flow, without inspiratory pause, and VT 10 mL·kg^{-1}. Six levels of TI/TTOT: 0.26, 0.33, 0.41, 0.50, 0.60 and 0.75 (inspiratory:expiratory time ratios: 1:2.9; 1:2; 1:1.4; 1:1; 1.5:1 and 3:1, respectively) with either no PEEP or 5 cmH$_2$O of PEEP were randomly applied to assess the effects on mucus

Table 2. The effects of duty cycle on mucus clearance and respiratory airflows

	Duty cycle		p-value
	0.25–0.41	**0.5–0.75**	
Mucus clearance analysis			
Mucus velocity[#] mm·min^{-1}	-0.22±1.71 (-5.78–2.42)	0.53±1.06 (-1.91-3.88)	0.0048
Incidence of mucus moving towards the glottis ⩽48 hours of MV[¶]	19/66 (28.79)	28/74 (37.84)	0.2858
Incidence of mucus moving towards the lungs ⩾48 hours of MV[¶]	38/68 (55.88)	27/71 (38.03)	0.0420
Respiratory airflow analysis[+]			
Inspiratory flow L·min^{-1}	19.8±4.4	10.8±2.6	<0.0001
PEF L·min^{-1}	43.3±7.1	43.8±6.7	0.2887
MEF L·min^{-1}	15.7±2.2	18.6±4.4	<0.0001
PEF-MIF difference L·min^{-1}	23.5±8.6	33.0±7.6	<0.0001
MEF-MIF difference L·min^{1}	-4.1±4.6	7.9±5.9	<0.0001
PEF-MIF ratio	2.3±0.7	4.3±1.2	<0.0001
MEF-MIF ratio	0.8±0.2	1.8±0.7	<0.0001

Data are presented as mean±SD (range), mean±SD or n/n (%), unless otherwise stated. The direction of mucus movement was described by a positive vector (towards the glottis) or negative vector (towards the lungs). MV: mechanical ventilation; PEF: peak expiratory flow; MEF: mean expiratory flow; MIF: mean inspiratory flow. [#]: 94 observations (tracked disks velocity means of the 4-day study for each animal and condition) were analysed. [¶]: 279 categorical observations (vectors of mucus velocities, toward either the glottis or the lungs, for each day, animal and condition) were analysed. Only occurrence of mucus moving toward the lungs is reported. [+]: 348 observations (respiratory parameters for each day, animal and condition) were analysed. Reproduced from [97] with permission from the publisher.

transport. As shown in figure 5, PEEP and the prolongation of TI/TTOT affected the expiratory–inspiratory flow bias. Interestingly, PEEP did not influence mucus clearance. Instead, prolongation of TI/TTOT improved mucus clearance. In particular, as reported in table 2, two clusters of mucus velocities were identified in this study, suggestive of a potential threshold effect on mucus clearance as TI/TTOT was prolonged beyond 0.41. Hence, TI/TTOT ⩾0.5 in comparison to TI/TTOT ⩽0.4 generated higher expiratory flow bias and mucus clearance was enhanced to 0.53±1.06 (range -1.91–3.88) from -0.21±1.71 (range -5.78–2.42) mm·min^{-1} (p=0.0048), respectively. The influence of airflow on mucus was particularly significant following 48 hours of MV and longer periods since the last tracheal aspiration, confirming that airflow particularly influences transport of thick retained mucus.

Importantly, despite consistent laboratory results, there is still great paucity of translational clinical studies in this field. In clinical practice, the same range of expiratory–inspiratory flow biases could be reproduced during volume-control ventilation, through modulation of several parameters such as VT, respiratory rate, inspiratory rise time and inspiratory pause time. Importantly, in comparison to the aforementioned studies conducted on healthy animals, in patients with injured poorly compliant lungs higher expiratory flow are developed. Consequently, minor changes of ventilatory parameters should be necessary to achieve expiratory–inspiratory flow biases that promote outward clearance. Importantly, the effects of pressure-limited modes of ventilation on airflow rates are more difficult to predict, because inspiratory flow rate is partly related to the mechanical properties of the respiratory system. Indeed, in a recent report by NTOUMENOPOULOS et al. [98] on 20 ICU patients, mainly ventilated in pressure support, airflow biases commonly reached levels presumably not sufficient to clear mucus.

Conclusions

The ETT, body position and ventilatory settings play a significant role in the pathogenesis of VAP. Several strategies have been developed to prevent VAP through modulation of these factors. In particular, improvements on the design and material of the ETT cuff; a body position that allows gravity-driven drainage of oropharyngeal and airways secretions; and adjustment of ventilatory settings to thwart pulmonary aspiration and improve respiratory defences could be translated in relevant clinical applications. Nevertheless, although a growing interest exists on the potential of these novel preventive strategies, further evidence, specifically from human studies, is necessary to comprehensively assess their benefits and ensure a clear comprehension of their limitations.

Statement of interest

G. Li Bassi has received honoraria for lectures and research from Covidien. A. Torres has received research grants and honoraria for lectures from Pfizer and Covidien. He has participated in the advisory boards of Astellas and Sanofi-Aventis.

References

1. America Thoracic Society. Guidelines for the management of adults with hospital-acquired, ventilator-associated, and healthcare-associated pneumonia. *Am J Respir Crit Care Med* 2005; 171: 388–416.
2. Rello J, Ollendorf DA, Oster G, *et al.* Epidemiology and outcomes of ventilator-associated pneumonia in a large US database. *Chest* 2002; 122: 2115–2121.
3. Kollef MH, Silver D, Murphy DM, *et al.* The effect of late-onset ventilator-associated pneumonia in determining patient mortality. *Chest* 1995; 108: 1655–1662.
4. Warren DK, Shukla SJ, Olsen MA, *et al.* Outcome and attributable cost of ventilator-associated pneumonia among intensive care unit patients in a suburban medical center. *Crit Care Med* 2003; 31: 1312–1317.
5. Safdar N, Crnich CJ, Maki DG. The pathogenesis of ventilator-associated pneumonia: its relevance to developing effective strategies for prevention. *Respir Care* 2005; 50: 725–739.
6. Berra L, Kolobow T. Ventilator-associated pneumonia or endotracheal tube-associated pneumonia or none of the above? Lessons learned from laboratory animal studies. *Anesthesiology* 2009; 111: 921–922.
7. Torres A, Serra-Batlles J, Ros E, *et al.* Pulmonary aspiration of gastric contents in patients receiving mechanical ventilation: the effect of body position. *Ann Intern Med* 1992; 116: 540–543.
8. Drakulovic MB, Torres A, Bauer TT, *et al.* Supine body position as a risk factor for nosocomial pneumonia in mechanically ventilated patients: a randomised trial. *Lancet* 1999; 354: 1851–1858.
9. Muscedere J, Rewa O, McKechnie K, *et al.* Subglottic secretion drainage for the prevention of ventilator-associated pneumonia: a systematic review and meta-analysis. *Crit Care Med* 2011; 39: 1985–1991.
10. Lacherade JC, De Jonghe B, Guezennec P, *et al.* Intermittent subglottic secretion drainage and ventilator-associated pneumonia: a multicenter trial. *Am J Respir Crit Care Med* 2010; 182: 910–917.
11. Carroll RG, McGinnis GE, Grenvik A. Performance characteristics of tracheal cuffs. *Int Anesthesiol Clin* 1974; 12: 111–141.
12. Dullenkopf A, Gerber A, Weiss M. Fluid leakage past tracheal tube cuffs: evaluation of the new Microcuff endotracheal tube. *Intensive Care Med* 2003; 29: 1849–1853.
13. Seegobin RD, van Hasselt GL. Aspiration beyond endotracheal cuffs. *Can Anaesth Soc J* 1986; 33: 273–279.
14. Pavlin EG, VanNimwegan D, Hornbein TF. Failure of a high-compliance low-pressure cuff to prevent aspiration. *Anesthesiology* 1975; 42: 216–219.
15. Kolobow T, Cressoni M, Epp M, *et al.* Comparison of a novel lycra endotracheal tube cuff to standard polyvinyl chloride cuff and polyurethane cuff for fluid leak prevention. *Respir Care* 2011; 56: 1095–1099.
16. Zanella A, Scaravilli V, Isgro S, *et al.* Fluid leakage across tracheal tube cuff, effect of different cuff material, shape, and positive expiratory pressure: a bench-top study. *Intensive Care Med* 2011; 37: 343–347.
17. Ouanes I, Lyazidi A, Danin PE, *et al.* Mechanical influences on fluid leakage past the tracheal tube cuff in a benchtop model. *Intensive Care Med* 2011; 37: 695–700.
18. Dave MH, Frotzler A, Weiss M. Closed tracheal suction and fluid aspiration past the tracheal tube. Impact of tube cuff and airway pressure. *Minerva Anestesiol* 2011; 77: 166–171.
19. Dave MH, Frotzler A, Madjdpour C, *et al.* Massive aspiration past the tracheal tube cuff caused by closed tracheal suction system. *J Intensive Care Med* 2011; 26: 326–329.
20. Dave MH, Koepfer N, Madjdpour C, *et al.* Tracheal fluid leakage in benchtop trials: comparison of static *versus* dynamic ventilation model with and without lubrication. *J Anesth* 2010; 24: 247–252.
21. Dave MH, Frotzler A, Spielmann N, *et al.* Effect of tracheal tube cuff shape on fluid leakage across the cuff: an *in vitro* study. *Br J Anaesth* 2010; 105: 538–543.
22. Pitts R, Fisher D, Sulemanji D, *et al.* Variables affecting leakage past endotracheal tube cuffs: a bench study. *Intensive Care Med* 2010; 36: 2066–2073.
23. Lucangelo U, Zin WA, Antonaglia V, *et al.* Effect of positive expiratory pressure and type of tracheal cuff on the incidence of aspiration in mechanically ventilated patients in an intensive care unit. *Crit Care Med* 2008; 36: 409–413.

24. Zanella A, Cressoni M, Epp M, *et al.* A double-layer tracheal tube cuff designed to prevent leakage: a bench-top study. *Intensive Care Med* 2008; 34: 1145–1149.
25. Winklmaier U, Wüst K, Schiller S, *et al.* Leakage of fluid in different types of tracheal tubes. *Dysphagia* 2006; 21: 237–242.
26. Young PJ, Pakeerathan S, Blunt MC, *et al.* A low-volume, low-pressure tracheal tube cuff reduces pulmonary aspiration. *Crit Care Med* 2006; 34: 632–639.
27. Blunt MC, Young PJ, Patil A, *et al.* Gel lubrication of the tracheal tube cuff reduces pulmonary aspiration. *Anesthesiology* 2001; 95: 377–381.
28. Asai T, Shingu K. Leakage of fluid around high-volume, low-pressure cuffs apparatus. A comparison of four tracheal tubes. *Anaesthesia* 2001; 56: 38–42.
29. Young PJ, Blunt MC. Compliance characteristics of the Portex Soft Seal Cuff improves seal against leakage of fluid in a pig trachea model. *Crit Care* 1999; 3: 123–126.
30. Young PJ, Blunt MC. Improving the shape and compliance characteristics of a high-volume, low-pressure cuff improves tracheal seal. *Br J Anaesth* 1999; 83: 887–889.
31. Young PJ, Ridley SA, Downward G. Evaluation of a new design of tracheal tube cuff to prevent leakage of fluid to the lungs. *Br J Anaesth* 1998; 80: 796–799.
32. Young PJ, Rollinson M, Downward G, *et al.* Leakage of fluid past the tracheal tube cuff in a benchtop model. *Br J Anaesth* 1997; 78: 557–562.
33. Miller MA, Arndt JL, Konkle MA, *et al.* A polyurethane cuffed endotracheal tube is associated with decreased rates of ventilator-associated pneumonia. *J Crit Care* 2011; 26: 280–286.
34. Nseir S, Zerimech F, De Jonckheere J, *et al.* Impact of polyurethane on variations in tracheal cuff pressure in critically ill patients: a prospective observational study. *Intensive Care Med* 2010; 36: 1156–1163.
35. Poelaert J, Depuydt P, De WA, *et al.* Polyurethane cuffed endotracheal tubes to prevent early postoperative pneumonia after cardiac surgery: a pilot study. *J Thorac Cardiovasc Surg* 2008; 135: 771–776.
36. Lorente L, Lecuona M, Jiménez A, *et al.* Influence of an endotracheal tube with polyurethane cuff and subglottic secretion drainage on pneumonia. *Am J Respir Crit Care Med* 2007; 176: 1079–1083.
37. Young PJ, Burchett K, Harvey I, *et al.* The prevention of pulmonary aspiration with control of tracheal wall pressure using a silicone cuff. *Anaesth Intensive Care* 2000; 28: 660–665.
38. Seegobin RD, van Hasselt GL. Endotracheal cuff pressure and tracheal mucosal blood flow: endoscopic study of effects of four large volume cuffs. *Br Med J* 1984; 288: 965–968.
39. Medina CR, Camargo JJ, Felicetti JC, *et al.* Post-intubation tracheal injury: report of three cases and literature review. *J Bras Pneumol* 2009; 35: 809–813.
40. Harris R, Joseph A. Acute tracheal rupture related to endotracheal intubation: case report. *J Emerg Med* 2000; 18: 35–39.
41. Hameed AA, Mohamed H, Al-Mansoori M. Acquired tracheoesophageal fistula due to high intracuff pressure. *Ann Thorac Med* 2008; 3: 23–25.
42. Rello J, Sonora R, Jubert P, *et al.* Pneumonia in intubated patients: role of respiratory airway care. *Am J Respir Crit Care Med* 1996; 154: 111–115.
43. Faris C, Koury E, Philpott J, *et al.* Estimation of tracheostomy tube cuff pressure by pilot balloon palpation. *J Laryngol Otol* 2007; 121: 869–871.
44. Fernandez R, Blanch L, Mancebo J, *et al.* Endotracheal tube cuff pressure assessment: pitfalls of finger estimation and need for objective measurement. *Crit Care Med* 1990; 18: 1423–1426.
45. Liu J, Zhang X, Gong W et al. Correlations between controlled endotracheal tube cuff pressure and postprocedural complications: a multicenter study. *Anesth Analg* 2010; 111: 1133–1137.
46. O'Donnell JM. A comparison of endotracheal tube cuff pressures using estimation techniques and direct intracuff measurement. *AANA J* 2004; 72: 250–251.
47. Vyas D, Inweregbu K, Pittard A. Measurement of tracheal tube cuff pressure in critical care. *Anaesthesia* 2002; 57: 275–277.
48. Valencia M, Ferrer M, Farre R, *et al.* Automatic control of tracheal tube cuff pressure in ventilated patients in semirecumbent position: a randomized trial. *Crit Care Med* 2007; 35: 1543–1549.
49. Duguet A, D'Amico L, Biondi G, *et al.* Control of tracheal cuff pressure: a pilot study using a pneumatic device. *Intensive Care Med* 2007; 33: 128–132.
50. Nseir S, Zerimech F, Fournier C, *et al.* Continuous control of tracheal cuff pressure and microaspiration of gastric contents in critically ill patients. *Am J Respir Crit Care Med* 2011; 184: 1041–1047.
51. Costerton JW, Stewart PS, Greenberg EP. Bacterial biofilms: a common cause of persistent infections. *Science* 1999; 21: 1318–1322.
52. Berra L, De ML, Yu ZX, *et al.* Endotracheal tubes coated with antiseptics decrease bacterial colonization of the ventilator circuits, lungs, and endotracheal tube. *Anesthesiology* 2004; 100: 1446–1456.
53. Inglis TJ, Millar MR, Jones JG, *et al.* Tracheal tube biofilm as a source of bacterial colonization of the lung. *J Clin Microbiol* 1989; 27: 2014–2018.
54. Ng KS, Kumarasinghe G, Inglis TJ. Dissemination of respiratory secretions during tracheal tube suctioning in an intensive care unit. *Ann Acad Med Singapore* 1999; 28: 178–182.
55. Adair CG, Gorman SP, Feron BM, *et al.* Implications of endotracheal tube biofilm for ventilator-associated pneumonia. *Intensive Care Med* 1999; 25: 1072–1076.

56. Olson ME, Harmon BG, Kollef MH. Silver-coated endotracheal tubes associated with reduced bacterial burden in the lungs of mechanically ventilated dogs. *Chest* 2002; 121: 863–870.

57. Berra L, Curto F, Li Bassi G, *et al.* Antibacterial-coated tracheal tubes cleaned with the Mucus Shaver: a novel method to retain long-term bactericidal activity of coated tracheal tubes. *Intensive Care Med* 2006; 32: 888–893.

58. Li Bassi G, Berra L, Kolobow T. Silver-coated endotracheal tubes: is the bactericidal effect time limited? *Crit Care Med* 2007; 35: 986.

59. Kolobow T, Berra L, Li Bassi G, *et al.* Novel system for complete removal of secretions within the endotracheal tube: the Mucus Shaver. *Anesthesiology* 2005; 102: 1063–1065.

60. Berra L, Corbeil C, Bittner EA, *et al.* A clinical assessment of the Mucus Shaver: a device to keep the endotracheal tube free from secretions. *Crit Care Med* 2012; 40: 119–124.

61. Kollef MH, Afessa B, Anzueto A, *et al.* Silver-coated endotracheal tubes and incidence of ventilator-associated pneumonia: the NASCENT randomized trial. *JAMA* 2008; 300: 805–813.

62. Afessa B, Shorr AF, Anzueto AR, *et al.* Association between a silver-coated endotracheal tube and reduced mortality in patients with ventilator-associated pneumonia. *Chest* 2010; 137: 1015–1021.

63. Shorr AF, Zilberberg MD, Kollef M. Cost-effectiveness analysis of a silver-coated endotracheal tube to reduce the incidence of ventilator-associated pneumonia. *Infect Control Hosp Epidemiol* 2009; 30: 759–763.

64. Ferrer M, Bauer TT, Torres A, *et al.* Effect of nasogastric tube size on gastroesophageal reflux and microaspiration in intubated patients. *Ann Intern Med* 1999; 130: 991–994.

65. Donowitz LG, Page MC, Mileur BL, *et al.* Alteration of normal gastric flora in critical care patients receiving antacid and cimetidine therapy. *Infect Control* 1986; 7: 23–26.

66. Hillman KM. Colonisation of the gastric contents in critically ill patients. *Acta Anaesthesiol Belg* 1983; 34: 191–192.

67. Heyland D, Mandell LA. Gastric colonization by gram-negative bacilli and nosocomial pneumonia in the intensive care unit patient. Evidence for causation. *Chest* 1992; 101: 187–193.

68. Torres A, El-Ebiary M, Gonzalez J, *et al.* Gastric and pharyngeal flora in nosocomial pneumonia acquired during mechanical ventilation. *Am Rev Respir Dis* 1993; 148: 352–357.

69. Bonten MJ, Gaillard CA, van Thiel FH, *et al.* The stomach is not a source for colonization of the upper respiratory tract and pneumonia in ICU patients. *Chest* 1994; 105: 878–884.

70. Bonten MJ, Bergmans DC, Ambergen AW, *et al.* Risk factors for pneumonia, and colonization of respiratory tract and stomach in mechanically ventilated ICU patients. *Am J Respir Crit Care Med* 1996; 154: 1339–1346.

71. Cardeñosa Cendrero JA, Sole-Violan J, Bordes Benitez A, *et al.* Role of different routes of tracheal colonization in the development of pneumonia in patients receiving mechanical ventilation. *Chest* 1999; 116: 462–470.

72. Feldman C, Kassel M, Cantrell J, *et al.* The presence and sequence of endotracheal tube colonization in patients undergoing mechanical ventilation. *Eur Respir J* 1999; 13: 546–551.

73. Li Bassi G, Torres A. Ventilator-associated pneumonia: role of positioning. *Curr Opin Crit Care* 2011; 17: 57–63.

74. Tablan OC, Anderson LJ, Besser R, *et al.* Guidelines for preventing health-care-associated pneumonia, 2003: recommendations of CDC and the Healthcare Infection Control Practices Advisory Committee. *MMWR Recomm Rep 2004; 53(RR-3):* 1–36.

75. Rotstein C, Evans G, Born A, *et al.* Clinical practice guidelines for hospital-acquired pneumonia and ventilator-associated pneumonia in adults. *Can J Infect Dis Med Microbiol* 2008; 19: 19–53.

76. Li Bassi G, Zanella A, Cressoni M, *et al.* Following tracheal intubation, mucus flow is reversed in the semirecumbent position: possible role in the pathogenesis of ventilator-associated pneumonia. *Crit Care Med* 2008; 36: 518–525.

77. Panigada M, Berra L, Greco G, *et al.* Bacterial colonization of the respiratory tract following tracheal intubation-effect of gravity: an experimental study. *Crit Care Med* 2003; 31: 729–737.

78. Mauri T, Berra L, Kumwilaisak K, *et al.* Lateral-horizontal patient position and horizontal orientation of the endotracheal tube to prevent aspiration in adult surgical intensive care unit patients: a feasibility study. *Respir Care* 2010; 55: 294–302.

79. Aly H, Badawy M, El-Kholy A, *et al.* Randomized, controlled trial on tracheal colonization of ventilated infants: can gravity prevent ventilator-associated pneumonia? *Pediatrics* 2008; 122: 770–774.

80. Manzano F, Fernandez-Mondejar E, Colmenero M, *et al.* Positive-end expiratory pressure reduces incidence of ventilator-associated pneumonia in nonhypoxemic patients. *Crit Care Med* 2008; 36: 2225–2231.

81. van Kaam AH, Lachmann RA, Herting E, *et al.* Reducing atelectasis attenuates bacterial growth and translocation in experimental pneumonia. *Am J Respir Crit Care Med* 2004; 169: 1046–1053.

82. Tilson MD, Bunke MC, Walker Smith GJ, *et al.* Quantitative bacteriology and pathology of the lung in experimental *Pseudomonas* pneumonia treated with positive end-expiratory pressure (PEEP). *Surgery* 1977; 82: 133–140.

83. Shennib H, Mulder DS, Chiu RC. The effects of pulmonary atelectasis and reexpansion on lung cellular immune defenses. *Arch Surg* 1984; 119: 274–277.

84. Charles PE, Martin L, Etienne M, *et al.* Influence of positive end-expiratory pressure (PEEP) on histopathological and bacteriological aspects of pneumonia during low tidal volume mechanical ventilation. *Intensive Care Med* 2004; 30: 2263–2270.

85. Ganz T. Antimicrobial polypeptides in host defense of the respiratory tract. *J Clin Invest* 2002; 109: 693–697.

86. Salathe M. Regulation of mammalian ciliary beating. *Annu Rev Physiol* 2007; 69: 401–422.
87. Yeates DB, Aspin N, Levison H, *et al*. Mucociliary tracheal transport rates in man. *J Appl Physiol* 1975; 39: 487–495.
88. Sackner MA, Rosen MJ, Wanner A. Estimation of tracheal mucous velocity by bronchofiberscopy. *J Appl Physiol* 1973; 34: 495–499.
89. Konrad F, Schreiber T, Brecht-Kraus D, *et al*. Mucociliary transport in ICU patients. *Chest* 1994; 105: 237–241.
90. Sackner MA, Hirsch J, Epstein S. Effect of cuffed endotracheal tubes on tracheal mucous velocity. *Chest* 1975; 68: 774–777.
91. Cole AM, Dewan P, Ganz T. Innate antimicrobial activity of nasal secretions. *Infect Immun* 1999; 67: 3267–3275.
92. Kim CS, Greene MA, Sankaran S, *et al*. Mucus transport in the airways by two-phase gas-liquid flow mechanism: continuous flow model. *J Appl Physiol* 1986; 60: 908–917.
93. Kim CS, Rodriguez CR, Eldridge MA, *et al*. Criteria for mucus transport in the airways by two-phase gas-liquid flow mechanism. *J Appl Physiol* 1986; 60: 901–907.
94. Kim CS, Iglesias AJ, Sackner MA. Mucus clearance by two-phase gas-liquid flow mechanism: asymmetric periodic flow model. *J Appl Physiol* 1987; 62: 959–971.
95. Volpe MS, Adams AB, Amato MB, *et al*. Ventilation patterns influence airway secretion movement. *Respir Care* 2008; 53: 1287–1294.
96. Benjamin RG, Chapman GA, Kim CS, *et al*. Removal of bronchial secretions by two-phase gas-liquid transport. *Chest* 1989; 95: 658–663.
97. Li Bassi G, Saucedo L, Marti J-D, *et al*. Effects of duty cycle and positive end-expiratory pressure on mucus clearance during mechanical ventilation. *Crit Care Med* 2011; [Epub ahead of print DOI: 10.1097/CCM.0b013e318236efb5].
98. Ntoumenopoulos G, Shannon H, Main E. Do commonly used ventilator settings for mechanically ventilated adults have the potential to embed secretions or promote clearance? *Respir Care* 2011; 56: 1887–1892.

Chapter 13

Predictors of weaning from mechanical ventilation

F. Laghi and D. Morales

Summary

The dangers of mechanical ventilation make it critical to wean patients at the earliest time possible. However, premature weaning trials trigger significant respiratory distress, which can cause setbacks in a patient's clinical course. Premature extubation is also a known risk. To reduce delayed weaning and premature extubation, a three-step diagnostic strategy has been suggested: 1) measurement of weaning predictors; 2) a trial of unassisted breathing (T-tube trial); and 3) a trial of extubation.

It is imperative not to defer this first step by waiting for a more difficult diagnostic test, such as a T-tube trial. To increase the likelihood that a patient will tolerate extubation, a positive result on a screening test (weaning predictor test) is followed by a confirmatory test (weaning trial).

Many difficult aspects of pulmonary pathophysiology encroach on weaning management. Accordingly, weaning commands sophisticated individualised care. Few other responsibilities of an intensivist require a more analytical effort and carry more promise for improving a patient's outcome than the application of physiological principles in the weaning of patients.

Keywords: Diagnostic tests, extubation, mechanical ventilation, monitoring, screening, weaning

Loyola University of Chicago Stritch School of Medicine, Division of Pulmonary and Critical Care Medicine, Edward Hines, Jr. VA Hospital, Hines, IL, USA.

Correspondence: F. Laghi, Loyola University of Chicago Stritch School of Medicine, Division of Pulmonary and Critical Care Medicine, Edward Hines, Jr. VA Hospital, 111N, 5th Avenue and Roosevelt Road, Hines, 60141, IL, USA. Email flaghi@lumc.edu

Eur Respir Mon 2012; 55: 169–190.
Printed in UK – all rights reserved
Copyright ERS 2012
European Respiratory Monograph
ISSN: 1025-448x
DOI: 10.1183/1025448x.10002611

Although mechanical ventilation can be lifesaving it is often associated with life-threatening complications [1]. Accordingly, when it can be performed safely, it is essential to discontinue mechanical ventilation at the earliest possible time. The process of discontinuing mechanical ventilation is known as weaning. Unfortunately, various investigators and clinicians can have different understandings for the word "weaning". For some, weaning is the gradual reduction in ventilator support in a patient recovering from respiratory failure; however, the patient is not yet ready for spontaneous respiration. For others, weaning is the act of disconnecting the patient from the ventilator support completely, whilst for others, weaning comprises of both the discontinuation from mechanical ventilation support system and extubation.

Seven stages of weaning

With the intension of bringing some order to this field, TOBIN and JUBRAN [2] proposed a framework that outlined the seven stages of weaning (fig. 1). According to the proposed seven-stage schematic system, stage 1 is pre-weaning, when patients are too ill to be considered ready for weaning, *e.g.* patients requiring high levels of oxygen and positive end-expiratory pressure (PEEP). All ventilated patients begin at stage 1. In some larger series, 13–26% of patients never get beyond stage 1 [3–5]. During stage 1, measurements of weaning predictors are inappropriate and potentially dangerous.

Stage 2 is the period of diagnostic triggering. This is the time in which a physician begins to think that the patient "might be ready" to come off the ventilator. Failure to engage in this period of diagnostic triggering may be the greatest impediment to prompt weaning [2]. In more than 75% of patients who are ventilated for a week, or longer, the ventilator can be successfully discontinued the same day weaning predictors are measured [6, 7]. This observation raises the possibility in many patients that mechanical ventilation could have been discontinued a day or so earlier if the physicians had thought sooner that the patient "might have been" ready to come off the ventilator.

Stage 3 is the time to obtain physiological measurements that serve as predictors (weaning predictors) and to interpret them in context with each patient's unique clinical condition. During stage 4 (weaning trial) ventilatory support is either gradually decreased over hours or days, *e.g.* there is a gradual reduction in pressure support ventilation (PSV) or it is removed abruptly and completely (T-tube trial). In stage 5, patients who succeeded the weaning trial are extubated. Patients who do not succeed the weaning trial are returned to ventilator support. Stages 6 and 7 apply to patients who after extubation perform poorly. Stage 6 is the continuation of ventilator support with noninvasive ventilation (NIV). Stage 7 is reintubation, which is usually accompanied by the reinstatement of mechanical ventilation [2].

This chapter will review the clinical use of predictors for weaning outcome. The techniques of weaning and extubation failure will be examined briefly along with the clinical use of predictors for extubation failure; a field of critical care that is still in its infancy. Areas of active research and controversial topics will be highlighted throughout this chapter.

Prediction of weaning outcome

Research on prediction of weaning outcome employs the tools of medical decision analysis. Therefore, before discussing weaning predictor tests, it is useful to review the principles of medical decision analysis.

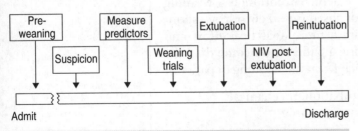

Figure 1. The seven stages of weaning. Stage 1 is pre-weaning, a stage that many patients never move beyond. Stage 2 is the period of diagnostic triggering, the time when a physician begins to think that their patient might be ready to come off the ventilator. Stage 3 is the time of measuring and interpreting weaning predictors. Stage 4 is the time of decreasing ventilator support (abruptly or gradually). Stage 5 is either extubation (of a weaning-success patient) or when mechanical ventilation is reinstated (in a weaning-failure patient). Stage 6 is the use of noninvasive ventilation (NIV) after extubation. Stage 7 is reintubation. Failure to appreciate stage 2 probably leads to the greatest delay in weaning. Reproduced from [2] with permission from the publisher.

Medical decision analysis

Diagnostic tests are designed to screen for a condition and to confirm the condition. The characteristics of screening tests and confirmatory tests differ and it is rare for a single diagnostic test to fulfil both functions [8].

The primary goal of weaning-predictor tests is screening [2]. A good weaning-predictor test, like any good screening test, should not miss a patient who has the condition under consideration, *i.e.* is ready for a weaning trial. This means that a good weaning-predictor test must have a low rate of false-negative results and, therefore, a high sensitivity (fig. 2) [2, 8]. A high rate of false-positive results (low specificity) is acceptable [2, 8].

The process of weaning involves the measurement of weaning predictors, a trial of weaning, and a trial of extubation (fig. 1) [2]. Each step in this sequence is a diagnostic test. Measurements of weaning predictors (screening tests) are used to diagnose readiness for a weaning trial. The trial of weaning (a confirmatory test for the screening tests) is used to screen for the readiness to extubate. Extubation (the confirmatory test for the weaning trial) is used to diagnose/screen for readiness to maintain spontaneous respiration. To apply diagnostic tests in sequence (screening or confirmatory) introduces critical confounders in the interpretation of studies designed to assess the reliability of a (pre-existing) predictor test. These confounders are spectrum bias, test-referral bias and base-rate fallacy [8, 9]. In the case of weaning, spectrum bias arises when the study population in a new investigation contains more (or fewer) sick patients than the population in which the diagnostic test was first developed [8, 9]. Test-referral bias arises when the results of the weaning predictor, which is being assessed, are used to choose patients for a reference-standard test, *i.e.* passing a weaning trial that leads to extubation [8, 9]. Base-rate fallacy occurs when physicians fail to take into account the pre-test probability of the disorder [9].

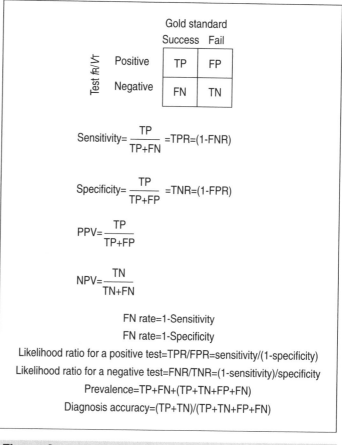

$$\text{Sensitivity} = \frac{TP}{TP+FN} = TPR = (1-FNR)$$

$$\text{Specificity} = \frac{TP}{TP+FP} = TNR = (1-FPR)$$

$$PPV = \frac{TP}{TP+FP}$$

$$NPV = \frac{TN}{TN+FN}$$

FN rate=1-Sensitivity
FN rate=1-Specificity
Likelihood ratio for a positive test=TPR/FPR=sensitivity/(1-specificity)
Likelihood ratio for a negative test=FNR/TNR=(1-sensitivity)/specificity
Prevalence=TP+FN+(TP+TN+FP+FN)
Diagnosis accuracy=(TP+TN)/(TP+TN+FP+FN)

Figure 2. A tabular display of the characteristics of diagnostic tests. Readings for respiratory frequency/tidal volume ratio (fR/Vt) ≤100 are classified as positive test results and readings >100 are classified as negative test results. The relationship of these binary results to the outcome of a T-tube weaning trial forms a decision matrix, which has four possible combinations. TP: true positive; test predicts weaning success and patient actually succeeds. TN: true negative; test predicts weaning failure and patient actually fails. FP: false positive; test predicts weaning success and patient actually fails. FN: false negative; test predicts weaning failure and patient actually succeeds. PPV: positive predicted value; NPV: negative predicted value; R: rate. Reproduced from [2] with permission from the publisher.

Pre-test probability is a physician's estimate for the likelihood of a particular condition (weaning outcome) before a diagnostic test is undertaken [2]. Post-test probability (typically expressed as a positive or negative predictive value) is the new likelihood after the test results are obtained (fig. 2). A good diagnostic tests achieves a marked increase (or decrease) in the post-test probability (over pre-test probability). For every test in every medical subspecialty, the magnitude of change between pre-test and post-test probability is determined by Bayes' theorem [9]. Three factors alone determine the magnitude of the pre- to post-test change: sensitivity, specificity and pre-test probability. It is commonly assumed that sensitivity and specificity remain constant for a test. In truth, test-referral bias, a common occurrence in studies of weaning tests, leads to major changes in sensitivity and specificity [8]. Likewise, major changes in pre-test probability arise as a consequence of spectrum bias [8]. All of these factors need to be carefully considered when reading a study that evaluates the reliability of a weaning-predictor test.

Weaning-predictor tests

Several weaning-predictor tests have been proposed and studied over the years. These tests include measurements of breathing patterns, pulmonary gas exchange, muscle strength and neuromuscular drive. Their goal is to safely speed up the weaning process.

Respiratory frequency/tidal volume ratio

The respiratory frequency/tidal volume ratio ($fR/V\text{T}$) is measured during 1 minute of spontaneous breathing (fig. 3) [10]. The $fR/V\text{T}$ can be recorded with a handheld spirometer after disconnecting the patient's endotracheal tube from the ventilator circuit [5]. Alternatively, $fR/V\text{T}$ can be recorded using a neumotachograph within the ventilator. In this case, physicians must take care to place the patient in the "flow-by" mode and they must ensure that PSV and continuous positive airway pressure (CPAP) are both set at zero [11]. However, it must be noted that even if a clinician uses "flow-by" with pressure support set at 0 cmH$_2$O, ventilators manufactured by some companies (*e.g.* Nellcor Puritan Bennett, Boulder, CO, USA and Siemens, Munich, Germany) will still provide assistance of 1.5 cmH$_2$O during inhalation. It is necessary to ensure these steps are performed to avoid the inaccurate prediction of weaning outcome [2]. For instance, the use of PSV at 5 or 10 cmH$_2$O decreases $fR/V\text{T}$ by 20–80% when compared with unassisted breathing [12–15]. The use of CPAP at 5 cmH$_2$O decreases $fR/V\text{T}$ by 20–50% when compared with unassisted breathing [11, 16, 17].

When recording $fR/V\text{T}$ it is important that the patient's breathing pattern achieves equilibrium before starting the measurement. Mechanical ventilation can depress respiratory motor output and, thus, apnoeic pauses and shallow breaths are common during the first minute after disconnecting a patient from the ventilator. To avoid this pitfall the clinician must wait until the patient has established a regular respiratory rhythm, a process that can take approximately 1 minute. When regular respiratory rhythm has been established the clinician can then measure $fR/V\text{T}$ over the subsequent minute.

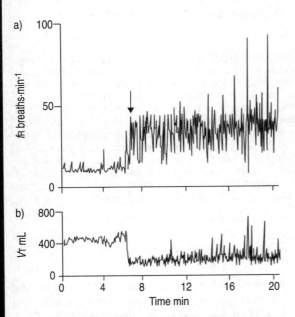

The higher the $fR/V\text{T}$, the more severe rapid and shallow breathing occurs and the greater the likelihood of unsuccessful weaning. An $fR/V\text{T}$ of 100 discriminates between successful and unsuccessful attempts at weaning [5]. The initial evaluation of $fR/V\text{T}$ during 1 minute of spontaneous breathing was reported in 1991 [5]. Since then, this test has been evaluated in more than 25 studies. Reported sensitivity ranges from 0.35 to 1.00 [9]. Specificity ranges from 0.00 to 0.89 [9]. At first glance, this wide scatter suggests that $fR/V\text{T}$ is an unreliable predictor for the outcome of weaning. However, many of the investigators ignored the possibility of test-referral bias and spectrum bias [2, 9]. These problems were compounded by an Evidence-Based Medicine Task Force set up by the American College of Chest Physicians (ACCP) [18], which in 2001 undertook a meta-analysis primarily based on

Figure 3. A time series of a breath-by-breath plot for a) respiratory frequency (*f*R) and b) tidal volume (*V*t) in a patient who failed a weaning trial. The arrow indicates the point of resuming spontaneous breathing. Rapid, shallow breathing developed almost immediately after discontinuation of the ventilator. Reproduced from [10] with permission form the publisher.

work performed by the McMaster University Evidence-based Practice Centre [19].

The Task Force calculated pooled likelihood ratios for fR/VT and judged the summated values to signify that fR/VT was not a reliable predictor of weaning success and recommended that clinicians should start the weaning process with a spontaneous breathing trial (a confirmatory test), and use the initial few minutes of the trial as a screening test [18, 19]. However, this recommendation was untenable for several reasons. First, the studies included in the meta-analysis exhibited significant heterogeneity in pre-test probability of successful outcome [9]. Such marked heterogeneity prohibits the undertaking of a reliable meta-analysis [20, 21]. When data from the studies (included in the meta-analysis) were entered into a Bayesian model with pre-test probability as the operating point, the reported positive predictive values were significantly correlated with the values predicted by the original report on fR/VT (r=0.86; p<0.0001) [5]. Likewise, reported negative predictive values were correlated with the values predicted (r=0.82; p<0.0001) (figs 4 and 5) [9].

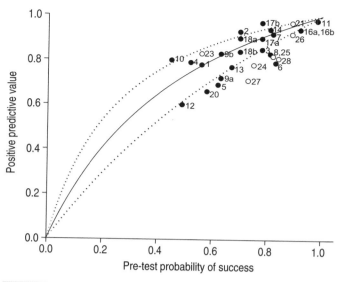

Figure 4. Observed positive predictive value (post-test probability of successful outcome) for respiratory frequency/tidal volume ratio (fR/VT) plotted against pre-test probability of weaning success. Studies 5, 6, 11, 18a, 18b and 24 include measurements of Bayes' formula obtained during pressure support. The study number refers to the study as cited in TOBIN and JUBRAN [9]. Studies 14 and 21 include measurements obtained in paediatric patients. Studies 7, 18a, 18b and 28 used fR/VT threshold values <65. ●: studies included in the American College of Chest Physicians (ACCP) Task Force meta-analysis [18]; ○: studies undertaken after publication of the ACCP Task Force report; ———: curve based on the sensitivity and specificity originally reported by YANG and TOBIN [5] and Bayes' formula for 0.01 unit increments in pre-test probability between 0.00 and 1.00; ┄┄┄┄: upper and lower 95% confidence intervals for the predicted relationship of the positive predictive values against pre-test probability. Data taken from [9].

Secondly, a spontaneous breathing trial in patients who are not ready for such a trial can cause cardiopulmonary stress [22, 23], which can be sufficient to trigger the release of interleukin (IL)-6, a major modulator of the stress response [24]. Thirdly, the recommendation to skip screening tests and begin with a spontaneous breathing trial is bound to foster delays in the removal of the ventilator [6, 7, 25]. Finally, this recommendation ignores extensive research in cognitive psychology that has revealed causes of faulty decision making [26, 27]. Psychologists have repeatedly shown that people make wrong decisions because they are overconfident in their judgments (e.g. deciding that a patient is not ready for a T-tube trial), and pay insufficient attention to prior probability [26, 27].

The primary task of a weaning-predictor test is screening, which requires a high sensitivity [2, 8]. The average sensitivity in all of the studies on fR/VT was 0.89 and 85% of the studies revealed a sensitivity greater than 0.90 [9]. This sensitivity compares well with commonly used diagnostic tests: creatine phosphokinase and troponin T for the diagnosis of acute myocardial infarction, sensitivity of 0.94 [2] and 0.98 [28], respectively; stress ECG for myocardial myocardial ischaemia 0.58 for females and 0.71 for males [29]; and sensitivity to diagnose endocarditis of less than 0.60–0.70 with transthoracic echocardiography and 0.75–0.95 with transesophageal echocardiography [30]. The sensitivity of a spontaneous breathing trial is unknown.

Since screening is the primary purpose of a weaning-predictor test, it is important that the test be performed early in a patient's ventilator course. However, figures 4 and 5 reveal that the pre-test probability of weaning success was 75% or higher in more than half of the studies undertaken on weaning-predictor tests. In other words, most physicians are postponing (inappropriately) the

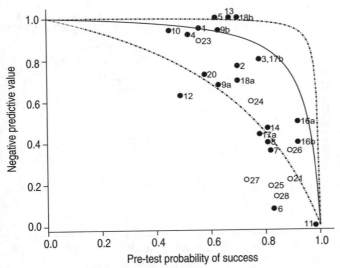

Figure 5. Negative predictive value (post-test probability of unsuccessful outcome) for respiratory frequency/tidal volume ratio (f_R/V_T) plotted against the pre-test probability of weaning success. The study number refers to the study as cited in TOBIN and JUBRAN [9]. Of note is study 11, which has a negative predictive value of 0.00 and specificity of 0.00. These values suggest that f_R/V_T is an unreliable test (and this will also be the natural conclusion reached by a meta-analysis of likelihood ratio). Instead, a negative predictive value of 0.00 and specificity of 0.00 are the values predicted for the pre-test probability of weaning success of 98.2% reported in study 11. ●: studies included in the American College of Chest Physicians (ACCP) Task Force's meta-analysis; ○: studies undertaken after publication of the ACCP Task Force's report; ——: curve based on the sensitivity and specificity originally reported by YANG and TOBIN [5] and Bayes' formula for 0.01 unit increments in pre-test probability between 0.00 and 1.00; ·········: upper and lower 95% confidence intervals for the predicted relationship of the negative predictive values against pre-test probability. Reproduced from [9] with permission from the publisher.

undertaking of weaning-predictor tests. A simple way for a physician to assess their own timeline for initiating weaning is to estimate the number of times they have obtained positive results on weaning-predictor tests over the preceding 6 months. If a physician, working in a typical medical intensive care unit (ICU), estimates that they obtained positive results 70% of the time or more, they should consider the possibility that they are being too slow in initiating weaning [2].

In 2006, TANIOS *et al.* [31] conducted an investigation to determine the effect of including f_R/V_T in a weaning protocol in 304 patients cared for in the ICUs of three hospitals. According to study design, patients in the f_R/V_T protocol group could proceed to a weaning trial (CPAP of $\leqslant 5$ cmH$_2$O and PS of $\leqslant 7$ cmH$_2$O) if they had a f_R/V_T of less than 106. Patients in the control group were weaned according to the physician's clinical judgment. The rate of extubation was the same in both groups, 82%. Duration of weaning was 1 day longer in the f_R/V_T protocol group than in the non-protocol group. The investigators concluded that f_R/V_T should not be used routinely in making the weaning decision as it prolongs weaning time.

The study has three major problems. First, the investigators assumed that physicians managing patients in the control group ignored f_R and V_T in deciding whether a patient should start weaning or not, something that is highly unlikely considering that physicians are well aware of the impact of breathing pattern on weaning. Secondly, the pre-test probability of weaning/extubation success was 82%. This high pre-test probability limits the likelihood that an f_R/V_T, or any other screening test, could show any benefit (fig. 5). Finally, in the research protocol of TANIOS *et al.* [31] patients who had an f_R/V_T of 105 or less progressed to a weaning trial, whereas patients with an f_R/V_T of 106 or higher were returned to the ventilator. This, of course, is what must be done when conducting a randomised controlled trial, *i.e.* no flexibility is permitted. However, in clinical practice, ventilator management should not be based on a one unit difference in a single measurement of an f_R/V_T.

Pulmonary gas exchange

Mechanical ventilation is virtually never discontinued in a patient who has severe hypoxaemia, such as arterial oxygen tension (P_{a,O_2}) <55 mmHg with an inspiratory oxygen fraction (F_{I,O_2}) >0.40. The $P_{a,O_2}/F_{I,O_2}$ ratio, the alveolar–arterial oxygen tension gradient (P_{A-a,O_2}) and the $P_{a,O_2}/P_{A-a,O_2}$ ratio are indices derived from arterial blood gas measurements proposed as predictors of weaning outcome. However, of these indices only $P_{a,O_2}/P_{A-a,O_2}$ has been prospectively evaluated and has performed poorly as a predictor of weaning outcome [5]. The study was marred by test-referral bias, *i.e.* patients with severe hypoxia were excluded from the study population. Therefore, it is not possible to conclude that the poor performance of $Pa,O_2/PA–a,O_2$ means that indices derived from arterial blood gas measurements are of no value in predicting weaning outcome. While threshold values of the efficiency of indices derived from arterial blood gas measurements cannot be recommended for weaning prediction, weaning attempts are not recommended in patients with borderline hypoxaemia.

Minute ventilation

Minute ventilation of less than 10 L·min^{-1} was a classic index used to predict a successful weaning outcome [32]. However, when prospectively assessed, minute ventilation has a high rate of false-negative and false-positive results and cannot be recommended as a predictor of weaning outcome [2].

Maximum inspiratory pressure

The use of maximum inspiratory pressure (PI,max) as a weaning predictor stems from a study by Sahn and Lakshminarayan [32]. They found that all patients with a PI,max value more negative than -30 cmH$_2$O were successfully weaned, whereas all patients with a PI,max less negative than -20 cmH$_2$O failed a weaning trial. In most successive investigations, these threshold values have shown poor sensitivity and specificity [5, 23, 33–36].

Vital capacity

The normal vital capacity (VC) is usually between 65 and 75 mL·kg^{-1}, and a value of 10 mL·kg^{-1} or more has been suggested to predict a successful weaning outcome [2]. In a study of 10 patients with Guillain–Barré syndrome, Chevrolet and Deleamont [37] reported that VC was helpful in guiding the weaning process. Patients with a VC of less than 7 mL·kg^{-1} were unable to tolerate 15 minutes of spontaneous breathing. As VC increased to greater than 15 mL·kg^{-1} with recovery from the illness, patients were safely extubated. Apart from unique circumstances, such as patients with Guillain–Barré syndrome, VC is rarely used as a weaning predictor and it is often unreliable [2].

Mouth occlusion pressure

Several investigators have evaluated the usefulness of mouth occlusion pressure at 100 ms ($P0.1$) as a predictor of weaning outcome [2]. In these studies, $P0.1$ values greater than 3.4 to 6.0 cmH$_2$O discriminated between weaning success and weaning failures [2]. However, other investigators have found $P0.1$ to be inaccurate [38]. One mechanism which could contribute to the poor performance of $P0.1$ is the limited reproducibility of the measurement. The within individual coefficient of variation of $P0.1$ is approximately 50% [39, 40] and the inter-individual coefficient of variation is as high as 60% [41].

B-type natriuretic peptides

The mechanical stretch of cardiomyocytes, caused by atrial or ventricular pressure overload, volume overload or both, triggers the release of pro-brain natriuretic peptide (pro-BNP), a prohormone. Pro-BNP is rapidly cleaved into a biologically active 32-amino acid carboxyl-terminal peptide (BNP) and its inactive 76-amino acid amino terminal (N-terminal) fragment (NT-proBNP) [42]. Several investigators have evaluated the accuracy of BNP and NT-proBNP in identifying the likelihood and presence of a cardiac cause for weaning failure. However, to date, there is substantial discrepancy in the results of studies assessing the capacity of natriuretic peptides to predict weaning outcome. For some investigators the change in a peptide concentration over the course of a weaning trial has the greatest predictive power [43], whilst for others the baseline values are more reliable [44], some report that BNP is more dependable than NT-proBNP [45], whereas others report the opposite [43]. In addition the threshold values that differentiate between weaning-success and weaning-failure patients has been known to differ greatly among investigations.

Gastric tonometry

The gastrointestinal mucosa becomes ischaemic early due to the development of either haemodynamic compromise or a redistribution of blood flow. One factor that leads to blood flow redistribution is an increase in respiratory muscle effort. Gastric tonometry is based on the principle that the carbon dioxide tension (PCO$_2$) of the fluid in the gastric lumen equilibrates with the PCO$_2$ of the mucosal layer, and that the recording of PCO$_2$ in gastric fluid provides a reliable estimate of the pH of the gut mucosa [46]. However, the assumption that PCO$_2$ in the gastric lumen is similar to that in the tissues of the gastric wall may not be true, especially in patients who experience an uneven distribution of gastric blood flow [2].

When assessing the accuracy of gastric tonometry as a predictor of weaning outcome some investigators found that the measurements discriminated between the weaning-success and the weaning-failure patient during mechanical ventilation [47, 48], whereas others did not [49–51]. If the ventilator was set at a level to achieve satisfactory muscle rest, it is difficult to see why gastric intra-mucosal pH should differ between the groups before the onset of spontaneous breathing. The studies reveal different levels of accuracy in predicting weaning outcome. The reported accuracy represents an overestimation, because none of the investigators divided their data sets into training and validation subsets. Several investigators commented that the technique was simple. Yet, it involves inserting a special intragastric tonometer, obtaining a radiograph to confirm location, the administration of histamine-2 receptor blockers, withholding enteral feeding, waiting sufficient time for satisfactory equilibration, and withdrawing and analysing a saline sample and an arterial blood gas [2].

Diaphragm ultrasonography

Diaphragmatic dysfunction is common in mechanically ventilated patients [33, 52]. M-mode ultrasonography is a promising and noninvasive technique to identify diaphragmatic dysfunction in these patients. Recently, KIM et al. [53] assessed the impact of diaphragmatic dysfunction in 88 patients who were deemed ready for a trial of spontaneous respiration, and had no history of diaphragmatic disease. Diaphragmatic dysfunction was defined as either a vertical excursion of the muscle of less than 10 mm or as paradoxic movements. 24 (29%) of the 82 eligible patients had evidence of diaphragmatic dysfunction. Compared with patients without dysfunction those with dysfunction had a longer weaning time (17 days versus 4 days, p<0.01) and total ventilation time (24 days versus 9 days, p<0.01). Future studies are necessary to assess the role of diaphragm ultrasonography in identifying patients at high risk of difficulty weaning.

Weaning trials

When a screening test is positive, e.g. low fR/VT, the physician proceeds to a confirmatory test e.g. PSV of 6–8 cm-H$_2$O or spontaneous respiration through a T-Tube [8]. The goal of a positive result from a confirmatory test (no respiratory distress at the conclusion of the PSV trial or T-tube trial) is to rule in a condition, i.e. in this case the increased likelihood that a patient would tolerate a trial of extubation [8]. An ideal confirmatory test has a very low rate of false-positive results, i.e. a high specificity [8]. To determine the specificity of a spontaneous breathing test it is required to extubate all patients who fail a weaning trial and to count how many require re-intubation [2]. Unfortunately, the specificity of a spontaneous breathing trial is not known. Indeed, its specificity will never be known, as it would require an unethical experiment, i.e. all patients who failed a weaning trial would have to be extubated and the number requiring reintubation would need to be counted without introducing confounders, such as the use of NIV for post-extubation respiratory distress [54].

The major weaning techniques used include T-tube trial, PSV, intermittent mandatory ventilation (IMV), or some combination of these three. Recently, positive-pressure NIV has been used to facilitate extubation in selected patients [55].

Intermittent mandatory ventilation

When IMV is used for weaning, the ventilator's mandatory rate is reduced in steps of one to three breaths per minute, and an arterial blood gas is obtained approximately 30 minutes after each rate change [56]. Unfortunately, when the ventilator's mandatory rate is titrated, in accordance with the arterial blood gases results, a false sense of security can occur. As few as two or three IMV breaths per minute can achieve acceptable blood gas results; however, these values provide no information regarding the patient's work of breathing [2]. At IMV rates of 14 breaths per minute, or fewer, the patient's work of breathing may be excessive [57, 58]. By providing inadequate respiratory muscle rest, IMV is likely to delay rather than facilitate weaning [7].

Pressure support ventilation

When PSV is used for weaning, the level of pressure is reduced gradually and titrated on the basis of the patient's f_R [59]. When the patient tolerates a minimal level of PSV, they are extubated. What constitutes a "minimal level of PSV" has never been defined [12]. For example, a PSV of 6 to 8 cmH$_2$O is widely used to compensate for the resistance imposed by the endotracheal tube and ventilator circuit [60]. It has been reasoned that a patient who can breathe comfortably at this level of PSV will be able to tolerate extubation. However, if the upper airway is swollen because an endotracheal tube has been in place for several days, the work produced by breathing through the swollen airway is approximately the same as that caused by breathing through an endotracheal tube [60]. Accordingly, any amount of PSV used could overcompensate and may give misleading information regarding the likelihood that a patient could tolerate an extubation.

A novel strategy of PSV weaning involves the use of a computer-driven, closed-loop, knowledge-based algorithm [61]. Studies conducted with this strategy have been published [24, 62] or are underway [63]. LELLOUCHE et al. [64] provide further details in their chapter.

T-tube trials

The use of repeated T-tube trials, several times a day, is the oldest method for conducting a weaning trial [65]. The patient receives an enriched supply of oxygen through a T-tube circuit. Initially 5–10 minutes in duration, T-tube trials are extended and repeated several times a day until the patient can sustain spontaneous ventilation for several hours. This approach has become unpopular because it requires considerable time on the part of intensive care staff.

Today, it is usual to perform a single daily T-tube trial, lasting for 30 to 120 minutes [66]. Performing single daily T-tube trials is as effective as performing such trials several times a day, but is much simpler [7]. If the trial is successful, the patient is extubated. If the trial is unsuccessful, the patient is given at least 24 hours of respiratory muscle rest with full ventilator support before another trial is performed.

Patients are judged to have failed a T-tube trial when they develop severe tachypnoea, increased accessory muscle activity, diaphoresis, facial signs of respiratory distress, oxygen desaturation, tachycardia, arrhythmias or hypotension. However, the degree of change in these variables can change from report to report. A standardised approach to patient monitoring during a T-tube trial does not exist. Indeed, there is no agreement as to whether the monitoring of any variable helps in deciding whether to continue a T-tube trial for an initially planned duration, prolong it or curtail it [2].

JUBRAN et al. [67] investigated whether repeated measurements of oesophageal pressure, throughout a trial of spontaneous breathing, might provide additional guidance for a single measurement obtained during the first minute of the trial. The group quantified the change in oesophageal pressure over the first 9 minutes of the trial using a multivariate, adaptive regression, spline procedure in 60 patients (31 patients in the training subgroup and 29 patients in the validation subgroup) (fig. 6). The study found that the oesophageal pressure–trend index had a sensitivity of 0.91 and a specificity of 0.89. Specifically, an oesophageal pressure–trend index reading of $\leqslant 0.44$ was 8.2 times more likely to occur in weaning failure than in weaning success patients. These data suggest that the continuous monitoring of

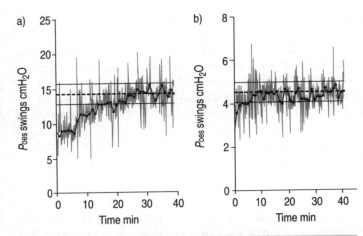

Figure 6. Time-series plot of swings in oesophageal pressure (P_{oes}) in a) a weaning failure patient and b) a weaning success patient, during a trial of spontaneous breathing. The time taken to reach $\pm 10\%$ of the final value for P_{oes} swings was 14 minutes for the failure patient and 6 minutes for the success patient. ●: 1-minute averages; ———: the average value for P_{oes} swings in the final minute of the trial; – – – –: $\pm 10\%$ of the final minute values for P_{oes} swings. a) Reproduced from [67] with permission from the publisher.

oesophageal pressure swings during a T-tube trial may provide additional guidance in patient management over tests used for deciding when to initiate weaning.

Noninvasive ventilation in weaning

Positive-pressure NIV has been used to facilitate extubation among intubated patients with chronic obstructive pulmonary disease (COPD) and acute hypercapnic respiratory failure [54, 68–70]. This is further discussed by FERRER *et al.* [55] in their chapter.

Comparison of weaning methods

Weaning methods are not equally effective. For example, the period of weaning can be three times as long with IMV when compared with T-tube trials [7] or PSV trials [6]. In a study involving patients with respiratory difficulties on weaning, T-tube trials halved the weaning time when compared with PSV [7]; in a different study the weaning time was found to be similar for both trial methods [6].

Weaning by protocol *versus* usual care

The use of human driven protocols for weaning *versus* usual care for weaning have been compared in six randomised controlled trials [3, 71–75]. The reports by NAMEN *et al.* [71], RANDOLPH *et al.* [72] and KRISHNAN *et al.* [73] show no advantage for a protocol approach. The reports by KOLLEF *et al.* [3], MARELICH *et al.* [74] and ELY *et al.* [75] are viewed as evidence for the superiority of a protocol approach to weaning.

However, in the trial by KOLLEF *et al.* [3], no advantage for weaning by protocol was observed in three of the four ICUs studied. In the fourth ICU, where a significant advantage for a protocol approach to weaning was observed, patients who had been assigned to usual care were significantly sicker than those patients who had been assigned to protocol management in that ICU. This confounding factor markedly weakens (if not destroys) any assertion that protocol weaning was superior.

MARELICH *et al.* [74] studied weaning by protocol in two ICUs, and found no significant advantage in either. The study by ELY *et al.* [75] did not consist of a straightforward comparison of protocol *versus* non-protocol care. All of the patients in the intervention arm were weaned by T-tube or flow-by trials, whereas 76% of the patients in the non-intervention arm were managed by IMV alone or in combination with PSV. Physiological studies and randomised trials have repeatedly shown that IMV is the least effective weaning modality [6, 7, 57, 58]. With this fundamental difference in the techniques, it is impossible to use data from this study to form a judgment concerning the efficacy of a protocol *per se*. Instead, the report of ELY *et al.* [75] can be viewed primarily as another study of IMV [2], confirming the reports of BROCHARD *et al.* [6] and ESTEBAN *et al.* [7] that IMV slows weaning.

The outcome of a protocol not to improve weaning is not surprising [2, 7]. A distinction needs to be made between the use of algorithms in research protocols and their subsequent application in everyday practice. As noted previously, the algorithm in a research protocol is specified with exacting precision.

For example, if $f_R/V_T \leqslant 100$ is the nodal point for advancement to a T-tube trial, then patients with an f_R/V_T of 100 will undergo the trial whereas patients with an f_R/V_T of 101 will return to mechanical ventilation for another 24 hours. However, an experienced physician should think it silly to comply with a protocol that decides an entire day of ventilator management is required based on a one unit difference in a single measurement of f_R/V_T (or any other weaning predictor) [76]. Instead, an intelligent physician customises the knowledge generated by research to the particulars of each patient. The intelligent application of physiological principles is likely to outperform an inflexible application of a protocol.

Weaning outcome and short- and long-term prognosis

The panellists of an International Consensus Conference on weaning from mechanical ventilation proposed that weaning should be categorised into three groups, according to the difficulty and duration of the weaning process [77]. According to the proposed classification, patients with "simple weaning" are those extubated at the first attempt of spontaneous breathing. Patients with "difficult weaning" are extubated within 7 days from the first trial of spontaneous breathing. Patients with "prolonged weaning" are those who fail at least three weaning attempts or who require more than 7 days of weaning. To date, four groups of investigators have assessed the usefulness of this classification in determining the outcome of patients who require mechanical ventilation. The investigators are concordant in reporting greater mortality [78–81], longer duration of mechanical ventilation [79, 80] and longer duration of stay in the ICU [78–81] with prolonged weaning. The last two findings are not surprising considering how the weaning categories are defined. Any other result would be counterintuitive [82]. In a retrospective study by Tonnelier *et al.* [78], long-term outcomes were assessed according to the new classification and no association between weaning group and 1-year mortality was found.

Extubation

Decisions made on weaning and extubations are commonly merged [1]. However, merging these two decisions can cause patient mismanagement [1]. When a patient tolerates a weaning trial without distress, a clinician feels reasonably confident that the patient will be able to sustain spontaneous ventilation after extubation. However, passing a weaning trial without distress is not the only consideration. The clinician also needs to consider whether the patient will be able to maintain a patent upper airway after extubation.

Removal of an endotracheal tube is typically performed under controlled conditions [1]. Once the patient has satisfactorily tolerated a weaning trial the enteral feeding is temporally withheld for approximately 4 hours. When possible, the head of the bed should be at a 30° to 90° angle from horizontal [83]. The endotracheal tube, mouth and upper airway are suctioned, paying attention to the collection of secretions above an inflated cuff. Inadequate clearing of secretions can result in post-extubation laryngospasm [83]. Some clinicians recommend keeping a suction catheter in place; aiming for the catheter to barely protrude from the distal end of the endotracheal tube. This step is taken in an attempt to capture any secretions sitting on top of an inflated cuff, which might fall into the airway after deflating the cuff. Some clinicians inflate the lungs with an Ambu Bag immediately before pulling out the endotracheal tube, in the expectation that the larger than usual ensuing exhalation will push secretions upwards and outwards [84]. The cuff is then deflated and the endotracheal tube is withdrawn. After removal of the endotracheal tube the patient is given supplemental oxygen, titrated to oxygen saturation; however, caution must be taken with a patient who is at risk of carbon dioxide retention. Patients may have impaired airway protection reflexes immediately after extubation [85, 86], and aspiration can be silent (*i.e.* aspiration without coughing) [87]. If speech is impaired for more than 24 hours, indirect laryngoscopy should be undertaken to assess vocal cord function. Oral intake should be delayed in patients who have been intubated for a prolonged period of time [85, 86].

In the hours following extubation, patients are carefully monitored for their ability to protect their upper airway and sustain ventilation. Most patients will display progressive improvement, allowing the discontinuation of supplemental oxygen and ultimate discharge from the ICU. However, it has been found that between 2% and 30% of patients experience respiratory distress in the post-extubation period [25, 51, 88–92]. Many of whom, but not all, require the reinsertion of the endotracheal tube and further mechanical ventilation [54]. These patients are commonly classified as extubation failures. In contrast with the relatively short time required to recognise that a patient is failing a weaning trial, the time course for the development of post-extubation distress extends over a longer time span. For example, in the study by EPSTEIN *et al.* [93], 33% of reintubations occurred within the first 12 hours post-extubation and 42% occurred after 24 hours.

Causes of post-extubation distress

The listed indications for reintubation vary considerably from study to study. Of these, post-extubation upper airway obstruction has attracted the most attention.

Post-extubation upper airway obstruction

Upper airway obstruction is one of the most urgent and potentially lethal medical emergencies. Complete airway obstruction, lasting for as little as 4 to 6 minutes, can cause irreversible brain damage [94]. The upper airway, which encompasses the passage between the nares and carina, can be obstructed by functional or anatomic causes. Among the first causes are vocal cord paralysis, paradoxical vocal cord motion and laryngospasm. Among the second are trauma (including arytenoid dislocation), burn, granulomas, infections, foreign bodies, tumours, tracheomalacia, compression caused by a haematoma in close proximity to the airway, and supraglottic, retroarytenoidal and subglottic oedema [1]. Oedema can develop as early as 6 hours after intubation [95]. A thinner mucosa covering the cartilage of the vocal processes, less resistance to trauma, and a smaller laryngeal diameter are probably responsible for the greater prevalence of laryngeal oedema in female than male patients [96–98]. Other risk factors associated with the development of laryngeal oedema include traumatic intubation, excessive tube size, excessive tube mobility secondary to insufficient fixation, a patient fighting against the tube or trying to speak, excessive pressure in the cuff, too frequent or too aggressive tracheal suctioning, occurrence of infections or hypotension, and the presence of a nasogastric tube that predisposes to gastro-oesophageal reflux [98–100]. It is also possible that a biochemical reaction between the tube material and the airway mucosa may cause laryngeal oedema [100]. Life threatening obstruction (functional and anatomic) can occur post-operatively in patients with redundant pharyngeal soft tissue (sleep apnoea) and loss of muscle tone related to post-anaesthetic state [94].

A number of investigators have reported that upper airway obstruction accounts for approximately 15% of patients requiring reintubation [66, 93, 101]. When upper airway obstruction occurs, it typically manifests within 3 to 12 hours after extubation [96, 99, 100]. Symptoms rarely occur until 75% of the upper airway lumen has been obliterated [102, 103]. Occasionally, symptoms may not occur until the diameter of the airway is reduced to 5 mm [104].

Upper airway obstruction causes stridor but only if the patient is capable of generating sufficient airflow. If airflow is insufficient, obstruction may cause hypercapnia, hypoxaemia or paradoxical breathing, but not stridor. Females are more susceptible to post-extubation stridor than males [96–98]. Among patients who develop stridor, 1–69% require reintubation [96, 97, 99, 105]. Many [93, 95, 96, 102], but not all [94], investigators have noted that the rate of post-extubation stridor increases in proportion to the duration of mechanical ventilation.

The first warning of airway obstruction in an unconscious patient may be failure of a jaw-thrust manoeuver to open the airway or the inability to ventilate with a bag valve. In a conscious patient, respiratory distress, stridor, altered voice (aphonia or dysphonia), snoring, dysphagia, odynophagia, prominence of neck veins, and neck and facial swelling may all indicate impending airway obstruction [94]. Patients may bring their hands to their neck, a sign of choking. Other signs include suprasternal and intercostal indrawing, and a reduction or absent air movement on auscultation. Wheezing may also be present. Thoraco–abdominal paradox may be prominent. Sympathetic discharge is high. Patients are diaphoretic, tachycardic and hypertensive. As asphyxia progresses, bradycardia, hypotension and death ensue [94]. Arterial blood gases are not particularly helpful, because they are not specific to airway patency [106]. They may show little change until a patient is in extremis [106].

Other causes of post-extubation distress

Conditions other than upper airway obstruction that cause post-extubation distress include respiratory failure, congestive heart failure, aspiration or excessive secretions, encephalopathy and other conditions [66, 93, 101].

Predictors of post-extubation distress

Because reintubation causes serious complications in some patients, attempts are made to predict its probable occurrence. A number of physiological variables have been evaluated for their ability to predict this likelihood (table 1). For some patients, the likelihood of reintubation is considered so high that a clinician may proceed to tracheotomy without first attempting extubation [1].

Ability to sustain spontaneous respiration

A true-positive result from a T-tube trial is defined as a patient who has tolerated the trial without distress, has undergone extubated, and does not require reintubation [1]. The usual rate of reintubation is 15–20% (sometimes lower), but higher reintubation rates have been reported by some investigators, i.e. 24% [107], 25% [50], 27% [51], 29% [90, 91] and 30% [56]. These false-positive test results (i.e. patients who tolerate the T-tube trial but require reintubation after extubation) mean that the positive predictive value and specificity of passing a T-tube trial in predicting that a patient will not require reintubation is less than 100%. To measure the false-negative rate (fig. 2) would require extubation patients who fail a T-tube trial, and counting how many do not require reintubation. For obvious ethical reasons, this number is not known. Given the natural caution of physicians, it can be confidently assumed that it is higher than 0%.

Weaning-predictor tests

Several investigators have examined the ability of weaning-predictor tests to predict the development of distress after extubation. The question posed is along these lines: "Does fR/V_T or some other predictor test, measured before a T-tube trial, predict the likelihood of reintubation?" To answer this question with scientific validity, it is imperative to avoid test referral bias. This can be avoided if the investigators take steps to ensure that physicians do not perform a T-tube trial, or are not taking the results of the T-tube trial into account, when deciding whether to extubate the patient in the study. In other words, a decision to extubate the patient must be taken before the T-tube trial, and must proceed even if the patient exhibits significant distress during the trial; a strategy which raises obvious ethical concerns.

ZEGGWAGH et al. [108] are the only group of investigators who assessed the ability of weaning-predictor tests to forecast development of distress after extubation without performing a weaning trial (after the weaning predictors had been recorded). The investigators prospectively studied 101 patients at the point at which their ICU physicians contemplated weaning. They measured a series of physiological

Table 1. Possible predictors of post-extubation distress

Ability to sustain spontaneous ventilation
Weaning-predictor tests
Cuff-leak test
Laryngeal ultrasound
Secretions and cough
Neurological assessment
Respiratory drive in the post-extubation period

Reproduced from [1] with permission from the publisher.

measurements during 2 minutes of spontaneous breathing. The results of these measurements were not communicated to the primary care team. The team then extubated the patients without first undertaking any form of weaning trial. The extubation decision was made by the ICU team, based on the following criteria: improvement or resolution of the condition precipitating the need for mechanical ventilation; good level of consciousness with cessation of all sedative agents; temperature less than 38°C; fR less than 35 breaths per minute; oxygen saturation greater than 90% on $FI,O_2 \leqslant 0.40$; haemodynamic stability; and the absence of electrolyte disorders, acid-base disturbance or anaemia (haemoglobin less than 10 g·dL^{-1}).

Reintubation was necessary in 37% of the patients. Several variables predicted the need for reintubation with a reasonable degree of accuracy. For example, fR/VT had a sensitivity of 0.77 and a specificity of 0.79, with an area under a receiver operating characteristic (ROC) curve of 0.81 ± 0.06; maximum expiratory pressure had a sensitivity of 0.52 and a specificity of 0.92, with an area under a ROC curve of 0.73 ± 0.07. The investigators developed a model based on three variables: fR/VT, maximum expiratory pressure, and VC. The area under the ROC curve for the model was 0.91 ± 0.04 for a development data series and 0.86 ± 0.06 for a validation data series. The accuracy of weaning predictors to predict the development of distress after extubation in the study by ZEGGWAGH et al. [108] contrasted sharply with their limited accuracy in studies where the investigators permitted a weaning trial, which altered physician's extubation decisions between measurement of the predictors and extubation [1]. This difference in diagnostic accuracy is probably due to test referral bias [2]. An important aspect of the study by ZEGGWAGH et al. [108] was that the results suggested undertaking a weaning trial before extubation was useful, i.e. the rate of reintubation was approximately double in the ZEGGWAGH et al. [108] study, compared with those reported in studies in which weaning trials preceded extubation [1].

Cuff-leak test

The presence of an endotracheal tube makes it extremely difficult to evaluate the structure and function of the airway before extubation. The amount of air leaking around the outside of an endotracheal tube on deflation of the balloon cuff has been used by a number of investigators to predict upper airway obstruction after extubation (fig. 7). The idea was first reported by ADDERLEY and MULLINS [109] who studied 31 planned extubations in 28 children with croup. After extubation, reintubation was required in 13% of children who had an audible leak (on coughing or when plateau pressure was 40 cmH$_2$O), and reintubation was required in 38% of the children without a leak. The cuff-leak test has since been evaluated by a number of investigators [97–100, 105, 110–114]. However, for several reasons it is difficult to provide general recommendations on how to perform, and how to interpret, a cuff-leak test [1]. Firstly, the method for performing the test has not been standardised. Secondly, the outcome criterion is not always clearly stated: rate of reintubation for any reason, occurrence of stridor of any severity, or occurrence of stridor that requires reintubation. Thirdly, the rates of stridor vary considerably among studies, suggesting that investigators used different criteria (admittedly, it is not obvious that severity of stridor can be graded in any reproducible manner). Fourthly, in

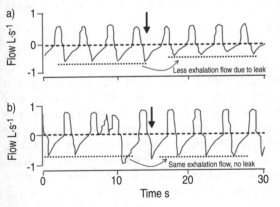

Figure 7. Tracings of inspiratory flow (upward lines) and expiratory flow (downward lines) in two patients before and after deflation of the cuff on the endotracheal tube (downward arrow). Patient (a) had a large leak (positive test result) and it was observed that after the deflation of the cuff the expiratory flow became substantially smaller than the inspiratory flow. Patient (b) had a small leak (less than 12% of inspired tidal volume; negative test result) and it was observed that the expiratory flow exhibited little if any decrease after cuff deflation in this patient. ·······: peak expiratory flow. Modified from [99].

some studies it is not clear whether the investigators carefully excluded reasons for reintubation other than stridor. If a patient is reintubated because of left ventricular failure, it is not logical to expect the cuff-leak test to predict such an event. Fifthly, the thresholds for defining a significant leak vary. Sixthly, calculations of test performance are over estimates, none of the investigators split their data set into training and validation subsets. Finally, in adult patients, small or absent cuff leaks do not necessarily translate into the development of stridor or the need for reintubation (and *vice versa*) [98, 100, 111]. In view of all the above observations, some investigators reason that, for adult patients, failing a cuff-leak test should not be used as an indicator for either delaying extubation or initiating other specific therapies [98, 111, 115], but as a possible indicator of increasing vigilance at the time of extubation [115]. Factors that may contribute to small or absent cuff leaks in a patient not developing post-extubation distress include: secretions located around the endotracheal tube, head and neck positioning, presence or absence of sedation, and large endotracheal tube relative to the size of the patient's larynx [98, 115].

Laryngeal ultrasound

In intubated patients, laryngeal ultrasonography can delineate the anatomical structures of the larynx and can record the shape and width of the air column (both within and around the endotracheal tube), which passes through the vocal cords [116]. Using laryngeal ultrasonography in 51 patients considered ready for extubation (four developed post-extubation stridor and two of them required reintubation), DING *et al.* [116] measured the difference in width of the column of air passing through the vocal cords when the cuff from the endotracheal tube was inflated and the corresponding value when the cuff was deflated (fig. 8). The results found that the smaller the difference in width, the greater the possibility for post-extubation stridor to occur [116]. However, as the authors of the study indicate, the study was not designed to assess the impact of secretions located around the endotracheal tube, the cross-sectional dimension of the endotracheal tube and wakefulness. Consequently, all patients were studied while sedated to avoid the confounding effect of cough on ultrasound signals, *i.e.* the column of air passing through the trachea [116]. Based on this single study, it is premature to recommend laryngeal ultrasonography as a screening tool before extubation.

Secretions and cough

A proportion of patients fail either a weaning attempt or an extubation attempt because of excessive airway secretions. This proportion varies among reports, largely because there is no consistent definition of "excessive secretions" or even on how to quantify secretions [1]. If one quantifies secretions according to the volume obtained by suctioning over a fixed time interval, a patient who coughs and expels secretions without difficulty may be classified as having a greater secretion problem than a patient who has thick viscid secretions that cannot be dislodged from the lower airways [1].

Investigators have evaluated measurements of secretions as predictors of post-extubation distress [101, 117–120]. KHAMIEES *et al.* [117] attempted to quantify cough strength by placing a white card 1–2 cm from the end of the endotracheal tube and requesting the patient to cough as many as three to four times just before extubation. Any wetness on the card was classified as a positive test (assessment was made by a single observer). This test was seen as a test of cough strength and not of the amount of secretions present. They studied 100 extubations in 91 patients; 18 patients were classified as extubation failures and 11 were reintubated within 72 hours of extubation (the criteria for classifying the other seven patients as extubation failures were not clarified). Extubation failure was three times more likely in patients with a negative white-card test (no secretions coughed onto the card). Three other measurements were also found to predict extubation. Failure was four times more likely among patients who had a weak or absent cough than in patients with a moderate or strong cough. Extubation failure was eight times more likely in patients classified as having moderate or abundant secretions by the nursing staff in the 4–6 hours preceding extubation than in patients with absent or mild secretions. Extubation failure was 16 times more likely among patients whose secretions required suctioning every 2 hours or less.

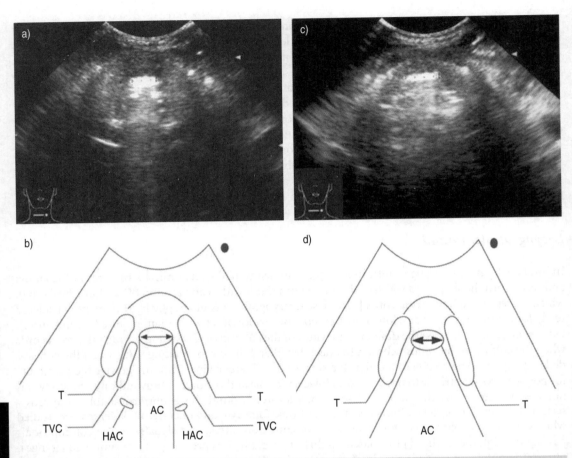

Figure 8. a, c) Laryngeal ultrasounds and b, d) schematic illustrations of an intubated patient who did not develop post-extubation stridor. When the balloon cuff on the endotracheal tube is inflated (a and b) the column of air (AC) passing through the true vocal cords (TVC) appears as a square. The hypoechoic true vocal cords can be seen on both sides of the column of air. The hyperechoic arytenoid cartilages (HAC) are located behind the true vocal cords and adjacent to the column of air. When the cuff is deflated (c and d) the column of air passing through the true vocal cords appears as a trapezoid and the width of the air column increases. In addition, the acoustic shadow of the laryngeal air column masks the hyperechoic arytenoid cartilages and part of the true vocal cords. Arrow indicates the width of the air column. T: thyroid cartilage. Reproduced from [116] with permission from the publisher.

SALAM *et al.* [118], from the same investigation group undertook a further study of predictors of reintubation in 88 patients who underwent 100 extubations (extubation failure was defined as reintubation). Reintubation within 72 hours was required in 16% of the patients. The cough peak flow was lower in reintubated patients than in patients successfully extubated (mean ± SE 58 ± 5 *versus* 80 ± 4 L·min^{-1}). A threshold peak flow of ≤60 L·min^{-1} had a sensitivity of 0.77, a specificity of 0.66, a likelihood ratio of 2.3 and a risk ratio of 4.8. The investigators also re-evaluated the white-card test described by KHAMIEES *et al.* [117], and found that it did not predict reintubation. Clearly, physicians in the study by SALAM *et al.* [118] had reduced the number of extubations attempted in patients with larger volumes of secretions. The physicians had altered their pretest probability of extubation failure based on the need for frequent suctioning. The physicians refused to advance such patients to extubation (test-referral bias) and, thus, the results of the study gave an erroneous impression that frequent suctioning is not a good predictor of reintubation. A limitation of the white-card test is that it will be negative in patients with a strong cough who have little or no secretions. The volume of secretions collected in the 2–3 hours prior to extubation was equivalent in reintubated and successfully extubated patients (mean ± SE 2.5 ± 0.9 *versus*

2.3 ± 0.4 mL·hour^{-1}). However, a threshold of greater than 2.5 mL·hour^{-1} did discriminate between the groups (sensitivity 0.71, specificity 0.62, likelihood ratio 1.9 and risk ratio 3.0).

Neurological assessment

Some ventilated patients demonstrate good respiratory function and tolerate a T-tube trial without distress, yet their physicians are reluctant to extubate them because they fear that the patients will not be able to protect their airway after extubation [1]. Inability to protect the airway can be caused, among other factors, by unsatisfactory neural control over the airway, such that the tongue may fall back and occlude the airway in the recumbent patient, or can be caused by impaired upper airway reflexes (increased risk of aspiration of secretions or of ingested food).

Concerns with protecting the airway often arise in patients with evidence of brain injury. Three groups of investigators, COPLIN et al. [119], NAMEN et al. [71] and SALAM et al. [118], have studied the role of brain function in patients being considered for extubation. The most careful study was by COPLIN et al. [119], who studied 136 brain-injury patients. Based on their data, COPLIN et al. [119] concluded that a depressed level of consciousness, quantified with the Glasgow Coma Scale score, and the absence of a gag reflex should not be used as the sole indication for prolonged intubation.

In contrast to COPLIN et al. [119], NAMEN et al. [71] concluded that a Glasgow Coma Scale score of $\geqslant 8$ helps in predicting successful extubation in brain injury patients. A fundamental problem with this second study is that half of the extubations were part of the withdrawal of life-support therapy (all these patients died). Because these patients were not reintubated, it appears that the authors classified them as extubation successes. Irrespective of how these patients were classified, it is impossible to interpret data on extubation predictors where half of the extubations arose from a decision to withdraw life support.

The studies of COPLIN et al. [119] and NAMEN et al. [71] were conducted in patients with brain injury, whereas SALAM et al. [114] studied neurological function as a predictor of reintubation in medical-cardiac ICU patients. Neurological performance was quantified by requesting patients to perform four simple tasks [121] these were to open their eyes, to follow an observer with their eyes, to grasp the observer's hand, and stick out their tongue. Reintubation within 72 hours was required in 16% of the patients. Patients tolerating extubation performed a higher number of tasks than the reintubated patients (mean $\pm$ SE 3.8 ± 0.1 versus 2.9 ± 0.5). Patients who were unable to complete all four tasks were 4.3 times more likely to require reintubation than patients who could complete all four tasks. The failure to perform any of the four tasks had a sensitivity of 0.42 and specificity of 0.91 in predicting reintubation.

Respiratory neuromuscular drive in the post-extubation period

Increased neuromuscular drive ($P_{0.1} > 5$ cmH$_2$O) 20 minutes into a T-tube weaning trial had been reported to predict the need for reintubation with a sensitivity of 0.87 and a specificity 0.91 [122]. In contrast to $P_{0.1}$ values recorded during a T-tube trial [122], measurements of $P_{0.1}$ during a PSV weaning trial are less accurate in predicting the need for reintubation [123]. In patients with COPD, an increase in $P_{0.1}$ 30 minutes after extubation (when compared with $P_{0.1}$ values before extubation) may predict the development of post-extubation distress [124]. Limitations of these studies include lack of prospective validation of $P_{0.1}$ thresholds and, for the latter study, the need to initiate NIV for the sole purpose of measuring $P_{0.1}$ in all extubated patients.

Conclusions

In conclusion, to reduce the possibility of delayed weaning or premature extubation, physicians should contemplate a three-step diagnostic strategy. First, use measurements of weaning predictors. Secondly, use a trial of unassisted breathing (T-tube trial). Thirdly use a trial of extubation. Each step consists of a diagnostic test, therefore, physicians must be aware of the scientific principles of diagnostic testing when they interpret the information produced by each step. The key point is for physicians to consider the possibility that a patient "just might" be able to tolerate weaning. Such diagnostic triggering is facilitated through the use of a screening test, and is the rationale for the measurements of weaning-predictor tests. A positive result on a screening test (weaning-predictor test) is followed by a confirmatory test (weaning trial), to increase the possibility that a patient will successfully tolerate extubation. It is important not to postpone the use of screening tests by waiting for a more complex diagnostic test, such as a T-tube trial. In contrast to our greater knowledge on prediction of weaning outcome, our knowledge on prediction of extubation outcome is still rudimentary.

The key points that should be taken from this chapter are as follows. 1) The dangers of mechanical ventilation make it critical to wean patients at the earliest possible time. 2) To reduce delayed weaning (and premature extubation) a three-step diagnostic strategy is suggested: measurements of weaning predictors, a trial of unassisted breathing (T-tube trial), and a trial of extubation. 3) Physicians must be aware of the principals involved in clinical decision making when interpreting the information generated by each of the above three step. 4) The critical stage is for the physician to consider the likelihood that a patient "just might" be capable to tolerate a weaning trial. Such diagnostic prompt is facilitated through use of a screening test *i.e.* weaning-predictor tests. 5) The sole purpose of weaning predictors is to act as a screening test, *i.e.* to alert a physician to consider performing a trial of unassisted breathing sooner than their custom. 6) It is imperative not to defer the consideration that a patient "just might" be capable of tolerating a weaning trial by waiting for a more difficult diagnostic test, such as a T-tube trial. 7) To increase the likelihood that a patient will tolerate extubation, a positive result on a screening test (weaning-predictor test) is followed by a confirmatory test (weaning trial). 8) Weaning methods are not equally effective: the period of weaning is as much as three times as long when progressively decreasing the mandatory rate of IMV as with T-tube trials or trials of PSV. 9) When planning extubation, failing a cuff-leak test should not be used as an indication for either delaying extubation or initiating other specific therapy but, possibly, as an indicator of increasing vigilance at the time of extubation.

Support statement

F. Laghi has received research grants from the Veterans Administration Research Service (Washington, DC, USA).

Statement of interest

None declared.

References
1. Laghi F. Weaning from mechanical ventilation. *In:* Gabrielli A, Layon AJ, Yu M, eds. Civetta, Taylor and Kirby's Critical Care. 4th Edn. Philadelphia, Lippincott Williams and Wilkins, 2009; pp. 1991–2028.
2. Tobin MJ, Jubran A. Weaning from mechanical ventilation. *In:* Tobin MJ, ed. Principles and Practice of Mechanical Ventilation. New York, McGraw-Hill, 2006; pp. 1185–1220.
3. Kollef MH, Shapiro SD, Silver P, *et al.* A randomized, controlled trial of protocol-directed *versus* physician-directed weaning from mechanical ventilation. *Crit Care Med* 1997; 25: 567–574.
4. Epstein SK. Etiology of extubation failure and the predictive value of the rapid shallow breathing index. *Am J Respir Crit Care Med* 1995; 152: 545–549.
5. Yang KL, Tobin MJ. A prospective study of indexes predicting the outcome of trials of weaning from mechanical ventilation. *N Engl J Med* 1991; 324: 1445–1450.
6. Brochard L, Rauss A, Benito S, *et al.* Comparison of three methods of gradual withdrawal from ventilatory support during weaning from mechanical ventilation. *Am J Respir Crit Care Med* 1994; 150: 896–903.
7. Esteban A, Frutos F, Tobin MJ, *et al.* A comparison of four methods of weaning patients from mechanical ventilation. Spanish Lung Failure Collaborative Group. *N Engl J Med* 1995; 332: 345–350.
8. Feinstein AR, ed. Clinical Epidemiology: the Architecture of Clinical Research. Philadelphia, W.B. Saunders Company, 1985.

9. Tobin MJ, Jubran A. Variable performance of weaning-predictor tests: role of Bayes' theorem and spectrum and test-referral bias. *Intensive Care Med* 2006; 32: 2002–2012.

10. Tobin MJ, Perez W, Guenther SM, *et al.* The pattern of breathing during successful and unsuccessful trials of weaning from mechanical ventilation. *Am Rev Respir Dis* 1986; 134: 1111–1118.

11. Patel KN, Ganatra KD, Bates JH, *et al.* Variation in the rapid shallow breathing index associated with common measurement techniques and conditions. *Respir Care* 2009; 54: 1462–1466.

12. Jubran A, Van de Graaff WB, Tobin MJ. Variability of patient-ventilator interaction with pressure support ventilation in patients with chronic obstructive pulmonary disease. *Am J Respir Crit Care Med* 1995; 152: 129–136.

13. Sassoon CS, Light RW, Lodia R, *et al.* Pressure-time product during continuous positive airway pressure, pressure support ventilation, and T-piece during weaning from mechanical ventilation. *Am Rev Respir Dis* 1991; 143: 469–475.

14. Brochard L, Pluskwa F, Lemaire F. Improved efficacy of spontaneous breathing with inspiratory pressure support. *Am Rev Respir Dis* 1987; 136: 411–415.

15. Tokioka H, Saito S, Kosaka F. Effect of pressure support ventilation on breathing patterns and respiratory work. *Intensive Care Med* 1989; 15: 491–494.

16. Tobin MJ, Jenouri G, Birch S, *et al.* Effect of positive end-expiratory pressure on breathing patterns of normal subjects and intubated patients with respiratory failure. *Crit Care Med* 1983; 11: 859–867.

17. El Khatib MF, Jamaleddine GW, Khoury AR, *et al.* Effect of continuous positive airway pressure on the rapid shallow breathing index in patients following cardiac surgery. *Chest* 2002; 121: 475–479.

18. MacIntyre NR, Cook DJ, Ely EW Jr, *et al.* Evidence-based guidelines for weaning and discontinuing ventilatory support: a collective task force facilitated by the American College of Chest Physicians; the American Association for Respiratory Care; and the American College of Critical Care Medicine. *Chest* 2001; 120: Suppl. 6, 375S–395S.

19. Meade M, Guyatt G, Cook D, *et al.* Predicting success in weaning from mechanical ventilation. *Chest* 2001; 120: Suppl. 6, 400S–424S.

20. Brand R, Kragt H. Importance of trends in the interpretation of an overall odds ratio in the meta-analysis of clinical trials. *Stat Med* 1992; 11: 2077–2082.

21. Schmid CH, Lau J, McIntosh MW, *et al.* An empirical study of the effect of the control rate as a predictor of treatment efficacy in meta-analysis of clinical trials. *Stat Med* 1998; 17: 1923–1942.

22. Jubran A, Mathru M, Dries D, *et al.* Continuous recordings of mixed venous oxygen saturation during weaning from mechanical ventilation and the ramifications thereof. *Am J Respir Crit Care Med* 1998; 158: 1763–1769.

23. Zakynthinos S, Routsi C, Vassilakopoulos T, *et al.* Differential cardiovascular responses during weaning failure: effects on tissue oxygenation and lactate. *Intensive Care Med* 2005; 31: 1634–1642.

24. Sellarés J, Loureiro H, Ferrer M, *et al.* The effect of spontaneous breathing on systemic interleukin-6 during ventilator weaning. *Eur Respir J* 2012; 39: 654-660.

25. Lellouche F, Mancebo J, Jolliet P, *et al.* A multicenter randomized trial of computer-driven protocolized weaning from mechanical ventilation. *Am J Respir Crit Care Med* 2006; 174: 894–900.

26. Slovic P, Fischhoff B, Lichtenstein S. Behavioral decision theory. *Ann Rev Psychol* 1977; 28: 39.

27. Tversky A, Kahneman D. Judgment under Uncertainty: Heuristics and Biases. *Science* 1974; 185: 1124–1131.

28. Engel G, Rockson SG. Rapid diagnosis of myocardial injury with troponin T and CK-MB relative index. *Mol Diagn Ther* 2007; 11: 109–116.

29. San Román JA, Vilacosta I, Castillo JA, *et al.* Selection of the optimal stress test for the diagnosis of coronary artery disease. *Heart* 1998; 80: 370–376.

30. Mylonakis E, Calderwood SB. Infective endocarditis in adults. *N Engl J Med* 2001; 345: 1318–1330.

31. Tanios MA, Nevins ML, Hendra KP, *et al.* A randomized, controlled trial of the role of weaning predictors in clinical decision making. *Crit Care Med* 2006; 34: 2530–2535.

32. Sahn SA, Lakshminarayan S. Bedside criteria for discontinuation of mechanical ventilation. *Chest* 1973; 63: 1002–1005.

33. Laghi F, Cattapan SE, Jubran A, *et al.* Is weaning failure caused by low-frequency fatigue of the diaphragm? *Am J Respir Crit Care Med* 2003; 167: 120–127.

34. Sassoon CS, Mahutte CK. Airway occlusion pressure and breathing pattern as predictors of weaning outcome. *Am Rev Respir Dis* 1993; 148: 860–866.

35. Fiastro JF, Habib MP, Shon BY, *et al.* Comparison of standard weaning parameters and the mechanical work of breathing in mechanically ventilated patients. *Chest* 1988; 94: 232–238.

36. Tahvanainen J, Salmenpera M, Nikki P. Extubation criteria after weaning from intermittent mandatory ventilation and continuous positive airway pressure. *Crit Care Med* 1983; 11: 702–707.

37. Chevrolet JC, Deleamont P. Repeated vital capacity measurements as predictive parameters for mechanical ventilation need and weaning success in the Guillain-Barré syndrome. *Am Rev Respir Dis* 1991; 144: 814–818.

38. Montgomery AB, Holle RH, Neagley SR, *et al.* Prediction of successful ventilator weaning using airway occlusion pressure and hypercapnic challenge. *Chest* 1987; 91: 496–499.

39. Brenner M, Mukai DS, Russell JE, *et al.* A new method for measurement of airway occlusion pressure. *Chest* 1990; 98: 421–427.

40. Burki NK. The effects of changes in functional residual capacity with posture on mouth occlusion pressure and ventilatory pattern. *Am Rev Respir Dis* 1977; 116: 895–900.

41. Lederer DH, Altose MD, Kelsen SG, *et al.* Comparison of occlusion pressure and ventilatory responses. *Thorax* 1977; 32: 212–220.

42. Vanderheyden M, Bartunek J, Goethals M. Brain and other natriuretic peptides: molecular aspects. *Eur J Heart Fail* 2004; 6: 261–268.

43. Grasso S, Leone A, De Michele M, *et al.* Use of N-terminal pro-brain natriuretic peptide to detect acute cardiac dysfunction during weaning failure in difficult-to-wean patients with chronic obstructive pulmonary disease. *Crit Care Med* 2007; 35: 96–105.

44. Mekontso-Dessap A, de Prost N, Girou E, *et al.* B-type natriuretic peptide and weaning from mechanical ventilation. *Intensive Care Med* 2006; 32: 1529–1536.

45. Zapata L, Vera P, Roglan A, *et al.* B-type natriuretic peptides for prediction and diagnosis of weaning failure from cardiac origin. *Intensive Care Med* 2011; 37: 477–485.

46. Brown SD, Gutierrez G. Gut mucosal pH monitoring. *In:* Tobin MJ, ed. Principles and Practice of Intensive Care Monitoring. New York, McGraw-Hill, 1998; pp. 351–368.

47. Mohsenifar Z, Hay A, Hay J, *et al.* Gastric intramural pH as a predictor of success or failure in weaning patients from mechanical ventilation. *Ann Intern Med* 1993; 119: 794–798.

48. Bouachour G, Guiraud MP, Gouello JP, *et al.* Gastric intramucosal pH: an indicator of weaning outcome from mechanical ventilation in COPD patients. *Eur Respir J* 1996; 9: 1868–1873.

49. Bocquillon N, Mathieu D, Neviere R, *et al.* Gastric mucosal pH and blood flow during weaning from mechanical ventilation in patients with chronic obstructive pulmonary disease. *Am J Respir Crit Care Med* 1999; 160: 1555–1561.

50. Uusaro A, Chittock DR, Russell JA, *et al.* Stress test and gastric-arterial PCO_2 measurement improve prediction of successful extubation. *Crit Care Med* 2000; 28: 2313–2319.

51. Maldonado A, Bauer TT, Ferrer M, *et al.* Capnometric recirculation gas tonometry and weaning from mechanical ventilation. *Am J Respir Crit Care Med* 2000; 161: 171–176.

52. Jaber S, Petrof BJ, Jung B, *et al.* Rapidly progressive diaphragmatic weakness and injury during mechanical ventilation in humans. *Am J Respir Crit Care Med* 2011; 183: 364–371.

53. Kim WY, Suh HJ, Hong SB, *et al.* Diaphragm dysfunction assessed by ultrasonography: influence on weaning from mechanical ventilation. *Crit Care Med* 2011; 39: 2627–2630.

54. Girault C, Bubenheim M, Abroug F, *et al.* Noninvasive ventilation and weaning in chronic hypercapnic respiratory failure patients: a randomized multicenter trial. *Am J Respir Crit Care Med* 2011; 184: 672–679.

55. Ferrer M, Sellares J, Torres A. NIV in withdrawal from mechanical ventilation. *Eur Respir Mon* 2012: 55; 191–205.

56. Sassoon CS. Intermittent mechanical ventilation. *In:* Tobin MJ, ed. Principles and Practice of Mechanical Ventilation. New York: McGraw-Hill, 2006; pp. 201–220.

57. Marini JJ, Smith TC, Lamb VJ. External work output and force generation during synchronized intermittent mechanical ventilation. Effect of machine assistance on breathing effort. *Am Rev Respir Dis* 1988; 138: 1169–1179.

58. Imsand C, Feihl F, Perret C, *et al.* Regulation of inspiratory neuromuscular output during synchronized intermittent mechanical ventilation. *Anesthesiology* 1994; 80: 13–22.

59. Brochard L. Pressure-support ventilation. *In:* Tobin MJ, ed. Principles and Practice of Mechanical Ventilation. New York, McGraw-Hill, 2006; pp. 221–250.

60. Straus C, Louis B, Isabey D, *et al.* Contribution of the endotracheal tube and the upper airway to breathing workload. *Am J Respir Crit Care Med* 1998; 157: 23–30.

61. Laghi F. Weaning: can the computer help? *Intensive Care Med* 2008; 34: 1746–1748.

62. Rose L, Presneill JJ, Johnston L, *et al.* A randomised, controlled trial of conventional *versus* automated weaning from mechanical ventilation using SmartCare/PS. *Intensive Care Med* 2008; 34: 1788–1795.

63. Burns KE, Meade MO, Lessard MR, *et al.* Wean Earlier and Automatically with New technology (the WEAN study): a protocol of a multicentre, pilot randomized controlled trial. *Trials* 2009; 10: 81.

64. Lellouche F, Bojmehrani A, Burns K. Mechanical ventilation with advanced closed-loop systems. *Eur Respir Mon* 2012: 55: 217–228.

65. Tobin MJ. Remembrance of weaning past: the seminal papers. *Intensive Care Med* 2006; 32: 1485–1493.

66. Esteban A, Alia I, Tobin MJ, *et al.* Effect of spontaneous breathing trial duration on outcome of attempts to discontinue mechanical ventilation. Spanish Lung Failure Collaborative Group. *Am J Respir Crit Care Med* 1999; 159: 512–518.

67. Jubran A, Grant BJ, Laghi F, *et al.* Weaning prediction: esophageal pressure monitoring complements readiness testing. *Am J Respir Crit Care Med* 2005; 171: 1252–1259.

68. Nava S, Ambrosino N, Clini E, *et al.* Noninvasive mechanical ventilation in the weaning of patients with respiratory failure due to chronic obstructive pulmonary disease. A randomized, controlled trial. *Ann Intern Med* 1998; 128: 721–728.

69. Ferrer M, Esquinas A, Arancibia F, *et al.* Noninvasive ventilation during persistent weaning failure: a randomized controlled trial. *Am J Respir Crit Care Med* 2003; 168: 70–76.

70. Ferrer M, Sellares J, Valencia M, *et al.* Non-invasive ventilation after extubation in hypercapnic patients with chronic respiratory disorders: randomised controlled trial. *Lancet* 2009; 374: 1082–1088.

71. Namen AM, Ely EW, Tatter SB, *et al.* Predictors of successful extubation in neurosurgical patients. *Am J Respir Crit Care Med* 2001; 163: 658–664.

72. Randolph AG, Wypij D, Venkataraman ST, *et al.* Effect of mechanical ventilator weaning protocols on respiratory outcomes in infants and children: a randomized controlled trial. *JAMA* 2002; 288: 2561–2568.

73. Krishnan JA, Moore D, Robeson C, *et al.* A prospective, controlled trial of a protocol-based strategy to discontinue mechanical ventilation. *Am J Respir Crit Care Med* 2004; 169: 673–678.

74. Marelich GP, Murin S, Battistella F, *et al.* Protocol weaning of mechanical ventilation in medical and surgical patients by respiratory care practitioners and nurses: effect on weaning time and incidence of ventilator-associated pneumonia. *Chest* 2000; 118: 459–467.

75. Ely EW, Baker AM, Evans GW, *et al.* The prognostic significance of passing a daily screen of weaning parameters. *Intensive Care Med* 1999; 25: 581–587.

76. Tobin MJ. Of principles and protocols and weaning. *Am J Respir Crit Care Med* 2004; 169: 661–662.

77. Boles JM, Bion J, Connors A, *et al.* Weaning from mechanical ventilation. *Eur Respir J* 2007; 29: 1033–1056.

78. Tonnelier A, Tonnelier JM, Nowak E, *et al.* Clinical relevance of classification according to weaning difficulty. *Respir Care* 2011; 56: 583–590.

79. Funk GC, Anders S, Breyer MK, *et al.* Incidence and outcome of weaning from mechanical ventilation according to new categories. *Eur Respir J* 2010; 35: 88–94.

80. Sellares J, Ferrer M, Cano E, *et al.* Predictors of prolonged weaning and survival during ventilator weaning in a respiratory ICU. *Intensive Care Med* 2011; 37: 775–784.

81. Penuelas O, Frutos-Vivar F, Fernandez C, *et al.* Characteristics and outcomes of ventilated patients according to time to liberation from mechanical ventilation. *Am J Respir Crit Care Med* 2011; 184: 430–437.

82. Laghi F. Stratification of difficulty in weaning. *Intensive Care Med* 2011; 37: 732–734.

83. de la Linde Valverde CM. La extubacion de la via aerea dificil [Extubation of the difficult airway]. *Rev Esp Anestesiol Reanim* 2005; 52: 557–570.

84. Gal TG. Airway management. *In:* Miller RD, ed. Miller's Anesthesia. 6th Edn. Philadelphia, Elsevier, Churchill Livingstone, 2005; pp. 1617–1652.

85. Leder SB, Cohn SM, Moller BA. Fiberoptic endoscopic documentation of the high incidence of aspiration following extubation in critically ill trauma patients. *Dysphagia* 1998; 13: 208–212.

86. El Solh A, Okada M, Bhat A, *et al.* Swallowing disorders post orotracheal intubation in the elderly. *Intensive Care Med* 2003; 29: 1451–1455.

87. Barquist E, Brown M, Cohn S, *et al.* Postextubation fiberoptic endoscopic evaluation of swallowing after prolonged endotracheal intubation: a randomized, prospective trial. *Crit Care Med* 2001; 29: 1710–1713.

88. Leitch EA, Moran JL, Grealy B. Weaning and extubation in the intensive care unit. Clinical or index-driven approach? *Intensive Care Med* 1996; 22: 752–759.

89. Conti G, Montini L, Pennisi MA, *et al.* A prospective, blinded evaluation of indexes proposed to predict weaning from mechanical ventilation. *Intensive Care Med* 2004; 30: 830–836.

90. Dojat M, Harf A, Touchard D, *et al.* Evaluation of a knowledge-based system providing ventilatory management and decision for extubation. *Am J Respir Crit Care Med* 1996; 153: 997–1004.

91. Cohen JD, Shapiro M, Grozovski E, *et al.* Automatic tube compensation-assisted respiratory rate to tidal volume ratio improves the prediction of weaning outcome. *Chest* 2002; 122: 980–984.

92. Esteban A, Frutos-Vivar F, Ferguson ND, *et al.* Noninvasive positive-pressure ventilation for respiratory failure after extubation. *N Engl J Med* 2004; 350: 2452–2460.

93. Epstein SK, Ciubotaru RL. Independent effects of etiology of failure and time to reintubation on outcome for patients failing extubation. *Am J Respir Crit Care Med* 1998; 158: 489–493.

94. Laghi F, Tobin MJ. Indications for mechanical ventilation. *In:* Tobin MJ, ed. Principles and Practice of Mechanical Ventilation. New York, McGraw-Hill, 2006; pp. 129–162.

95. Hartley M, Vaughan RS. Problems associated with tracheal extubation. *Br J Anaesth* 1993; 71: 561–568.

96. Darmon JY, Rauss A, Dreyfuss D, *et al.* Evaluation of risk factors for laryngeal edema after tracheal extubation in adults and its prevention by dexamethasone. A placebo-controlled, double-blind, multicenter study. *Anesthesiology* 1992; 77: 245–251.

97. Ho LI, Harn HJ, Lien TC, *et al.* Postextubation laryngeal edema in adults. Risk factor evaluation and prevention by hydrocortisone. *Intensive Care Med* 1996; 22: 933–936.

98. Kriner EJ, Shafazand S, Colice GL. The endotracheal tube cuff-leak test as a predictor for postextubation stridor. *Respir Care* 2005; 50: 1632–1638.

99. Jaber S, Chanques G, Matecki S, *et al.* Post-extubation stridor in intensive care unit patients. Risk factors evaluation and importance of the cuff-leak test. *Intensive Care Med* 2003; 29: 69–74.

100. De Bast Y, De Backer D, Moraine JJ, *et al.* The cuff leak test to predict failure of tracheal extubation for laryngeal edema. *Intensive Care Med* 2002; 28: 1267–1272.

101. Smina M, Salam A, Khamiees M, *et al.* Cough peak flows and extubation outcomes. *Chest* 2003; 124: 262–268.

102. Dane TE, King EG. A prospective study of complications after tracheostomy for assisted ventilation. *Chest* 1975; 67: 398–404.

103. Pearson FG, Goldberg M, da Silva AJ. Tracheal stenosis complicating tracheostomy with cuffed tubes. Clinical experience and observations from a prospective study. *Arch Surg* 1968; 97: 380–394.

104. Stauffer JL, Olson DE, Petty TL. Complications and consequences of endotracheal intubation and tracheotomy. A prospective study of 150 critically ill adult patients. *Am J Med* 1981; 70: 65–76.

105. Sandhu RS, Pasquale MD, Miller K, *et al.* Measurement of endotracheal tube cuff leak to predict postextubation stridor and need for reintubation. *J Am Coll Surg* 2000; 190: 682–687.

106. Khosh MM, Lebovics RS. Upper airway obstruction. *In:* Parrillo JE, Dellinger PR, eds. Critical Care Medicine. Principles of Diagnosis and Management in the Adult. St. Louis, Mosby, 2001; pp. 808–825.

107. Torres A, Gatell JM, Aznar E, *et al.* Re-intubation increases the risk of nosocomial pneumonia in patients needing mechanical ventilation. *Am J Respir Crit Care Med* 1995; 152: 137–141.

108. Zeggwagh AA, Abouqal R, Madani N, *et al.* Weaning from mechanical ventilation: a model for extubation. *Intensive Care Med* 1999; 25: 1077–1083.

109. Adderley RJ, Mullins GC. When to extubate the croup patient: the "leak" test. *Can J Anaesth* 1987; 34: 304–306.

110. Miller RL, Cole RP. Association between reduced cuff leak volume and postextubation stridor. *Chest* 1996; 110: 1035–1040.

111. Engoren M. Evaluation of the cuff-leak test in a cardiac surgery population. *Chest* 1999; 116: 1029–1031.

112. Cheng KC, Hou CC, Huang HC, *et al.* Intravenous injection of methylprednisolone reduces the incidence of postextubation stridor in intensive care unit patients. *Crit Care Med* 2006; 34: 1345–1350.

113. Prinianakis G, Alexopoulou C, Mamidakis E, *et al.* Determinants of the cuff-leak test: a physiological study. *Crit Care* 2005; 9: R24–R31.

114. Chung YH, Chao TY, Chiu CT, *et al.* The cuff-leak test is a simple tool to verify severe laryngeal edema in patients undergoing long-term mechanical ventilation. *Crit Care Med* 2006; 34: 409–414.

115. Deem S. Limited value of the cuff-leak test. *Respir Care* 2005; 50: 1617–1618.

116. Ding LW, Wang HC, Wu HD, *et al.* Laryngeal ultrasound: a useful method in predicting post-extubation stridor. A pilot study. *Eur Respir J* 2006; 27: 384–389.

117. Khamiees M, Raju P, DeGirolamo A, *et al.* Predictors of extubation outcome in patients who have successfully completed a spontaneous breathing trial. *Chest* 2001; 120: 1262–1270.

118. Salam A, Tilluckdharry L, Amoateng-Adjepong Y, *et al.* Neurologic status, cough, secretions and extubation outcomes. *Intensive Care Med* 2004; 30: 1334–1339.

119. Coplin WM, Pierson DJ, Cooley KD, *et al.* Implications of extubation delay in brain-injured patients meeting standard weaning criteria. *Am J Respir Crit Care Med* 2000; 161: 1530–1536.

120. Vallverdu I, Calaf N, Subirana M, *et al.* Clinical characteristics, respiratory functional parameters, and outcome of a two-hour T-piece trial in patients weaning from mechanical ventilation. *Am J Respir Crit Care Med* 1998; 158: 1855–1862.

121. Kress JP, O'Connor MF, Pohlman AS, *et al.* Sedation of critically ill patients during mechanical ventilation. A comparison of propofol and midazolam. *Am J Respir Crit Care Med* 1996; 153: 1012–1018.

122. Capdevila XJ, Perrigault PF, Perey PJ, *et al.* Occlusion pressure and its ratio to maximum inspiratory pressure are useful predictors for successful extubation following T-piece weaning trial. *Chest* 1995; 108: 482–489.

123. Fernandez R, Raurich JM, Mut T, *et al.* Extubation failure: diagnostic value of occlusion pressure (P0.1) and P0.1-derived parameters. *Intensive Care Med* 2004; 30: 234–240.

124. Hilbert G, Gruson D, Portel L, *et al.* Airway occlusion pressure at 0.1 s (P0.1) after extubation: an early indicator of postextubation hypercapnic respiratory insufficiency. *Intensive Care Med* 1998; 24: 1277–1282.

Chapter 14

NIV in withdrawal from mechanical ventilation

M. Ferrer*,#,¶, J. Sellares*,#,¶ and A. Torres*,#,¶

Summary

Patients with chronic airflow obstruction and difficult or prolonged weaning are at increased risk for prolonged invasive mechanical ventilation. Several randomised controlled trials, mainly conducted in patients who had pre-existing lung disease, have shown that the use of noninvasive ventilation (NIV) in order to advance extubation in patients with difficult and prolonged weaning can result in reduced periods of endotracheal intubation, complication rates and improved survival. Patients in these studies were haemodynamically stable, with a normal level of consciousness, no fever and a preserved cough reflex. The use of NIV in the management of mixed populations with respiratory failure after extubation, including small proportions of chronic respiratory patients, did not show clinical benefits. By contrast, NIV immediately after extubation is effective in avoiding respiratory failure following extubation and improving survival in patients at risk for this complication, particularly those with chronic respiratory disorders, cardiac co-morbidity and hypercapnic respiratory failure. Finally, both continuous positive airway pressure and NIV can improve clinical outcomes in patients with post-operative acute respiratory failure, particularly abdominal and thoracic surgery.

Keywords: Difficult weaning, extubation, noninvasive ventilation, post-operative respiratory failure, prolonged weaning, respiratory failure

*Respiratory Intensive Care Unit, Thorax Institute, Hospital Clínic, #Institut d'Investigacions Biomèdiques August Pi i Sunyer (IDIBAPS), and ¶Centro de Investigación Biomédica en Red de Enfermedades Respiratorias (CIBERES), Barcelona, Spain.

Correspondence: M. Ferrer, Servei de Pneumologia, Hospital Clinic, Villarroel 170, 08036 Barcelona, Spain.
Email miferrer@clinic.ub.es

Eur Respir Mon 2012; 55: 191–205.
Printed in UK – all rights reserved
Copyright ERS 2012
European Respiratory Monograph
ISSN: 1025-448x
DOI: 10.1183/1025448x.10002711

Mechanical ventilation using an artificial airway is a life-saving procedure used in the management of critically ill patients with severe respiratory failure, but this is associated with multiple complications, mainly an increased risk of nosocomial pneumonia with a high mortality rate [1].

Noninvasive ventilation (NIV) has been used in different indications during withdrawal of mechanical ventilation to: 1) advance extubation in patients with difficult or prolonged weaning; 2) avoid re-intubation in patients who have developed post-extubation respiratory failure; and

3) prevent the development of post-extubation respiratory failure. The role of NIV in all of these indications will be reviewed, including the post-operative period.

Weaning from mechanical ventilation

Weaning from mechanical ventilation consists of measures aimed to achieve successful disconnection of patients from the ventilator. This is a challenging period that represents 40–50% of the duration of mechanical ventilation [2–5], with increasing burden on the healthcare system related to prolonged mechanical ventilation [6]. Different approaches have been proposed to optimise the weaning process [7, 8], including weaning protocols [4, 9, 10], automated systems [11], daily spontaneous breathing trials (SBTs) [12] and pressure support ventilation (PSV) [13]. In spite of this, it is estimated that 20–30% of the patients cannot be extubated in the first weaning attempt [3, 7].

An International Consensus Conference on weaning from mechanical ventilation [7] proposed a new classification based on the difficulty and duration of the weaning period. 1) Simple weaning: patients who proceed from initiation of weaning to extubation on the first attempt without difficulty. 2) Difficult weaning: patients who failed initial weaning and required up to three SBTs or up to 7 days from the first SBT to achieve successful weaning. 3) Prolonged weaning: patients who failed at least three weaning attempts or required more than 7 days of weaning after the first SBT. Although it was estimated that prolonged weaning was associated with the lowest survival [7, 14], this classification was based solely on experts' opinion. The International Consensus Conference recommended further research on a carefully tested and investigated group of patients who had undergone weaning, and stressed the need for studies assessing the outcome of patients with difficult and prolonged weaning [7].

A recent study in medical and surgical intensive care units (ICUs) showed that prolonged weaning was associated with increased mortality and morbidity [15]. However, the proportion of difficult and prolonged weaning is low in general ICU populations [3, 7]. Moreover, factors associated with prolonged weaning were not assessed in that study [15]. A subsequent study in a respiratory ICU, a specific setting with higher proportions of difficult and prolonged weaning, compared the clinical characteristics and outcomes of patients with simple, difficult and prolonged weaning, and determined the predictive factors associated with prolonged weaning and its potential association

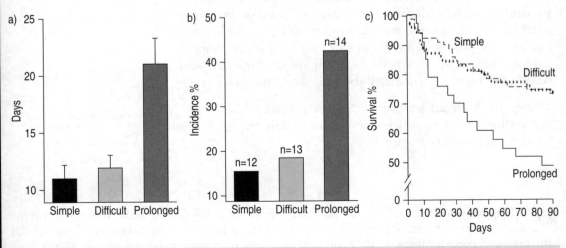

Figure 1. a) Length of intensive care unit (ICU) stay, b) incidence of ventilator-associated pneumonia (VAP) and c) Kaplan–Meier survival curves 90 days after the start of the weaning process for patients with simple, difficult and prolonged weaning. The length of ICU stay and the incidence of VAP were higher, and the survival probability lower, in the prolonged weaning group. No differences were observed between patients with simple and difficult weaning. a) p<0.001, b) p=0.005, c) p=0.019. c) Data taken from [16].

with mortality [16]. This study found that, because of similar characteristics and outcomes, the differentiation between simple and difficult weaning had no relevant clinical consequences in a respiratory ICU, while patients with prolonged weaning had the worst outcomes (fig. 1) [16]. Hypercapnia at the end of spontaneous breathing predicted prolonged weaning and worse survival in this study (fig. 2). Consequently, this finding should alert clinicians to implement measures aimed at reducing the need for prolonged mechanical ventilation and improving weaning outcome.

The main recommendations of the International Consensus Conference [7] were as follows. 1) Patients should be categorised into the three groups based on the difficulty and duration of the weaning process. 2) Weaning should be considered as early as possible. 3) An SBT is the major diagnostic test to determine whether patients can be successfully extubated. 4) The initial trial should last for 30 minutes and consist of either T-tube breathing or low levels of pressure support. 5) Pressure support or assist control ventilation modes should be favoured in patients failing an initial trial. 6) NIV techniques should be considered in selected patients to shorten the duration of intubation but should not be routinely used as a tool for extubation failure.

Pathophysiological mechanisms of difficult and prolonged weaning

Patients with unsuccessful weaning from mechanical ventilation are likely to develop a rapid and shallow breathing pattern during an SBT [17]. In chronic obstructive pulmonary disease (COPD) patients, failure in the transition from positive pressure ventilation to spontaneous breathing is associated with increased workload of the respiratory muscles, progressively higher levels of dynamic lung elastance, intrinsic positive end-expiratory pressure (PEEP), inspiratory resistance and work of breathing [18]. In ventilator-dependent patients with COPD or after cardiac surgery, the presence of a high drive to breathe and an imbalance between the increased workload and reduced inspiratory muscle strength causes respiratory distress and hypercapnia. All of these changes are not present when patients successfully tolerate an SBT.

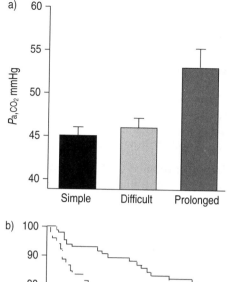

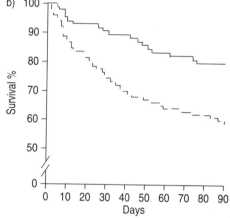

Figure 2. Relationship between increased arterial carbon dioxide tension (P_{a,CO_2}) and outcomes during weaning. a) P_{a,CO_2} at the end of the first spontaneous breathing trial in patients with simple, difficult and prolonged weaning. The P_{a,CO_2} was higher in patients with prolonged weaning, p=0.001. b) Kaplan–Meier survival curves 90 days after the start of the weaning process for patients with hypercapnia (- - - -) and normocapnia (——) at the end of the first spontaneous breathing trial. The survival probability was lower for patients with hypercapnia, p=0.002. Data taken from [16].

The cardiovascular response to the switch from positive pressure ventilation to spontaneous breathing is also important in order to achieve successful weaning. An increase in the venous return to the right ventricle and, consequently, a leftward shift of the ventricular septum caused by the ventricular interdependence and the large negative deflections in intrathoracic pressure due to the inspiratory threshold load may increase left ventricular afterload [19]. An inappropriate cardiovascular response to these changes with left ventricular dysfunction and increased pulmonary artery occlusion pressure may occur during weaning failure [19]. Weaning failure is also associated with decreased mixed venous oxygen saturation during spontaneous breathing [20], reflecting the inability of the cardiovascular system to compensate the increased systemic oxygen demands when spontaneous breathing is initiated. Conversely, in successfully weaned patients, mixed venous oxygen tension or saturation was shown to remain unchanged or to be increased during spontaneous breathing, compared with positive pressure ventilation [20–22].

Rationale for the use of NIV during difficult and prolonged weaning

The rationale for using NIV in facilitating weaning may be related to the ability of NIV to offset several pathophysiological mechanisms associated with unsuccessful weaning from mechanical ventilation, such as the increased workload of the respiratory muscles and the development of a rapid and shallow breathing pattern.

In non-intubated COPD patients with acute hypercapnia, NIV is effective in reducing the work of breathing and the large negative deflections in intrathoracic pressure [23]. In this study, an additive effect of both positive pressure ventilation (as inspiratory support) and external PEEP (to counterbalance inspiratory PEEP) was shown. The mechanisms of short-term improvement of hypoxaemia and hypercapnia with NIV in these patients appear to be related to increased alveolar ventilation secondary to attainment of a slower and deeper breathing pattern, with no changes in the ventilation–perfusion mismatch [24]. Similarly, in intubated patients without COPD and SBT failure, the rapid and shallow pattern of breathing improved after extubation with NIV support [25]. In patients affected by chronic respiratory disorders not ready to sustain totally spontaneous breathing, PSV delivered through the endotracheal tube and noninvasively after extubation is equally effective in reducing the work of breathing and improving arterial blood gases, compared with spontaneous breathing during a T-piece trial [26].

The use of NIV during difficult and prolonged weaning

Shortening weaning and avoiding re-intubation should be the primary end-point when NIV is indicated in patients with unsuccessful weaning from mechanical ventilation, as stated in an International Consensus Conference [27].

The first randomised controlled trial for the application of NIV in difficult weaning was performed in a select group of 50 intubated COPD patients with severe hypercapnic respiratory failure who had recovered from an exacerbation within 48 hours after mechanical ventilation was initiated but had failed an SBT with a T-piece [28]. In this study, patients were randomly allocated to be extubated and supported with noninvasive PSV or to remain intubated and ventilated with PSV, following a conventional weaning approach. Patients who were extubated and received NIV remained ventilated and admitted to the ICU for significantly shorter periods, had a lower incidence of nosocomial pneumonia as well as a higher 60-day survival rate. Moreover, noninvasive PSV was as effective as invasive PSV in maintaining the levels of arterial carbon dioxide tension (Pa,CO_2) and arterial pH in both groups. The authors concluded that the reduction of the period of endotracheal intubation was the main cause of decreased incidence of ventilator-associated complications and mortality.

Another randomised controlled trial assessing the efficacy of NIV during difficult weaning was performed in 33 intubated patients with acute-on-chronic respiratory failure after a single weaning trial failure with hypercapnic respiratory failure [29]. Patients were randomly allocated to remain intubated with PSV or to be extubated with noninvasive PSV. This study showed that NIV allowed a reduction of the endotracheal mechanical ventilation period of 3 days on average, but the total duration of ventilatory support related to weaning was longer in patients who were extubated with NIV. In this study, after the first few days following extubation, NIV was administered in most of the patients, especially during the night, mainly as a "preventative" tool rather than a necessity. Despite the fact that there was a trend towards lower incidence of complications to endotracheal mechanical ventilation and weaning, these differences were not significant, in part, because of the small sample size. No trend in improvement in the ICU stay and survival was observed. As in the previous study, both noninvasive and endotracheal PSV achieved similar improvement in the gas exchange compared with the SBT. Another study with similar design, but performed in a mixed population with difficult weaning, showed that extubation with NIV support resulted in lower incidence of pneumonia and tracheostomy, compared with patients following a conventional weaning approach, without changes in the length of ICU stay and mortality [30].

The effect of NIV during prolonged weaning has been studied in 43 patients who failed an SBT for three consecutive days [31]. Of these patients, 33 had underlying chronic respiratory disorders. Again, patients were randomly allocated to be extubated with NIV or to remain intubated following a conventional weaning approach. In this study, NIV resulted in a reduction of the endotracheal and total mechanical ventilation period, ICU and hospital stays, incidence of nosocomial pneumonia and septic shock/multiple organ failure and the need of tracheotomy to facilitate weaning, as well as an improvement in survival, both in the ICU and at 90 days. The marked efficacy of NIV in this study can be explained because the included patients were very difficult to wean. In this study, the differences between both groups occurred only in patients with underlying chronic respiratory disorders, whilst only a moderate trend to a lower period of ventilatory support and ICU stay was shown in patients from the NIV group without chronic respiratory disorders, with no trend to improve the incidence of complications or survival. Despite the fact that clear conclusions were able to be reached in a small number of these patients, these findings suggest that the efficacy of NIV during prolonged weaning would be limited only to patients with underlying chronic airflow obstruction, as shown in a systematic review on the use of NIV during weaning [32]. However, studies with larger populations of patients with prolonged weaning are needed to confirm this hypothesis.

A recent systematic review and meta-analysis on the use of NIV to wean critically ill adult patients off mechanical ventilation identified several additional randomised clinical trials published or presented as abstracts [33]. This study showed a consistent positive effect of NIV on mortality and ventilator-associated pneumonia, although the net clinical benefits remain to be fully elucidated (table 1). This study also recommended that NIV should preferentially be used in patients with COPD in a highly monitored environment. A recent study has emphasised that COPD is the population most likely to benefit from NIV in facilitating difficult and prolonged weaning [34].

Limitations of the use of NIV during weaning

In patients with difficult and prolonged weaning, evidence from randomised controlled trials has shown that the use of NIV in advancing extubation results in variable benefits in terms of reduced periods of endotracheal intubation and, in some, the rates of complications and survival. However, all these studies, and the conclusions drawn from them, are related to selected populations of patients with underlying chronic airflow obstruction and hypercapnic respiratory failure, haemodynamic stability, normal consciousness, absence of fever, and preserved cough reflex. Moreover, although a recent systematic review identified 12 randomised clinical trials that assessed the efficacy of NIV in these patients with 530 patients included, only three of these trials, with 126 patients included, were published in high quartile peer-review journals [33].

Table 1. Summary estimates of the effect of noninvasive ventilation to wean critically ill adults off invasive ventilation

Outcome	Summary estimate (95% CI)	p-value
Mortality[#]	0.55 (0.38–0.79)	0.001
VAP[#]	0.29 (0.19–0.45)	<0.001
Weaning failures[#]	0.72 (0.37–1.42)	0.34
Length of stay		
ICU[¶]	-6.3 (-8.8– -3.8)	<0.001
Hospital[¶]	-7.2 (-10.8– -3.6)	<0.001
Duration of MV		
Total[¶]	-5.6 (-9.5– -1.8)	0.004
Related to weaning[¶]	-0.9 (-3.2–1.4)	0.42
Endotracheal[¶]	-7.8 (-11.3– -4.3)	<0.001
Adverse effects		
Re-intubation[#]	0.73 (0.40–1.34)	0.31
Tracheostomy[#]	0.16 (0.04–0.75)	0.020
Arrhythmia[#]	1.05 (0.17–6.67)	0.96

VAP: ventilator-associated pneumonia; ICU: intensive care unit; MV: mechanical ventilation. [#]: relative risk; [¶]: weighted mean difference. Data taken from [33].

Because between dependence on the ventilator must be distinguished from the dependence on endotracheal intubation, when the process of mechanical ventilation withdrawal is initiated, it is necessary to evaluate: 1) the need of ventilatory support with an SBT; and 2) whether the artificial airway is needed or not. The beneficial effects of NIV as a weaning supporting technique can be expected only when an initial weaning attempt has failed (ventilator dependence) but there is no need for an artificial airway. The main reasons for failure of NIV are the lack of co-operation, excessive secretions, severe strength-load imbalance and haemodynamic instability, which can be corrected by protection of the airways and proper medical therapy. In general, it is estimated that approximately 30–35% of intubated COPD patients with hypercapnic respiratory failure needing progressive withdrawal of mechanical ventilation are not likely to benefit from NIV, but large-scale studies are needed to confirm these estimations.

Respiratory failure after extubation

Re-intubation, which occurs in 6–23% of cases within 48–72 hours after planned extubation [35–37], is a relevant consequence of respiratory failure after extubation [38]. The pathophysiology of respiratory failure after extubation includes upper airway obstruction, inadequate cough, excess respiratory secretions, encephalopathy and cardiac dysfunction [37, 39–41]. Among others, neurological impairment, older age, severity of illness, cardiac failure, longer duration of ventilation prior to extubation, anaemia and the use of continuous sedation have been identified as risk factors for extubation failure [14, 35, 37]. Although the need for re-intubation may be a marker of increased severity of illness, this is an independent risk factor for nosocomial pneumonia [42], and mortality and increased hospital stay [35]. Therefore, in addition to an accurate prediction of extubation outcome, strategies for preventing the development of respiratory failure after extubation and subsequent re-intubation are needed.

NIV in the management of respiratory failure after extubation

The clinical benefits of NIV in the management of patients who have been extubated but have developed respiratory failure after extubation are not encouraging. NIV was considered a promising therapy after extubation failure in order to avoid re-intubation in an International Consensus Conference [27]. This information was based on the findings of physiological or noncontrolled clinical studies. A physiological study in non-COPD patients who had persistent acute respiratory failure (ARF) after early extubation showed that the use of NIV improved pulmonary gas exchange and breathing pattern, decreased the intrapulmonary shunt fraction and decreased the work of breathing [25]. A clinical study compared 30 COPD patients in whom NIV was initiated when they developed extubation failure, if they did not have any criteria for re-intubation, with a retrospective historical control group of 30 patients [43]. The group of patients treated with NIV had lower rates of re-intubation and shorter duration of mechanical ventilation with no differences in the mortality rates, compared with patients from the control group. The main limitation of this study was the use of historically matched controls, with the possible bias implicated. This trial emphasised the need of future randomised controlled trials assessing the application of NIV in post-extubation failure.

However, two randomised clinical trials did not show benefits from NIV in avoiding re-intubation in patients who have developed respiratory failure after extubation [38, 44]. The first trial assessed 358 patients who underwent a planned extubation and selected 81 patients that developed post-extubation respiratory distress [44]. Respiratory distress was defined as a respiratory rate >30 breaths·min^{-1}, an increase in respiratory rate of >50% from baseline, use of accessory muscles of respiration or abdominal paradox. Patients were randomly allocated to be treated with NIV or conventional approach. This trial failed in finding significant differences in terms of rates of re-intubation, duration of mechanical ventilation, hospital and ICU stays, and survival. It is remarkable that only 11% of patients included in this study had a diagnosis of COPD because, after the first year, patients with an acute exacerbation of COPD were excluded because evidence from the randomised trial strongly supported the use of noninvasive positive pressure ventilation (NPPV) for these patients and, therefore, because NIV was applied when these patients developed respiratory distress.

A more recent multicentre international randomised controlled study confirmed the results of the previous study [38]. Among 980 patients from ICUs in different countries, 221 patients who developed respiratory failure after extubation were randomly allocated to receive NIV (114 patients) or standard medical therapy (107 patients). There were no statistical differences in rate of re-intubation (48% in both groups) and length of hospital stay. The most striking outcome of this study was a higher ICU mortality in patients treated with NIV (25% *versus* 14%, p=0.048), predominantly because the mortality rate among the patients who required re-intubation and received NIV was higher than that of the re-intubated patients from the control group. The time from extubation to re-intubation, an independent risk factor for increased mortality in re-intubated patients [45], was longer in patients who received NIV (p=0.02) in this study [38]. Similar to the previous trial, only 10% of patients included in this study had the diagnosis of COPD. Another relevant feature of this trial is that patients from the standard medical therapy group could be re-intubated or cross over to the NIV group if they met the predefined criteria for re-intubation. Thus, 28 (26%) patients from this group crossed over to receive NIV. This subset of patients had a lower rate of re-intubation (25%) compared with the overall population, as well as lower mortality in the ICU (11%) compared with the remaining patients. Finally, *post hoc* analysis performed in the 23 patients diagnosed with COPD showed that the rate of re-intubation was lower among those who received NIV, compared with the standard medical therapy group (50% *versus* 67%, p=0.67), although the small size of this sample did not allow any conclusions to be obtained.

NIV in the prevention of respiratory failure after extubation

Despite the disappointing results of the previous studies, there are some points to comment on. First, it is important to appreciate the low amount of COPD patients enrolled in these studies [38, 44]; taking into account that the clearest evidence on the efficacy of NIV is demonstrated in this population [46]. Secondly, the longer time from extubation to re-intubation is significantly associated with a worse outcome [45]. Since NIV has not demonstrated to avert re-intubation once patients have developed respiratory failure after extubation, and the delay in re-intubation is associated with poor outcome, a strategy based on the early use of NIV during the initial periods after extubation seems more appropriate in order to avert respiratory failure following extubation in patients at risk for this complication.

A randomised trial assessed the role of the early application of bi-level positive airway pressure on the outcome of extubation in ventilator weaning [47]. 93 extubated patients, 56 with planned and 37 with unplanned extubation, were randomly allocated to be extubated with early use of NIV just after extubation or conventional management. There were 24 COPD patients in the NIV group and 19 in the conventional therapy group. This study did not show any significant benefit of NIV in averting re-intubation. A possible reason for this lack of benefit of NIV could be that there was not a good criteria selection of patients due to the high proportion of unplanned extubation, which was the main determinant of poor outcome.

More recent randomised controlled studies assessed the efficacy of the early application of NIV after a planned extubation in selected patients at increased risk of developing respiratory failure after extubation. An Italian multicentre trial enrolled 97 consecutive patients mechanically ventilated for more than 48 hours who were considered at risk if they had one of the following criteria: hypercapnia; congestive heart failure; ineffective cough and excessive tracheobronchial secretions; more than one failure of a weaning trial; more than one comorbid condition; and upper airway obstruction [48]. After a successful weaning trial, 48 patients were randomised to receive NIV for at least 8 hours a day for the first 48 hours, and 49 patients received standard medical therapy. Patients who received NIV had a lower rate of re-intubation, compared with

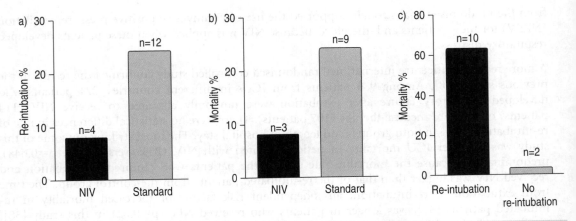

Figure 3. Effect of noninvasive ventilation (NIV) on a) the re-intubation rate and b, c) intensive care unit (ICU) mortality following planned extubation in patients who underwent a successful spontaneous breathing trial but who were at increased risk for extubation failure. In this study, re-intubation was significantly associated with increased ICU mortality (c). a) p=0.027, b) p=0.064, c) p<0.001. Data taken from [48].

those who received standard medical therapy (p=0.027) (fig. 3). In this study, the need for re-intubation was associated with a higher risk of mortality, and the use of NIV resulted in a reduction of the risk of ICU mortality (-10%, p>0.01). The authors concluded that NIV was more effective than standard medical therapy in preventing post-extubation respiratory failure in a population considered at risk for this complication.

Another randomised clinical trial was conducted in 162 patients mechanically ventilated for at least 48 hours who tolerated SBT through a T-piece [49]. Patients were considered at risk for respiratory failure after extubation if they had at least one of the following criteria: age >65 years, cardiac failure as the cause of intubation or increased severity, assessed by an APACHE (Acute Physiology And Chronic Health Evaluation) II score >12 on the day of extubation [35]. 79 patients were randomly allocated after extubation to receive NIV continuously during 24 hours, and 83 patients received conventional management. 51% of patients had underlying chronic respiratory disorders, mainly COPD or chronic bronchitis. Respiratory failure after extubation was less frequent in the NIV group (p=0.029) (fig. 4). Patients from the two groups who developed respiratory failure after extubation but did not meet the criteria for immediate re-intubation could receive NIV as rescue therapy in order to avoid re-intubation. Consequently, NIV as rescue therapy resulted in avoiding re-intubation in four out of four patients from the NIV group and nine out of 19 patients from the control group. For this reason, the rate of re-intubation was not significantly lower in the NIV group. The ICU mortality (two patients (3%) *versus* 12 patients (14%); p=0.015) was lower in the NIV group, but the hospital and 90-day survival was similar among patients from the two groups. More interestingly, the authors did a separate analysis of patients with and without hypercapnia (P_{a,CO_2} >45 mmHg) during the SBT. This analysis showed that the ICU and hospital mortality, as well as the 90-day survival, improved significantly only in the subset of patients with hypercapnia during spontaneous breathing (fig. 4). Among hypercapnic patients, 48 out of 49 had underlying chronic respiratory disorders, and the proportion of cardiac disorders was also high. The authors concluded that the beneficial effects of NIV in hypercapnic patients should be confirmed in a future clinical trial in this specific population.

After these findings, the same authors conducted a new randomised clinical trial specifically in patients with chronic respiratory disorders and hypercapnia during a successful SBT, with the same study design [50]. Again, the rate of cardiac comorbidity was high in this population (43%). The results from this study again confirm that the use of NIV immediately after extubation results in decreased incidence of respiratory failure after extubation (p<0.001) (fig. 5) and improved 90-day survival (p=0.015), compared with the conventional management with oxygen (Venturi

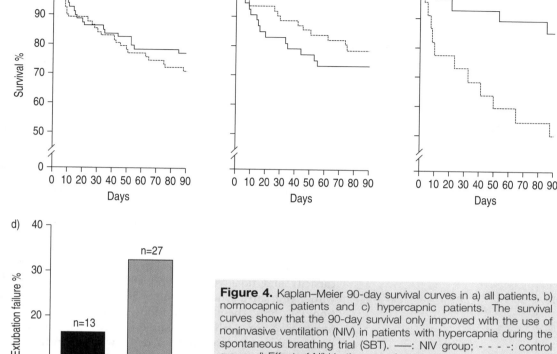

Figure 4. Kaplan–Meier 90-day survival curves in a) all patients, b) normocapnic patients and c) hypercapnic patients. The survival curves show that the 90-day survival only improved with the use of noninvasive ventilation (NIV) in patients with hypercapnia during the spontaneous breathing trial (SBT). ——: NIV group; - - - -: control group. d) Effect of NIV in the rate of extubation failure after planned extubation in patients who underwent a successful SBT but were at increased risk for extubation failure. a) p=0.397, b) p=0.429, c) p=0.006, d) p=0.029. Reproduced from [49] with permission from the publisher.

mask) after extubation. NIV (adjusted OR 0.17, 95% CI 0.06–0.44; p<0.001) was independently associated with lower risk for respiratory failure after extubation in this study.

The benefits of NIV in the prevention of respiratory failure after extubation were also documented in severely obese patients in a case–control study [51]. In this study, the benefits in survival were also restricted to hypercapnic patients only.

A very recent multicentre randomised controlled trial has investigated the effectiveness of NIV as an early weaning and extubation technique in difficult-to-wean patients with chronic hypercapnic respiratory failure [52]. This study enrolled 208 intubated patients who failed an SBT and randomly assigned them to three groups: 1) conventional invasive weaning, 2) extubation followed by standard oxygen therapy, or 3) extubation followed by NIV. The primary end-point was re-intubation within 7 days after extubation. This study did not report differences in the re-intubation rate between the three weaning strategies. However, the weaning failure rates, which included post-extubation respiratory failure, re-intubation or death occurrence within 7 days after extubation, was significantly lower for patients extubated with NIV, compared with the other groups. Moreover, the duration of intubation was lower for the two weaning strategies that consisted of extubation with or without NIV. The authors concluded that, although the re-intubation rate did not change, NIV decreased the intubation duration and might improve the weaning results in difficult-to-wean patients with chronic hypercapnic respiratory failure by reducing the risk of post-extubation respiratory failure.

In summary, these studies suggest that the early use of NIV in avoiding respiratory failure after extubation is useful in selected patients, particularly those with chronic respiratory disorders, cardiac comorbidity and hypercapnic respiratory failure. A very recent report has confirmed that

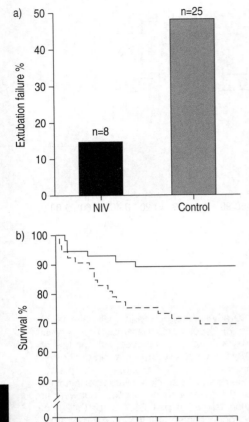

Figure 5. a) Effect of noninvasive ventilation (NIV) on the rate of extubation failure and b) Kaplan–Meier 90-day survival curves after planned extubation in patients with chronic respiratory disorders who underwent a successful spontaneous breathing trial and had hypercapnia in arterial blood gases. ——: NIV group; - - - -: control group. a) p<0.001, b) p=0.015. Data taken from [50].

mechanically ventilated patients aged >65 years with underlying chronic cardiac or respiratory disease are at high risk for extubation failure and subsequent pneumonia and death [53]. Therefore, the routine implementation of this strategy in the management of mechanically ventilated patients with chronic respiratory or cardiac disorders is advisable. By contrast, to date, no evidence exists on the benefits of NIV in avoiding re-intubation in mixed populations who have already developed post-extubation respiratory failure.

ARF in the post-operative period

The respiratory function may be substantially modified during the post-operative period. Anaesthesia, post-operative pain and surgery, particularly when the site of the surgery approaches the diaphragm, often induces respiratory modifications such as hypoxaemia, pulmonary volume decrease (vital capacity, functional residual capacity and tidal volume) and atelectasis associated with a restrictive syndrome and a diaphragm dysfunction [54, 55]. These modifications of the respiratory function occur early after surgery, and diaphragm dysfunction may last up to 7 days, with important deterioration in arterial oxygenation [56, 57]. Moreover, swallowing disorders and vomiting may cause aspiration during the post-operative period. Maintenance of adequate oxygenation in the post-operative period is of major importance, especially when pulmonary complications such as ARF occur [58].

Physiological effects of NIV and continuous positive airway pressure on post-operative respiratory failure

Both NIV and continuous positive airway pressure (CPAP) are frequently used in these clinical situations. Imaging studies have shown that the use of NIV may increase lung aeration and decrease the amount of atelectasis during the post-operative period of patients undergoing major abdominal surgery.

Physiological studies have shown that CPAP is effective in improving arterial oxygenation after extubation without adverse haemodynamic effects during post-operative periods of cardiac or thoracic surgery [59]. However, this study demonstrated that 9–10 cmH$_2$O is the minimally effective level of positive airway pressure for this purpose, since lower levels of airway pressure are not appropriately transmitted to the tracheal and thoracic cavity. The same authors had demonstrated that nasal CPAP improved arterial oxygenation and avoided re-intubation in 90% of cases in patients who had worsening of arterial oxygenation after elective surgery [60]. Similarly, a physiological study in patients submitted to elective lung resection showed that, compared with standard medical therapy, the addition of NIV resulted in improved arterial oxygenation without changes in arterial carbon dioxide levels, dead space and pleural leaks [61]. By contrast, physiological studies in patients extubated after elective cardiac surgery have shown that NIV caused haemodynamic changes, with improvement in the cardiac index, without changes in systemic and pulmonary artery pressure or in arterial oxygenation [62].

In obese patients with restrictive ventilatory disorder undergoing gastroplasty, nasal NIV during the post-operative period improved the diaphragm dysfunction and accelerated recovery of patients [63]. In a similar population of morbidly obese patients with known obstructive sleep apnoea undergoing laparoscopic bariatric surgery, NIV given immediately after extubation significantly improved spirometric lung function at 1 hour and 1 day post-operatively, compared with nasal CPAP started in the post-anaesthesia care unit [64].

NIV and CPAP in the management and prevention of post-operative respiratory failure

A case–control study showed that patients with post-operative ARF after oesophagectomy treated with NIV had lower rates of re-intubation, development of acute respiratory distress syndrome (ARDS) and anastomosis leakage, as well as shorter length of ICU stay, compared with historic controls treated conventionally [65]. A prospective observational study in patients who had ARF after abdominal surgery showed that the use of NIV resulted in avoidance of intubation in 67% of cases [66]. Patients who required intubation had worse arterial oxygenation and more extended bilateral pulmonary infiltrates than those who escaped from intubation. In this study, arterial oxygenation and tachypnoea improved only in the non-intubated patients, with a reduction in the hospital length of stay and mortality, compared with the intubated patients.

Several randomised clinical trials have assessed the efficacy of NIV and CPAP in the management and prevention of post-operative ARF of different cause. In patients with solid organ transplantation and post-operative ARF, NIV improved arterial oxygenation and decreased the need for tracheal intubation, compared with conventional treatment [67].

A study in patients who developed ARF during the post-operative period of lung cancer resection demonstrated that NIV was effective in decreasing the needs for tracheal intubation and improving hospital mortality [68]. More recently, a prospective survey confirmed the feasibility and efficacy of NIV in ARF following lung resection [69]. In a similar population of patients undergoing lung resection surgery, the use of prophylactic NIV during the pre- and post-operative period resulted in less incidence of post-operative atelectasis, improvement of arterial blood gases and pulmonary volumes, as well as in shorter length of hospital stay [70]. However, the efficacy of NIV in these studies seems to be related to the underlying disease of patients rather than the post-operative respiratory complications.

The prophylactic use of nasal CPAP in the post-operative period in patients undergoing elective thoracic-abdominal aortic surgery decreased the incidence of pulmonary complications, such as severe hypoxaemia, atelectasis, pneumonia and re-intubation and length of hospital stay [71]. The same group obtained similar benefits with the administration of prophylactic nasal CPAP following cardiac surgery, with improved arterial oxygenation, reduced incidence of pulmonary complications including pneumonia and re-intubation rate, and reduced readmission rate to the ICU [72].

Another randomised controlled trial in patients with ARF after major abdominal surgery compared the use of CPAP and oxygen therapy [73]. This study showed that CPAP reduced the rate of tracheal intubation, compared with oxygen therapy (1% *versus* 10%, respectively; p=0.005), as well as other severe complications, although the reduction of hospital mortality was not significant.

In summary, both CPAP and NIV improve the physiological mechanisms of post-operative ARF, with partial compensation of the affected respiratory function by reducing the work of breathing, improvement of alveolar recruitment with better oxygenation and ventilation, and reduction of the left ventricular after load increasing cardiac output and improving haemodynamics. The evidence suggests that CPAP and NIV are effective strategies to improve clinical outcomes in patients with post-operative ARF, particularly those with abdominal and thoracic surgery. This results in reduction of intubation rates, nosocomial infections, length of stay, morbidity and

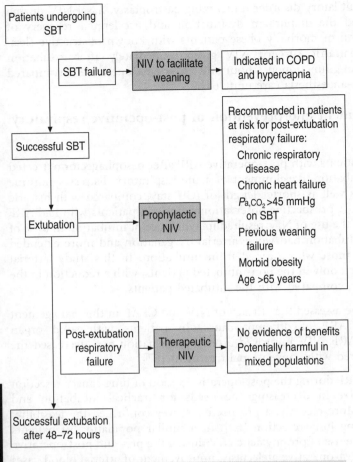

Figure 6. Schematic representation of the application of noninvasive ventilation (NIV) during the different phases of ventilator withdrawal. SBT: spontaneous breathing trial; COPD: chronic obstructive pulmonary disease; P_{a,CO_2}: arterial carbon dioxide tension. Data taken from [34].

mortality [58, 74]. However, it is recommended that before initiating NIV, any surgical complication must be treated.

Conclusions

NIV has been used during weaning from mechanical ventilation. This is consistently effective in advancing extubation and decreasing complications associated with prolonged invasive ventilation in intubated patients with chronic respiratory disorders and difficult or prolonged weaning. There is also evidence on the efficacy of NIV in preventing extubation failure and improving outcome in patients with chronic respiratory or cardiac diseases who present with hypercapnic respiratory failure during an SBT. By contrast, NIV is not effective in preventing re-intubation and may be even harmful in a mixed population who develop extubation failure. A schematic representation of the application of NIV during the different phases of ventilator withdrawal is shown in figure 6. The use of CPAP or NIV may improve the outcome of patients with post-operative ARF, particularly those with abdominal and thoracic surgery.

Statement of interest

A. Torres has received research grants and honoraria for lectures and research from Pfizer and Covidien. He has participated in the advisory boards of Astellas and Sanofi-Aventis.

References

1. Torres A, Aznar R, Gatell JM, *et al.* Incidence, risk, and prognosis factors of nosocomial pneumonia in mechanically ventilated patients. *Am Rev Respir Dis* 1990; 142: 523–528.
2. Esteban A, Alia I, Ibañez J, *et al.* Modes of mechanical ventilation and weaning. A national survey of Spanish hospitals. *Chest* 1994; 106: 1188–1193.
3. Esteban A, Ferguson ND, Meade MO, *et al.* Evolution of mechanical ventilation in response to clinical research. *Am J Respir Crit Care Med* 2008; 177: 170–177.
4. Ely EW, Baker AM, Dunagan DP, *et al.* Effect on the duration of mechanical ventilation of identifying patients capable of breathing spontaneously. *N Engl J Med* 1996; 335: 1864–1869.
5. Esteban A, Anzueto A, Frutos F, *et al.* Characteristics and outcomes in adult patients receiving mechanical ventilation: a 28-day international study. *JAMA* 2002; 287: 345–355.
6. Zilberberg MD, de Wit M, Pirone JR, *et al.* Growth in adult prolonged acute mechanical ventilation: implications for healthcare delivery. *Crit Care Med* 2008; 36: 1451–1455.

7. Boles J-M, Bion J, Connors A, *et al.* Weaning from mechanical ventilation. *Eur Respir J* 2007; 29: 1033–1056.
8. Tobin MJ, Jubran A. Discontinuation of mechanical ventilation. *In:* Tobin MJ, ed. Principles and Practice of Mechanical Ventilation. 2nd Edn. New York, McGraw-Hill Inc., 2006; pp. 1185–1220.
9. Vitacca M, Vianello A, Colombo D, *et al.* Comparison of two methods for weaning patients with chronic obstructive pulmonary disease requiring mechanical ventilation for more than 15 days. *Am J Respir Crit Care Med* 2001; 164: 225–230.
10. Kollef MH, Shapiro SD, Silver P, *et al.* A randomized, controlled trial of protocol-directed *versus* physician-directed weaning from mechanical ventilation. *Crit Care Med* 1997; 25: 567–574.
11. Burns KE, Lellouche F, Lessard MR. Automating the weaning process with advanced closed-loop systems. *Intensive Care Med* 2008; 34: 1757–1765.
12. Esteban A, Frutos F, Tobin MJ, *et al.* A comparison of four methods of weaning patients from mechanical ventilation. *N Engl J Med* 1995; 323: 345–350.
13. Brochard L, Rauss A, Benito S, *et al.* Comparison of three methods of gradual withdrawal from ventilatory support during weaning from mechanical ventilation. *Am J Respir Crit Care Med* 1994; 150: 896–903.
14. Vallverdú I, Calaf N, Subirana M, *et al.* Clinical characteristics, respiratory functional parameters, and outcome of a two-hour T-piece trial in patients weaning from mechanical ventilation. *Am J Respir Crit Care Med* 1998; 158: 1855–1862.
15. Funk G-C, Anders S, Breyer M-K, *et al.* Incidence and outcome of weaning from mechanical ventilation according to new categories. *Eur Respir J* 2010; 35: 88–94.
16. Sellares J, Ferrer M, Cano E, *et al.* Predictors of prolonged weaning and survival during ventilator weaning in a respiratory ICU. *Intensive Care Med* 2011; 37: 775–784.
17. Tobin MJ, Perez W, Guenther SM, *et al.* The pattern of breathing during successful and unsuccessful trials of weaning from mechanical ventilation. *Am Rev Respir Dis* 1986; 134: 1111–1118.
18. Jubran A, Tobin MJ. Pathophysiologic basis of acute respiratory distress in patients who fail a trial of weaning from mechanical ventilation. *Am J Respir Crit Care Med* 1997; 155: 906–915.
19. Lemaire F, Teboul J, Cinotti L, *et al.* Acute left ventricular dysfunction during unsuccessful weaning from mechanical ventilation. *Anesthesiology* 1988; 69: 171–179.
20. Jubran A, Mathru M, Dries D, *et al.* Continuous recordings of mixed venous oxygen saturation during weaning from mechanical ventilation and the ramifications thereof. *Am J Respir Crit Care Med* 1998; 158: 1763–1769.
21. Torres A, Reyes A, Roca J, *et al.* Ventilation–perfusion mismatching in chronic obstructive pulmonary disease during ventilator weaning. *Am Rev Respir Dis* 1989; 140: 1246–1250.
22. Ferrer M, Iglesia R, Roca J, *et al.* Pulmonary gas exchange response to weaning with pressure-support ventilation in exacerbated COPD patients. *Intensive Care Med* 2002; 28: 1595–1599.
23. Appendini L, Patessio A, Zanaboni S, *et al.* Physiologic effects of positive end-expiratory pressure and mask pressure support during exacerbations of chronic obstructive pulmonary disease. *Am J Respir Crit Care Med* 1994; 149: 1069–1076.
24. Diaz O, Iglesia R, Ferrer M, *et al.* Effects of noninvasive ventilation on pulmonary gas exchange and hemodynamics during acute hypercapnic exacerbations of chronic obstructive pulmonary disease. *Am J Respir Crit Care Med* 1997; 156: 1840–1845.
25. Kilger E, Briegel J, Haller M, *et al.* Effects of noninvasive positive pressure ventilatory support in non-COPD patients with acute respiratory insufficiency after early extubation. *Intensive Care Med* 1999; 25: 1374–1380.
26. Vitacca M, Ambrosino N, Clini E, *et al.* Physiological response to pressure support ventilation delivered before and after extubation in patients not capable of totally spontaneous autonomous breathing. *Am J Respir Crit Care Med* 2001; 164: 638–641.
27. International Consensus Conferences in Intensive Care Medicine: noninvasive positive pressure ventilation in acute respiratory failure. *Am J Respir Crit Care Med* 2001; 163: 283–291.
28. Nava S, Ambrosino N, Clini E, *et al.* Noninvasive mechanical ventilation in the weaning of patients with respiration failure due to chronic obstructive pulmonary disease. A randomized, controlled trial. *Ann Intern Med* 1998; 128: 721–728.
29. Girault C, Daudenthun I, Chevron V, *et al.* Noninvasive ventilation as a systematic extubation and weaning technique in acute-on-chronic respiratory failure. A prospective, randomized controlled study. *Am J Respir Crit Care Med* 1999; 160: 86–92.
30. Trevisan CE, Vieira SR. Noninvasive mechanical ventilation may be useful in treating patients who fail weaning from invasive mechanical ventilation: a randomized clinical trial. *Crit Care* 2008; 12: R51.
31. Ferrer M, Esquinas A, Arancibia F, *et al.* Noninvasive ventilation during persistent weaning failure. A randomized controlled trial. *Am J Respir Crit Care Med* 2003; 168: 70–76.
32. Burns KE, Adhikari NK, Meade MO. A meta-analysis of noninvasive weaning to facilitate liberation from mechanical ventilation. *Can J Anaesth* 2006; 53: 305–315.
33. Burns KE, Adhikari NK, Keenan SP, *et al.* Use of non-invasive ventilation to wean critically ill adults off invasive ventilation: meta-analysis and systematic review. *BMJ* 2009; 338: b1574.
34. Ferreyra G, Fanelli V, Del SL, *et al.* Are guidelines for non-invasive ventilation during weaning still valid? *Minerva Anestesiol* 2011; 77: 921–926.
35. Epstein SK, Ciubotaru RL, Wong J. Effect of failed extubation on the outcome of mechanical ventilation. *Chest* 1997; 112: 186–192.

36. Esteban A, Alía I, Tobin MJ, *et al.* Effect of spontaneous breathing trial duration on outcome of attempts to discontinue mechanical ventilation. *Am J Respir Crit Care Med* 1999; 159: 512–518.

37. Epstein SK. Decision to extubate. *Intensive Care Med* 2002; 28: 535–546.

38. Esteban A, Frutos-Vivar F, Ferguson ND, *et al.* Noninvasive positive-pressure ventilation for respiratory failure after extubation. *N Engl J Med* 2004; 350: 2452–2460.

39. Khamiees M, Raju P, DeGirolamo A, *et al.* Predictors of extubation outcome in patients who have successfully completed a spontaneous breathing trial. *Chest* 2001; 120: 1262–1270.

40. Smina M, Salam A, Khamiees M, *et al.* Cough peak flows and extubation outcomes. *Chest* 2003; 124: 262–268.

41. Salam A, Tilluckdharry L, Amoateng-Adjepong Y, *et al.* Neurologic status, cough, secretions and extubation outcomes. *Intensive Care Med* 2004; 30: 1334–1339.

42. Torres A, Gatell JM, Aznar E, *et al.* Re-intubation increases the risk of nosocomial pneumonia in patients needing mechanical ventilation. *Am J Respir Crit Care Med* 1995; 152: 137–141.

43. Hilbert G, Gruson D, Portel L, *et al.* Noninvasive pressure support ventilation in COPD patients with postextubation hypercapnic respiratory insufficiency. *Eur Respir J* 1998; 11: 1349–1353.

44. Keenan SP, Powers C, McCormack DG, *et al.* Noninvasive positive-pressure ventilation for postextubation respiratory distress: a randomized controlled trial. *JAMA* 2002; 287: 3238–3244.

45. Epstein SK, Ciubotaru RL. Independent effects of etiology of failure and time of reintubation on outcome for patients failing extubation. *Am J Respir Crit Care Med* 1998; 158: 489–493.

46. Mehta S, Hill NS. Noninvasive ventilation. *Am J Respir Crit Care Med* 2001; 163: 540–577.

47. Jiang JS, Kao SJ, Wang SN. Effect of early application of biphasic positive airway pressure on the outcome of extubation in ventilator weaning. *Respirology* 1999; 4: 151–155.

48. Nava S, Gregoretti C, Fanfulla F, *et al.* Noninvasive ventilation to prevent respiratory failure after extubation in high-risk patients. *Crit Care Med* 2005; 33: 2465–2470.

49. Ferrer M, Valencia M, Nicolas JM, *et al.* Early noninvasive ventilation averts extubation failure in patients at risk: a randomized trial. *Am J Respir Crit Care Med* 2006; 173: 164–170.

50. Ferrer M, Sellares J, Valencia M, *et al.* Non-invasive ventilation after extubation in hypercapnic patients with chronic respiratory disorders: randomised controlled trial. *Lancet* 2009; 374: 1082–1088.

51. El Solh AA, Aquilina A, Pineda L, *et al.* Noninvasive ventilation for prevention of post-extubation respiratory failure in obese patients. *Eur Respir J* 2006; 28: 588–595.

52. Girault C, Bubenheim M, Abroug F, *et al.* Non-invasive ventilation and weaning in chronic hypercapnic respiratory failure patients: a randomized multicenter trial. *Am J Respir Crit Care Med* 2011; 184: 672–679.

53. Thille AW, Harrois A, Schortgen F, *et al.* Outcomes of extubation failure in medical intensive care unit patients. *Crit Care Med* 2011; 39: 2612–2618.

54. Magnusson L, Spahn DR. New concepts of atelectasis during general anaesthesia. *Br J Anaesth* 2003; 91: 61–72.

55. Eichenberger A, Proietti S, Wicky S, *et al.* Morbid obesity and postoperative pulmonary atelectasis: an underestimated problem. *Anesth Analg* 2002; 95: 1788–1792.

56. Simonneau G, Vivien A, Sartene R, *et al.* Diaphragm dysfunction induced by upper abdominal surgery. Role of postoperative pain. *Am Rev Respir Dis* 1983; 128: 899–903.

57. Warner DO. Preventing postoperative pulmonary complications: the role of the anesthesiologist. *Anesthesiology* 2000; 92: 1467–1472.

58. Jaber S, Michelet P, Chanques G. Role of non-invasive ventilation (NIV) in the perioperative period. *Best Pract Res Clin Anaesthesiol* 2010; 24: 253–265.

59. Kindgen-Milles D, Buhl R, Loer SA, *et al.* Nasal CPAP therapy: effects of different CPAP levels on pressure transmission into the trachea and pulmonary oxygen transfer. *Acta Anaesthesiol Scand* 2002; 46: 860–865.

60. Kindgen-Milles D, Buhl R, Gabriel A, *et al.* Nasal continuous positive airway pressure: a method to avoid endotracheal reintubation in postoperative high-risk patients with severe nonhypercapnic oxygenation failure. *Chest* 2000; 117: 1106–1111.

61. Aguilo R, Togores B, Pons S, *et al.* Noninvasive ventilatory support after lung resectional surgery. *Chest* 1997; 112: 117–121.

62. Hoffmann B, Jepsen M, Hachenberg T, *et al.* Cardiopulmonary effects of non-invasive positive pressure ventilation (NPPV) – a controlled, prospective study. *Thorac Cardiovasc Surg* 2003; 51: 142–146.

63. Joris JL, Sottiaux TM, Chiche JD, *et al.* Effect of bi-level positive airway pressure (BiPAP) nasal ventilation on the postoperative pulmonary restrictive syndrome in obese patients undergoing gastroplasty. *Chest* 1997; 111: 665–670.

64. Neligan PJ, Malhotra G, Fraser M, *et al.* Noninvasive ventilation immediately after extubation improves lung function in morbidly obese patients with obstructive sleep apnea undergoing laparoscopic bariatric surgery. *Anesth Analg* 2010; 110: 1360–1365.

65. Michelet P, D'Journo XB, Seinaye F, *et al.* Non-invasive ventilation for treatment of postoperative respiratory failure after oesophagectomy. *Br J Surg* 2009; 96: 54–60.

66. Jaber S, Delay JM, Chanques G, *et al.* Outcomes of patients with acute respiratory failure after abdominal surgery treated with noninvasive positive pressure ventilation. *Chest* 2005; 128: 2688–2695.

67. Antonelli M, Conti G, Bufi M, *et al.* Noninvasive ventilation for treatment of acute respiratory failure in patients undergoing solid organ transplantation. *JAMA* 2000; 283: 235–241.

68. Auriant I, Jallot A, Hervé P, *et al.* Noninvasive ventilation reduces mortality in acute respiratory failure following lung resection. *Am J Respir Crit Care Med* 2001; 164: 1231–1235.

69. Lefebvre A, Lorut C, Alifano M, *et al.* Noninvasive ventilation for acute respiratory failure after lung resection: an observational study. *Intensive Care Med* 2009; 35: 663–670.

70. Perrin C, Jullien V, Venissac N, *et al.* Prophylactic use of noninvasive ventilation in patients undergoing lung resectional surgery. *Respir Med* 2007; 101: 1572–1578.

71. Kindgen-Milles D, Muller E, Buhl R, *et al.* Nasal-continuous positive airway pressure reduces pulmonary morbidity and length of hospital stay following thoracoabdominal aortic surgery. *Chest* 2005; 128: 821–828.

72. Zarbock A, Mueller E, Netzer S, *et al.* Prophylactic nasal continuous positive airway pressure following cardiac surgery protects from postoperative pulmonary complications: a prospective, randomized, controlled trial in 500 patients. *Chest* 2009; 135: 1252–1259.

73. Squadrone V, Coha M, Cerutti E, *et al.* Continuous positive airway pressure for treatment of postoperative hypoxemia: a randomized controlled trial. *JAMA* 2005; 293: 589–595.

74. Chiumello D, Chevallard G, Gregoretti C. Non-invasive ventilation in postoperative patients: a systematic review. *Intensive Care Med* 2011; 37: 918–929.

Chapter 15

Tracheostomy in mechanical ventilation

P. Terragni*, A. Trompeo#, C. Faggiano* and V.M. Ranieri*

Summary

Endotracheal intubation is commonly used for airway control, while tracheostomy is a procedure indicated for patients who suffer from respiratory failure and need prolonged mechanical ventilation. Between 6% and 11% of mechanically ventilated patients receive a tracheostomy that allows for a lower sedation and shorter weaning time leading to a reduction in intensive care unit (ICU) and hospital stay. The technique and timing of tracheostomy are still controversial in the literature. Percutaneous dilational tracheostomy techniques, performed at the bedside in the ICU, are widely used, but there are still patients (with severe coagulation disorders or cervical spine injury) who can benefit from the surgical "minimally invasive" techniques. The correct timing is also under debate but, excluding patients with severe brain or cervical spine injury, we can reasonably affirm that tracheostomy should not be performed earlier than 2 weeks following respiratory failure.

Keywords: Endotracheal intubation, percutaneous dilational tracheostomy, surgical tracheostomy, timing, tracheostomy, ventilator-associated pneumonia

*Dipartimento di Discipline Medico Chirurgiche, Università di Torino, Azienda Ospedaliero-Universitaria San Giovanni Battista di Torino, and #Dipartimento di Medicina degli Stati Critici, Azienda Ospedaliero-Universitaria San Giovanni Battista di Torino, Turin, Italy.

Correspondence: P. Terragni, Dept of Anesthesia and Intensive Care Medicine, University of Turin, S. Giovanni Battista Molinette Hospital, Corso Dogliotti 14, 10126 Turin, Italy.
Email pierpaolo.terragni@unito.it

Eur Respir Mon 2012; 55: 206–216.
Printed in UK – all rights reserved
Copyright ERS 2012
European Respiratory Monograph
ISSN: 1025-448x
DOI: 10.1183/1025448x.10002811

Tracheostomy is one of the most common procedures in the intensive care unit (ICU) because it facilitates airway management in long-term mechanical ventilation. In comparison with endotracheal intubation (ETI), other advantages of mechanical ventilation are improved patient comfort, greater airway security, lower respiratory resistance and faster weaning from mechanical ventilation with less need for sedation, reduced incidence of laryngeal ulceration, facilitation of patient communication and easier nursing with improved pulmonary toilet.

Nonetheless, tracheostomy practice remains controversial. The procedure is not without risk and several complications have been reported, such as stomal infections, fistulas, bleeding, pneumomediastinum, pneumothorax and, rarely, death.

The introduction of the percutaneous tracheostomy technique in 1985 by CIAGLIA et al. [1], as an alternative to the surgical approach, generated a lot of interest regarding the indication and most appropriate use of this valuable procedure.

Unresolved questions include the appropriate indications and most suitable technique, and complications and timing of the procedure; a proper timing effect on outcome is still unclear because guidelines regarding clinical practice and current evidence remain limited and conflicting [2, 3].

The only indications are those of the National Association of Medical Directors of Respiratory Care (NAMDRC), who recommend performing tracheostomy in patients requiring mechanical ventilation for more than 21 days after admission [4]. The American Association for Respiratory Care/American College of Chest Physicians/American College of Critical Care Medicine Task Force has made no specific recommendation about tracheostomy timing, but suggests the procedure be used in patients with expected prolonged mechanical ventilation [5].

History

Tracheostomy is one of the oldest surgical procedures. The first description of surgical tracheostomy dates back to the Bronze Age with the first report of throat incision. In Egypt, Imhotep (2600 BC), the father of modern medicine, described a tracheostomy performed in a case of upper airways obstruction with cauterisation to avoid bleeding.

Over many centuries tracheostomy has become a routine procedure for airways management. There was a unanimous opinion on the indications for the surgical procedure that included obstruction of the upper airways, such as abscesses, oedema, foreign bodies and tumours.

At the end of the 1500s, thanks to the progress of anatomy and surgery, tracheostomy became generally accepted as the last life-saving method in certain syndromes. The reason for the increase in acceptance of this technique was the explosion of the first major epidemic of diphtheria, which started in Spain and France before spreading to Italy and other European countries.

During the 19th century, the interest in tracheostomy procedures increased following the death in 1807 of Napoleon Bonaparte's nephew from diphtheria. At this time mortality from the procedure was considered acceptable if 25% of the patients survived.

Between the end of the 19th and the first half of the 20th century, new tracheostomy applications were discovered; preventive treatment began to be used during routine surgery demolition not only on the larynx but also on the cervicocephalic.

In the first half of the 20th century, several devices were suggested to facilitate the procedure and reduce the incidence of complications by focusing on the preparation of stoma [6]. In the 1960s, tracheostomy began to be applied to neurological and pneumological patients because they were known to have damage from tracheal intubation due to prolonged bed rest.

Recently, indications, complications and correlation with ETI have been clearly outlined. Thus, tracheostomy has found its place. The new percutaneous techniques and the development of synthetic materials with the use of low-pressure/high-volume cuffs have improved the procedure of tracheostomy and reduced complications (*e.g.* stenosis and erosion of large blood vessels).

Tracheostomy indications

The main clinical indications for tracheostomy are: 1) prolonged mechanical ventilation; 2) upper airway obstruction, also secondary to trauma or surgery in the face/neck region; 3) airway protection against inhalation; and 4) the need for less sedation and analgesia [7]. In all of these cases intubation is the most appropriate initial treatment approach that later supports tracheostomy.

Benefits of tracheostomy

Tracheostomy offers many clinical and practical benefits to patients who suffer from respiratory failure and need prolonged mechanical ventilation; the safe anchor of the tracheostomy tube reduces the risk of dislocation in the bronchial area and accidental extubation, which represents a dramatic event in patients dependent on mechanical ventilation [8]. Moreover, head and neck motions can displace the tracheal cannula less easily leading to reduced lesions due to abrasion on tracheal mucosa and laryngeal damage.

Tracheostomy allows draining and aspirating secretions, mainly in patients affected by bronchorrhea, facilitating pulmonary toilet and oral hygiene. It seems to improve patient comfort, and reduces the pain on swallowing and salivary stagnation in the larynx. It allows earlier and easier mobilisation of the patient, making oral feeding possible and shortening the residence time of nasogastric tubes [9, 10]. Due to the many aids available at present, the quality of relationships with relatives and nurses is improved due to the ability of patients to communicate.

Compared to intubation, the tracheostomy cannula reduces airflow resistance and facilitates weaning from artificial ventilation due to: the direct approach to the trachea; an internal diameter greater than the translaryngeal diameter; a shorter length; and the absence of multiple curves. It also allows for a faster resumption of the autonomy of respiratory function with reduced use of sedatives and, as a result, a decreased number of days on mechanical ventilation, a reduced length of stay in the ICU and decreased use of resources [7, 9, 11, 12].

Complications

Tracheostomy leads to many complications that can be of varying severity, with a global incidence (which includes all techniques) of 6–60%. The frequency and severity depend on the specific approach, the skill and experience of the operator and the anatomical and pathophysiological factors of the patient related to the degree of organ dysfunction (especially related to the respiratory and coagulation system).

There are a large number of uncontrolled case series reporting percutaneous dilational tracheostomy (PDT) complications. There are also few prospectively collected comparative studies of PDT and surgical tracheostomy complications and of the different PDT methods.

The meta-analysis by FREEMAN et al. [13], which examined the PDT technique of CIAGLIA et al. [1] and GRIGGS et al. [14], showed that percutaneous techniques are generally associated with lower rates of stomal bleeding, infection and post-operative complications if compared to surgical tracheostomy.

In a randomised trial with double-blinded follow-up on percutaneous translaryngeal tracheostomy (TLT) *versus* surgical tracheostomy, ANTONELLI et al. [15] found that the main advantage of TLT over surgical tracheostomy was a somewhat lower bleeding rate; however, there was no evidence that TLT increased the risk of bacteraemia caused by the spread of upper respiratory tract microbes. In addition, the long-term effects (physical and emotional) were similar with the two procedures [15].

In reference to the problem regarding the setting of tracheostomy, in a systematic review by DELANEY et al. [16], PDT appeared to be equivalent to surgical tracheostomy for the overall incidence of clinically relevant bleeding, major periprocedural and long-term complications, but subgroup analysis revealed that PDT was superior to surgical tracheostomy when the surgical tracheostomy was performed in the operating theatre. The results indicated that PDT, performed electively in the ICU, that is the most frequent applied solution in order to avoid critical patients transferring, should be the method of choice for performing tracheostomies in critically ill adult patients.

According to the outcome of recent studies, the rate of early complications is lower in patients subjected to PDT than in those with surgical tracheostomy [17]. Experience and operator preference should determine the choice. There are few situations in which one technique should be chosen over the other: for example, obese patients present a higher complication rate with either surgical tracheostomy or PDT, but the seriousness and frequency may be higher with PDT [18].

Moreover, surgical tracheostomy has changed over time. Today, surgeons use a minimally invasive technique that is very similar to PDT in order to avoid tracheal ring fracture with a complete control of bleeding, even in patients receiving heparin treatment. The classification of tracheostomy complications is based on the time between procedure and onset, being: 1) intra-operative, and 2) post-operative (early and late) complications.

Intra-operative complications

Intra-operative complications occur during the procedure. From prospective controlled trials comparing surgical tracheostomy with PDT, the percentage of intra-operative complication was in favour of PDT with low risk of minor and major bleeding, pneumothorax, accidental decannulation, subcutaneous emphysema and infection of the stoma; otherwise, there was an increase in some PDT-related complications, such as difficulty in tracheal cannula insertion, false placement, hypoxia, loss of airways and death [13, 19].

In general, complications reported in meta-analysis can be divided into minor and serious events. 1) Minor: changes in blood pressure and desaturation during the procedure, aspiration, and failure of the chosen technique to achieve successful airway control. 2) Serious: these are very rare and are represented by death, cardiac arrest, hypertensive pneumothorax, haemorrhage caused by lesions of jugular anterior veins (due to sectioning of the hystmus of the thyroid), tracheo-oesophageal fistula (due to the lesion of posterior wall of trachea), and lesion of recurrent nerve [20].

Lesions of the tracheal posterior wall and tracheal rupture represent the most frequent complications during the execution of the PDT when compared to those associated with the surgical techniques. Severe haemorrhage is less frequent. Techniques for tracheostomy are evolving and improving. At present, more procedures are performed using a number of PDT techniques at the patient's bedside in the ICU, with the bronchoscope vision support that provides safer procedures and makes the statistics presented in literature regarding complications less applicable to current clinical practice.

Post-operative early complications

These complications are caused by technical procedures and post-operative management errors and include: haemorrhage, subcutaneous emphysema, dislocation or obstruction of the tube, possible creation of a false path and stoma infection (skin or deep tissue).

Post-operative late complications

A meta-analysis of trials (1985–1996) comparing surgical tracheostomy to PDT found more frequent perioperative complications with the percutaneous approach but more post-operative complications with surgery [20]. The clinical relevance of late complications is considerable, as their manifestations range from minimally symptomatic to the failure to wean patients from the ventilator (tracheal stenosis) to life-threatening haemorrhage (tracheo-innominate fistula). The onset does not have a precise chronological correlation with the execution of the procedure. Many potential long-term complications of translaryngeal intubation and tracheostomy are similar and overlapping. Although most patients who have undergone these procedures tend to tolerate them without difficulties, significant morbidity and mortality may occur. Identifying the exact cause of the complication may not be possible at times, due to the multiple risk factors involved in the pathogenesis [21]. It is difficult to separate out the effects of preceding prolonged oro-tracheal intubation and tracheostomy intubation on complications. ETI itself may lead to either tracheal stenosis or tracheomalacia with chondritis, mucosal and sub mucosal ulceration or necrosis.

Late complications are represented by: tracheal narrowing; granuloma; vascular erosion; tracheomalacia; tracheo-oesophageal, tracheo-cutaneous or trachea-artery anonymous fistula; aspiration and pulmonary infection. Some of these complications can be silent. However, the anonymous artery lesion results in necrosis due to cannula compression, leading to very severe haemorrhage with 100% mortality rate. Treatment modalities vary depending upon the nature of the complication. For tracheal stenosis, which is the most frequent complication, a multi-disciplinary approach utilising bronchoscopy, laser, airway stents and tracheal surgery is most effective [22].

Tracheomalacia is another complication, resulting from tracheal ischaemic injury due to compression of the cannula balloon (when over-inflated) or by the cannula itself, which is followed by chondritis and necrosis of supporting tracheal cartilage. In this case, due to loss of airway support and absence of a positive pressure, tracheal airways collapse during expiration, generating a flow limitation and air trapping with retained respiratory secretions.

The effect of pars membranacea displacement can also occlude the lower border of the tube making ventilation difficult, resulting in increased flow resistances and high airway peak pressure. This problem is very common after extended periods of management with a balloon-fitted tube. There is also the risk of tracheo-oesophageal fistula due to ischaemia if the hyperinflated balloon is also involved in front of the nasogastric tube; in these cases it is essential to make a gastrostomy to avoid the trauma of pars membranacea. In the acute setting, tracheomalacia may present as failure to wean from mechanical ventilation. In these cases bronchoscopy or a computed tomography (CT) scan are necessary to reveal the presence of expiratory collapse of the trachea [23].

In an observational, long-term, follow-up study of PDT (performed with the Griggs technique), STEELE *et al.* [24] described a moderate tracheal dilatation in 30% of patients assessed with a spiral CT scan.

The approach to tracheomalacia depends upon the severity of expiratory upper airway obstruction: in most cases the best action is to eliminate the inflated balloon. The specific treatment includes placement of a longer tracheostomy tube to bypass the malacic region or to place a tracheal stent. In more severe cases, therapeutic options are resection or tracheoplasty [22].

Timing of tracheostomy

Tracheostomy is mainly used to replace ETI in patients requiring prolonged mechanical ventilation. The use of the procedure increased in recent years by nearly 200%; however, there is considerable variability in the time that is considered optimal for performing tracheostomy [25].

From observational data, between 6% and 11% of patients with mechanical ventilation receive a tracheostomy [11, 26]. Older guidelines recommended performing the procedure after 3 weeks of ETI, but only if extubation did not occur by day 21 [4]. However, defining and predicting the need for prolonged mechanical ventilation has always been a major methodological challenge. It is very difficult to prospectively identify patients who will require prolonged mechanical ventilation and who should potentially benefit from tracheostomy.

Detection of clinical features at day 7, such as a positive end-expiratory pressure of 10 cmH$_2$O or the absence of radiographic improvement and >50% of lung fields with radiographic alveolar infiltrates, could, with low sensitivity and higher specificity, predict the need for intubation beyond 14 days [27].

It is better to avoid an unnecessary procedure on patients who are close to extubation or in moribund patients, than to find those who might benefit from tracheostomy airways access. Recently, it has been suggested that tracheostomy should be considered within 2–10 days of intubation: observational studies reported that early tracheotomies may be associated with better comfort due to reduced oropharyngeal and laryngeal stimulation, lower sedation and possibly delirium. Other advantages, including improved pulmonary toilet and decreased resistance to breathing, accelerated weaning, decreased risk of ventilator-associated pneumonia (VAP) and, perhaps, shorted duration of mechanical ventilation [9, 28]. However, randomised controlled trials have failed to confirm this observation.

Rumbak et al. [29] reported data in favour of patients presenting with a tracheostomy within 2 days of hospital admission with reduction of mortality rate, occurrence of pneumonia and length of ICU stay compared with tracheostomy performed after 14 to 16 days of ETI. However, Blot et al. [3] did not find a difference in mortality, duration of mechanical ventilation, ICU stay and incidence of infections between patients randomised to receive a tracheostomy within 4 days following onset of mechanical ventilation and those randomised to maintain ETI for at least 14 days.

Recently, Terragni et al. [30] presented the results of a multicentre randomised controlled trial (Early vs Late Tracheotomy study (ELT)) performed in 12 Italian ICUs with 600 adult patients. 209 patients were randomised to receive early tracheostomy performed after 6–8 days of ETI (145 received tracheostomy) and 210 to receive late tracheostomy after 13–15 days of ETI (119 received tracheostomy). The enrolled patients were without lung infection, had been ventilated for 24 hours, had a Simplified Acute Physiology II Score of 35–65, and had a Sequential Organ Failure Assessment score of $\geqslant 5$.

The primary end-point was the incidence of VAP and secondary end-points included the number of ventilator-free days, number of ICU-free days, and the number of patients in each group who were still alive at 28 days.

VAP was observed in 30 (14%) patients in the early tracheostomy group and in 44 (21%) patients in the late tracheostomy group but without statistical significance (p=0.07). During the 28 days immediately following randomisation, the hazard ratio of developing VAP was 0.66 and the hazard ratios of remaining connected to the ventilator or in the ICU were 0.70 and 0.73, respectively. The hazard ratio of dying was 0.80 [30].

The authors concluded that early tracheostomy compared to late tracheostomy did not result in a statistically significant improvement in incidence of VAP. The algorithm for predicting which patients required prolonged mechanical ventilation is a step forward and could be adopted into clinical practice to help identify prognosis.

Moreover this trial should convince clinicians that routine early tracheostomy will most likely not lead to reduced VAP, shorter hospital stay or lower mortality. Most importantly, it shows that performing tracheostomy for perceived weaning failure must be tempered by the knowledge that many patients will improve with additional time [31].

The ELT study was also confirmed by the recent study of Trouillet et al. [32], which investigated the timing of tracheostomy in 216 cardiac surgery patients. The authors compared the outcome of severely ill patients who required prolonged mechanical ventilation and who were randomly assigned to early (immediate) percutaneous tracheostomy or prolonged intubation (15 days after randomisation). Early tracheostomy provided no benefit in terms of mechanical ventilation duration and hospital length of stay, mortality rate or infectious complications [32]. The subcategory of trauma patients with or without neurological injury deserves a separate discussion. However, in patients with severe multi-trauma and/or head injury with low Glasgow coma score, early tracheostomy, often within 3–4 days of intubation resulted in some benefit.

The Eastern Association for the Surgery of Trauma recommend early tracheostomy (level III) in trauma patients with respiratory failure or neurological impairment without head injuries who are anticipated to require mechanical ventilation for at least 7 days, because it may decrease the total days of mechanical ventilation and ICU stay, and may decrease the rate of pneumonia [33].

Neurological patients might benefit from continued intubation through prevention of aspiration because of their limited ability to clear secretions, but it has been shown that prolonged intubation in traumatic brain injury is associated with a high incidence of pneumonia [34]. Conversely, early tracheostomy after trauma reduces ICU length of stay, days of mechanical ventilation and incidence of VAP [35]. Koh et al. [36] confirmed that patients undergoing early elective tracheostomy had shorter ICU stays than patients who were treated with extubation trials before tracheostomy. Kluger et al. [37] found a lower incidence of pneumonia when early tracheostomy was performed in patients with brain injuries. QURESHI et al. [38] reported that an aggressive policy regarding tracheostomy was justified in patients with infratentorial lesions because of the low rate of successful extubation.

Although early tracheostomy in selected neurological patients may reduce the length of ICU stay and pulmonary morbidity, the initial 7–10 days following acute brain injury coincide with the greatest incidence of intracranial hypertension; the appropriate timing for tracheostomy in this group of patients must be considered in view of the risk for severe intracranial hypertension. In summary, the critical issue in developing effective ventilatory management strategies in patients with acute brain injury remains the identification of those who are more likely to require long-term ventilatory support and determination of the optimal timing for tracheostomy [39].

Techniques

There are many ways to perform a tracheostomy. A common classification of techniques is represented by PDT and surgical tracheostomy.

Percutaneous dilational tracheostomy

PDT is an invasive procedure in which the placement of a tracheostomy tube is achieved after establishing a tracheal stoma through dilation, rather than surgical creation of a stoma. Dedicated procedure kits include needles, guidewire and dilators. Easy access to bronchoscopy and airway management equipment is necessary.

Two dedicated operators need to be present for this procedure: one performs the procedure and the other manages the airway and endotracheal tube. The second operator should be prepared to perform bronchoscopy, if necessary.

Several techniques, with slight variations from one another, are described herein. Generally, the patient is in the supine position with the neck slightly extended. Ventilation should be controlled and the inspiratory oxygen fraction changed to 1.0%. Landmarks, represented by the tracheal cartilages, are identified and the area is then prepared and draped.

In 1985, CIAGLIA et al. [1] first described the use of a guidewire and serial dilation technique for PDT. The new method was a combination of the percutaneous nephrostomy multiple-dilator placement technique with a variant of vascular access, as described in 1953 by SELDINGER [40]. During the past decade, PDT popularity has grown dramatically and the incidence of tracheostomy for prolonged mechanical ventilation has increased over time [25]. Initially, PDT was reserved for patients with few risk factors and favourable neck anatomy; however, growing experience shows that indications for PDT expanded and the interest for surgical tracheostomy decreased. Several variants on PDT have been developed in the years since the first description by CIAGLIA et al. [1].

In 1990, GRIGGS et al. [14] described the guidewire dilator forceps technique (Portex Ltd, Hythe, UK), an improvement of the Rapitrach method, in which forceps were inserted along the guidewire and opened to the size of the skin incision to dilate the trachea.

This technique is still used for its simplicity. After tracheal puncture with an 18-gauge needle with a catheter, the needle is removed and the guidewire is introduced through the catheter. Then, forceps are introduced over the guidewire and the handle of the forceps are opened. Bronchoscopic monitoring is necessary during the procedure to avoid injury of the posterior tracheal wall (fig. 1).

The initial serial dilator technique of CIAGLIA et al. [1] was revised in 1999 by BYHAHN et al. [41] to use a single tapered dilator with a hydrophilic coating, permitting complete tracheal dilatation in a single step, known as the Blue Rhino (Cook Critical Care, Bloomington, IN, USA). Subsequent trials have confirmed the advantages of this technique.

In 1997, FANTONI and RIPAMONTI [42] described a TLT method (Covidien, St Louis, MO, USA) that did not require external compression of the trachea, with the dilator passing from inside to outside the trachea; however, an endotracheal tube change during the procedure for airway control and the management of mechanical ventilation is necessary.

In 2005, the PercuTwist method (Rüsch GmbH, Kernen, Germany) was devised, which uses a screw-like device to open the trachea wall, preventing loss of tracheal lumen view during bronchoscopy and minimising the risk of posterior tracheal wall injury [43].

The Ciaglia Blue Dolphin® system (Cook Ireland Ltd, Limerick, Ireland) was introduced in 2008. This system is a balloon dilation-PDT technique, which is primarily used with radial force to widen the tracheostoma in a single-step dilatation, minimising bleeding, injury to tracheal rings and achieving good cosmetic results after decannulation [44].

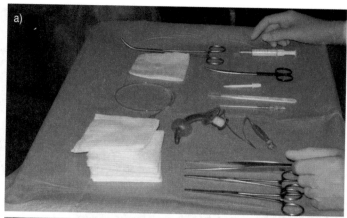
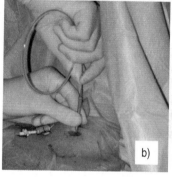
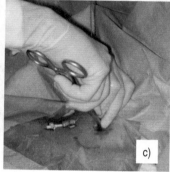

Figure 1. a) The Griggs technique with guidewire dilator forceps (Portex Ltd, Hythe, UK). b) The guidewire is introduced through the catheter; its insertion into the trachea is verified with the bronchoscope. c) The forceps are then introduced over the guidewire and the handles are opened with bronchoscopic monitoring to avoid injury of the posterior tracheal wall.

Currently, the Blue Rhino technique is the most widely used in North America, while in Europe the availability of different techniques means the use of procedure differs from centre to centre.

Surgical technique

Surgical tracheostomy is usually performed at the bedside in the ICU, even if this is a more difficult setting, e.g. due to lighting, suction, sterility and coagulation not being optimal. Only in selected cases may it be performed in the operating room, especially in patients undergoing surgery of the face/neck region at the same time.

Usually airways are secured by a cuffed endotracheal tube in general anaesthesia, but in case there is a need to keep the patient awake, surgeons can proceed with the tracheostomy following local anaesthesia and mild sedation.

During the procedure the patient's shoulders are elevated and the head extended (unless cervical disease or injury is present), elevating the larynx and exposing the upper part of the trachea. A local vasoconstrictor is administered into the skin and deeper tissues to reduce bleeding. Lower cricoid cartilage border the suprasternal notch and the second and third tracheal rings are identified and marked on the skin. The skin must then be cut with a transverse or vertical incision (1.5–2 cm). Following this the operator proceeds with dissection of the platysma being careful to avoid the thyroid isthmus and vascular structures. Haemostasis is performed with electocautery, which controls bleeding and means that the procedure can be performed in patients with

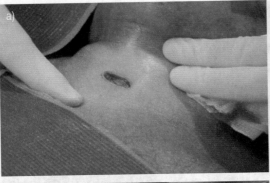
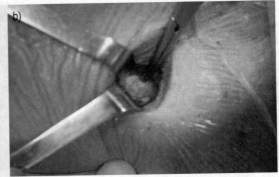
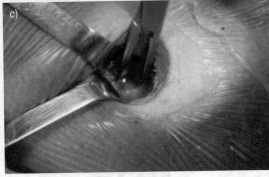

Figure 2. The mini-invasive surgical treatment of tracheal entry. a) It presents an open access without sutures similar to percutaneous dilational tracheostomy techniques. b) The thyroid can be retracted superiorly to reveal the access to the trachea. c) A small incision between the second and third tracheal ring creates a stable tract for tube insertion.

coagulation deficiency. Muscles are retracted laterally to expose the underlying thyroid gland and the trachea.

If the thyroid isthmus is identified in the upper part during blunt dissection, it can be retracted superiorly to gain access to the trachea. If the thyroid isthmus overlies the second and third rings it must be dissected to make the tracheal window available.

The surgical treatment of tracheal entry can be either minimally invasive, in the form of tracheostomy similar to PDT with an open access without sutures (fig. 2), or invasive by making a true stoma by removing the anterior part of the tracheal wall with a ring flap sutured to the skin. The sutures can be used to identify the trachea and reinsert the cannula when displaced.

After performing surgical tracheostomy or PDT, the trachea is not stable for at least 4–5 days so the cannula is at risk of dislocation.

Conclusions

ETI is the most common procedure for airways control in patients requiring mechanical ventilation. Between 6% and 11% of mechanically ventilated patients receive a tracheostomy after a median of 9–12 days; however, there is significant variability around patient selection, technical procedure and timing. The main benefits of tracheostomy are: less need for deeper sedation; shorter weaning time with an increase of ventilator-free days; and shorter ICU and hospital length of stay. Techniques for tracheostomy are constantly evolving and improving.

Various devices have been developed to minimise risks and improve procedure simplicity at the bedside in the ICU; however, the operator's skilled experience and the degree of patient complexity influence the choice of the specific technique performed in each case.

The determining factors in deciding whether to use surgical tracheostomy or PDT in particular pathological conditions include available resources, experienced clinicians and patient factors. Regarding timing, no algorithms are able to predict prolonged mechanical ventilation, except for the severity indexes. The clinician's ability to predict this duration is low, especially in the early stage of disease; therefore, the question of timing could be a question of indication.

Except for patients with severe traumatic brain injury or cervical spine injury who are likely to benefit from earlier tracheostomy, we can reasonably assert that, generally, in critically ill patients 2 weeks are risk free for decision making and selecting the best airway management in patients requiring prolonged mechanical ventilation.

Statement of interest

V.M. Ranieri is a member of the advisory board for Hemodec.

References

1. Ciaglia P, Firsching R, Syniec C. Elective percutaneous dilatational tracheostomy. A new simple bedside procedure; preliminary report. *Chest* 1985; 87: 715–719.
2. Griffiths J, Barber VS, Morgan L, *et al.* Systematic review and meta-analysis of studies of the timing of tracheostomy in adult patients undergoing artificial ventilation. *BMJ* 2005; 330: 1243.
3. Blot F, Similowski T, Trouillet JL, *et al.* Early tracheotomy *versus* prolonged endotracheal intubation in unselected severely ill ICU patients. *Intensive Care Med* 2008; 34: 1779–1787.
4. Plummer AL, Gracey DR. Consensus conference on artificial airways in patients receiving mechanical ventilation. *Chest* 1989; 96: 178–180.
5. MacIntyre NR, Cook DJ, Ely EW Jr, *et al.* Evidence-based guidelines for weaning and discontinuing ventilatory support: a collective task force facilitated by the American College of Chest Physicians, the American Association for Respiratory Care, and the American College of Critical Care Medicine. *Chest* 2001; 120: Suppl. 6, 375S–395S.
6. Szmuk P, Ezri T, Evron S, *et al.* A brief history of tracheostomy and tracheal intubation, from the Bronze Age to the Space Age. *Intensive Care Med* 2008; 34: 222–228.
7. Flaatten H, Gjerde S, Heimdal JH, *et al.* The effect of tracheostomy on outcome in intensive care unit patients. *Acta Anaesthesiol Scand* 2006; 50: 92–98.
8. Kollef MH, Ahrens TS, Shannon W. Clinical predictors and outcomes for patients requiring tracheostomy in the intensive care unit. *Crit Care Med* 1999; 27: 1714–1720.
9. Moller MG, Slaikeu JD, Bonelli P, *et al.* Early tracheostomy *versus* late tracheostomy in the surgical intensive care unit. *Am J Surg* 2005; 189: 293–296.
10. Blot F, Melot C. Indications, timing, and techniques of tracheostomy in 152 French ICUs. *Chest* 2005; 127: 1347–1352.
11. Frutos-Vivar F, Esteban A, Apezteguia C, *et al.* Outcome of mechanically ventilated patients who require a tracheostomy. *Crit Care Med* 2005; 33: 290–298.
12. Heffner JE. The role of tracheotomy in weaning. *Chest* 2001; 120: Suppl. 6, 477S–481S.
13. Freeman BD, Isabella K, Lin N, *et al.* A meta-analysis of prospective trials comparing percutaneous and surgical tracheostomy in critically ill patients. *Chest* 2000; 118: 1412–1418.
14. Griggs WM, Worthley LI, Gilligan JE, *et al.* A simple percutaneous tracheostomy technique. *Surg Gynecol Obstet* 1990; 170: 543–545.
15. Antonelli M, Michetti V, Di Palma A, *et al.* Percutaneous translaryngeal *versus* surgical tracheostomy: a randomized trial with 1-yr double-blind follow-up. *Crit Care Med* 2005; 33: 1015–1020.
16. Delaney A, Bagshaw SM, Nalos M. Percutaneous dilatational tracheostomy *versus* surgical tracheostomy in critically ill patients: a systematic review and meta-analysis. *Crit Care* 2006; 10: R55.
17. Durbin CG Jr. Early complications of tracheostomy. *Respir Care* 2005; 50: 511–515.
18. Byhahn C, Lischke V, Meininger D, *et al.* Peri-operative complications during percutaneous tracheostomy in obese patients. *Anaesthesia* 2005; 60: 12–15.
19. Holdgaard HO, Pedersen J, Jensen RH, *et al.* Percutaneous dilatational tracheostomy *versus* conventional surgical tracheostomy. A clinical randomised study. *Acta Anaesthesiol Scand* 1998; 42: 545–550.
20. Dulguerov P, Gysin C, Perneger TV, *et al.* Percutaneous or surgical tracheostomy: a meta-analysis. *Crit Care Med* 1999; 27: 1617–1625.
21. Sue RD, Susanto I. Long-term complications of artificial airways. *Clin Chest Med* 2003; 24: 457–471.
22. Epstein SK. Late complications of tracheostomy. *Respir Care* 2005; 50: 542–549.
23. Aquino SL, Shepard JA, Ginns LC, *et al.* Acquired tracheomalacia: detection by expiratory CT scan. *J Comput Assist Tomogr* 2001; 25: 394–399.
24. Steele AP, Evans HW, Afaq MA, *et al.* Long-term follow-up of Griggs percutaneous tracheostomy with spiral CT and questionnaire. *Chest* 2000; 117: 1430–1433.
25. Cox CE, Carson SS, Holmes GM, *et al.* Increase in tracheostomy for prolonged mechanical ventilation in North Carolina, 1993–2002. *Crit Care Med* 2004; 32: 2219–2226.

26. Freeman BD, Borecki IB, Coopersmith CM, *et al.* Relationship between tracheostomy timing and duration of mechanical ventilation in critically ill patients. *Crit Care Med* 2005; 33: 2513–2520.

27. Heffner JE, Zamora CA. Clinical predictors of prolonged translaryngeal intubation in patients with the adult respiratory distress syndrome. *Chest* 1990; 97: 447–452.

28. Durbin CG Jr. Indications for and timing of tracheostomy. *Respir Care* 2005; 50: 483–487.

29. Rumbak MJ, Newton M, Truncale T, *et al.* A prospective, randomized, study comparing early percutaneous dilational tracheotomy to prolonged translaryngeal intubation (delayed tracheotomy) in critically ill medical patients. *Crit Care Med* 2004; 32: 1689–1694.

30. Terragni PP, Antonelli M, Fumagalli R, *et al.* Early *vs* late tracheotomy for prevention of pneumonia in mechanically ventilated adult ICU patients: a randomized controlled trial. *JAMA* 2010; 303: 1483–1489.

31. Scales DC, Ferguson ND. Early *vs* late tracheotomy in ICU patients. *JAMA* 2010; 303: 1537–1538.

32. Trouillet JL, Luyt CE, Guiguet M, *et al.* Early percutaneous tracheotomy *versus* prolonged intubation of mechanically ventilated patients after cardiac surgery: a randomized trial. *Ann Intern Med* 2011; 154: 373–383.

33. Holevar M, Dunham JC, Brautigan R, *et al.* Practice management guidelines for timing of tracheostomy: the EAST Practice Management Guidelines Work Group. *J Trauma* 2009; 67: 870–874.

34. Hsieh AH, Bishop MJ, Kubilis PS, *et al.* Pneumonia following closed head injury. *Am Rev Respir Dis* 1992; 146: 290–294.

35. Armstrong PA, McCarthy MC, Peoples JB. Reduced use of resources by early tracheostomy in ventilator-dependent patients with blunt trauma. *Surgery* 1998; 124: 763–766.

36. Koh WY, Lew TW, Chin NM, *et al.* Tracheostomy in a neuro-intensive care setting: indications and timing. *Anaesth Intensive Care* 1997; 25: 365–368.

37. Kluger Y, Paul DB, Lucke J, *et al.* Early tracheostomy in trauma patients. *Eur J Emerg Med* 1996; 3: 95–101.

38. Qureshi AI, Suarez JI, Parekh PD, *et al.* Prediction and timing of tracheostomy in patients with infratentorial lesions requiring mechanical ventilatory support. *Crit Care Med* 2000; 28: 1383–1387.

39. Mascia L, Corno E, Terragni PP, *et al.* Pro/con clinical debate: tracheostomy is ideal for withdrawal of mechanical ventilation in severe neurological impairment. *Crit Care* 2004; 8: 327–330.

40. The Seldinger technique. Reprint from Acta Radiologica 1953. *AJR Am J Roentgenol* 1984; 142: 5–7.

41. Byhahn C, Lischke V, Halbig S, *et al.* Ciaglia Blue Rhino: Ein weiterentwickeltes Verfahren der perkutanen Dilatationstracheotomie. Technik und erste klinische Ergebnisse [Ciaglia blue rhino: a modified technique for percutaneous dilatation tracheostomy. Technique and early clinical results]. *Anaesthesist* 2000; 49: 202–206.

42. Fantoni A, Ripamonti D. A non-derivative, non-surgical tracheostomy: the translaryngeal method. *Intensive Care Med* 1997; 23: 386–392.

43. Westphal K, Maeser D, Scheifler G, *et al.* PercuTwist: a new single-dilator technique for percutaneous tracheostomy. *Anesth Analg* 2003; 96: 229–232.

44. Zgoda MA, Berger R. Balloon-facilitated percutaneous dilational tracheostomy tube placement: preliminary report of a novel technique. *Chest* 2005; 128: 3688–3690.

Chapter 16

Mechanical ventilation with advanced closed-loop systems

F. Lellouche*, A. Bojmehrani* and K. Burns#

Summary

Automated mechanical ventilation using advanced closed loops is anticipated to assume a larger role in supporting critically ill patients in intensive care units (ICU) in the future, for several reasons. They have the potential to improve knowledge transfer by continuously implementing automated protocols while improving patient outcomes. Additionally, closed-loop systems may provide a partial solution to address forecasted clinician shortages by reducing ICU-related costs, time spent on mechanical ventilation, and staff workload. At present, few systems that automate medical reasoning with advanced closed loops are commercially available. Preliminary studies evaluating first generation automated weaning systems and fully automated ventilation are promising. These closed-loop programmes will be refined as the technology improves and clinical experience with these products increases.

Keywords: Automated weaning, closed-loop systems, fully automated mechanical ventilation, healthcare costs, knowledge transfer, mechanical ventilation

*Centre de Recherche de l'Institut Universitaire de Cardiologie et de Pneumologie de Québec, Université Laval, Quebec, QC, and #Critical Care Dept, Saint-Michael's Hospital, Toronto University, Toronto, ON, Canada.

Correspondence: F. Lellouche, Centre de Recherche de l'Institut Universitaire de Cardiologie et de Pneumologie de Québec, 2725, chemin Sainte-Foy, G1V4G5, Québec, QC, Canada. Email francois.lellouche@criucpq. ulaval.ca

Eur Respir Mon 2012; 55: 217–228.
Printed in UK – all rights reserved
Copyright ERS 2012
European Respiratory Monograph
ISSN: 1025-448x
DOI: 10.1183/1025448x.10002911

Automated ventilation systems are likely to be used with increasing frequency in the future. The key reasons to promote the use of automated systems include difficulties in transferring knowledge into clinical practice [1, 2], anticipated discrepancies between demand (the number of patients requiring mechanical ventilation) and supply (the number of skilled clinicians available to manage these complex patients) [3–6] and escalating healthcare costs [7–9]. Intensive care unit (ICU) costs consume up to 20% of healthcare resources [10] and these costs are largely driven by mechanically ventilated patients [8], especially those requiring prolonged mechanical ventilation [9, 11]. Automated ventilation systems provide a partial solution to the aforementioned problems. In this chapter, we discuss currently available systems and ideas for new automated systems.

Automating knowledge transfer

Nearly half of all critically ill patients do not receive the recommended care in the USA [12]. While links between care processes and outcomes are just beginning to be investigated, it is speculated that inconsistencies in healthcare delivery, results in increased morbidity, mortality and costs. This is particularly true in critically ill patients where baseline mortality is high and interventions may have a large impact on mortality. In the USA, it has been estimated that within the ICU setting, failure to use recommended interventions may result in 170,000 preventable deaths [13]. Moreover, despite research studies demonstrating efficacy, investigators have shown that new therapies do not become widely clinically implemented until 20 years later [14]. Knowledge transfer is a key step limiting the uptake of new knowledge into clinical practice [15, 16]. Many barriers exist in implementing newly acquired knowledge into the clinical realm including conservatism, clinician lack of awareness and an inability to overcome inertia of prior practices [1, 15, 17, 18]. In addition, implementation of new recommendations or guidelines for clinical care imposes a significant workload on clinicians who must keep up with current guidelines [18, 19] and this requires dedicated time for continuing medical education [20].

In the field of mechanical ventilation several investigators have asked why ICU physicians are reluctant to clinically apply knowledge coming from research [21–24]. RUBENFELD [25] asked a clear question: why don't we do what we are supposed to do? Compliance with recommended practices including limiting tidal volume (V_T) in managing patients with acute respiratory distress syndrome (ARDS) [18, 26–32] and performance of daily screening to identify weaning candidates [33–35] are suboptimal. In ARDS patients, practice changes were demonstrated in ARDSnet centres [36], while in real life many patients with ARDS are still ventilated without a lung-protective, low V_T strategy [37]. Many of these processes, including weaning, lend themselves to automation [38]. Automated protocols may succeed where protocols implemented by clinicians have failed [29, 39]. One example is SmartCare™ (also known as NeoGanesh or "knowledge-based weaning system"), a first generation advanced closed-loop system for weaning critically ill patients from mechanical ventilation [40, 41]. More recently, a fully automated system of mechanical ventilation (Intellivent™; Hamilton Medical AG, Bonaduz, Switzerland) was released with promising results [42]. In this chapter, we will focus on two commercially available systems. 1) SmartCare™ (Evita Ventilator; Dräger Medical Inc., Lübeck, Germany), a knowledge-based weaning system with embedded artificial intelligence [43, 44]. This system can automatically implement a weaning protocol based on knowledge from the weaning literature. 2) Adaptive Support Ventilation™ (ASV) (Hamilton Medical AG)[45] and its more advanced feature Intellivent™, designed to be a fully automated system for delivering mechanical ventilation that incorporates complex physiological principles [46, 47]. This system automatically implements protective ventilation tailored to the patients' respiratory mechanics and promotes assisted ventilation as soon as patients are able to breathe on their own.

Reducing the gap between supply and demand

The outcome of critically ill patients has been shown to be directly linked to staff workload [48–51]. Although a marked increase in mechanical ventilation utilisation is expected in the coming years [3, 4, 52] the training of skilled clinicians who are able to care for these patients (mainly intensivists, anaesthesiologists, pneumologists and respiratory therapists) has not grown commensurately [3]. NEEDHAM et al. [4] projected that the number of patients requiring mechanical ventilation in Ontario (Canada) will increase by 80% over the next 15 years compared with the year 2000. The projected increase can largely be explained by the demographics of the population in developed countries, the increasing middle sector ("baby boomer") cohort of the population [4] and the increase in mean duration of mechanical ventilation [53]. These projections have been affirmed by a study published in 2008 [52]. This study projects that in 2020 the number of patients receiving prolonged ventilation (>96 hours) will more than double compared with the number in the year 2000. Moreover, the prolonged ventilation subgroup is expected to represent one-third of adults on mechanical ventilation and consume two-thirds of hospital resources. Prolonged mechanical ventilation is a key driver of ICU costs [8, 11], and reducing the duration of mechanical ventilation is an important goal of critical care medicine [7, 8].

ANGUS et al. [3] forecasted that the shortage of clinicians taking care of patients requiring mechanical ventilation would begin in approximately 2008, with a progressive worsening of the situation thereafter. The personnel shortage will occur amidst heightened awareness of medical errors [54–57] and of the severe "burnout syndrome" among critical care physicians [58, 59] and nurses [60, 61]. DONCHIN et al. [62] noted that the average number of activities performed by critical care clinicians per patient per day was 178 with a mean of 1.7 errors per patient per day. Among these activities, those related to respiration were the most frequent (26% of all activities), with errors related to data entry being the most common and errors related to respiratory system being the next most frequent (23% of all errors).

Automated systems may aid in reducing the gap between physician availability and need by aiding in the management of simple and repetitive ventilator tasks. Preliminary evaluations detailed below demonstrate that several automated systems have the potential to be at least as efficient as clinicians with fewer ventilator settings required by clinicians [42, 63–66].

Automated systems have the potential to reduce costs associated with mechanical ventilation. Investigators have demonstrated a reduced duration of mechanical ventilation and ICU length of stay with SmartCare^{TM} [64] and a reduced requirement for interventions made by clinicians with ASV [42, 67, 68]. Although no study examined the impact of automation on costs, it is expected that reduced ICU length of stay and workload will be associated with substantial cost savings.

Automated ventilation: where are we now?

The idea of automation during mechanical ventilation is not new [69] but recent technological improvements enable its clinical application with current commercially available ventilators. Automation of different aspects of mechanical ventilation is of growing interest among research groups and ventilator manufacturers [70]. Many computerised decision support systems have been developed for the management of mechanical ventilation [71–74]. However, these systems require clinician validation and function as open loops. Meanwhile, several automated mechanical ventilation systems have been developed using advanced closed-loop technology [75–85] but only a few are commercially available. Both SmartCare^{TM} and ASV/Intellivent^{TM} integrate knowledge from physiological studies and randomised trials into closed-loop systems.

SmartCare^{TM} continuously applies a weaning protocol in pressure support (PS) mode. The system aims to maintain the patients in a "comfort zone" of respiration by adapting the level of PS provided to spontaneously breathing patients and automatically initiates spontaneous breathing trials (SBT) in patients meeting predefined criteria. The system averages three respiratory parameters (respiratory rate, V_T and end-tidal CO_2 ($ETCO_2$)) every 2–5 minutes to arrive at a respiratory diagnosis which determines the next course of action (e.g. reduce/increase the PS or perform a SBT etc.) (fig. 1). The objective of the system is to let the patient breathe freely with a respiratory rate that can range from 15 to 30 breaths·min^{-1} (alternatively, 34 breaths·min^{-1} with neurologic disease), a V_T above a minimum threshold (minimum V_T=250 mL if the weight of the patient is <55 kg or minimum V_T=300 mL in other cases) and an $ETCO_2$ below a maximum threshold (max $ETCO_2$=55 mmHg or max $ETCO_2$=65 mmHg for patients with chronic obstructive pulmonary disease). When a patient's ventilatory parameters fall within these constraints, the SmartCare^{TM} diagnoses a normal ventilatory state. However, if the patient's ventilatory parameters fall outside of these constraints, the system adjusts the level of pressure support ventilation (PSV) provided to attain these targets (fig. 2). Specifically, the SmartCare^{TM} system will increase the PS delivered in response to tachypnoea and lower the PS delivered in response to bradypnoea with low $ETCO_2$.

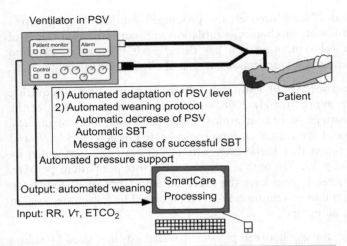

Figure 1. NeoGanseh/SmartCare™ working principles. Average values of three ventilatory parameters are used by the system to adapt the level of pressure support (PS) delivered during ventilation in pressure support ventilation (PSV) mode: respiratory rate (RR), tidal volume (V_T) and end-tidal CO_2 (ETCO$_2$). The two main functions of the system are to: 1) automatically adjust the level of assistance provided in PS mode to maintain the patient in a "comfort zone" (automatic PS); and 2) automatic implementation of a weaning protocol, progressive reduction of the level of assistance and assessment of the readiness to be separated from the ventilator with automated spontaneous breathing trials (SBTs). Finally, when the patient successfully passes an automated SBT, a message is displayed by the ventilator to inform the clinician that the patient can be extubated if other usual extubation criteria are present (secretions, neurological status, cough, haemodynamic stability). The computer represented here is now embedded in the ventilator.

SmartCare™ attempts to reproduce medical reasoning used by clinicians during weaning [40, 44] and adapts the ventilator support more frequently than can be achieved by clinicians [86]. Recent investigations have demonstrated that SmartCare™ can reduce weaning time, the total duration of mechanical ventilation and ICU length of stay [63, 64, 87]. We conducted the first randomised controlled multicentre study comparing automated weaning to usual care [64]. 144 adult patients were included and we showed that automated weaning reduced the duration of weaning (5 *versus* 3 days, p=0.01) and the duration of mechanical ventilation (12 *versus* 7.5 days) without an increased rate of re-intubation (23% in the control group *versus* 16% in the automated weaning group, p=0.4). Furthermore, the ICU length of stay was reduced from 15.5 to 12 days in the automated group (p=0.02) and there was a trend towards less patients with prolonged mechanical ventilation. ROSE *et al.* [65] in a single centre randomised trial compared the weaning conducted with SmartCare™ to usual management conducted by trained nurses in a highly staffed ICU with a 1:1 nurse to patient ratio. This study included 102 patients and failed to demonstrate any difference between the automated weaning system and the weaning conducted by the nurses. The time to successful extubation was similar (43 *versus* 40 hours, p=0.6), but there was a trend towards delayed "time to separation" (*i.e.* equivalent to a positive weaning trial) favouring the usual care group (20 *versus* 8 hours, p=0.3). This was probably due to high levels of positive end-expiratory pressure (PEEP) used during the weaning process (~10 cmH$_2$O), which impeded the automated system to conduct automated weaning trials. With the version of SmartCare™ used in this study, an SBT evaluation could only be made if the level of PEEP was ≤5 cmH$_2$O. SCHÄDLER *et al.* [66] conducted an evaluation comparing SmartCare™ to protocolised weaning in post-surgical patients requiring more than 9 hours of mechanical ventilation. They included 300 patients in the study and found no significant difference between the weaning strategies. The total duration of mechanical ventilation was mean ± SD 94 ± 144 hours with SmartCare™ and 118 ± 165 hours in the control group (p=0.12). In the subgroup of patients who underwent cardiac surgery, the weaning time was reduced with SmartCare™. More recently, we conducted a multicentre randomised pilot study in Canada (the WEAN study) comparing SmartCare™ to a paper-based weaning protocol in nine adult ICUs [88]. The protocol used in the control group was the same in all centres and was based on current weaning recommendations and current practice patterns in Canada [89]. We demonstrated good compliance for the weaning and sedation protocols in both groups (primary end-point of the study) and a reduction in the duration of weaning and ICU length of stay following randomisation favouring the automated weaning [63]. Interestingly, fewer patients required tracheotomy and fewer patients had prolonged mechanical ventilation with SmartCare™. Although the study was not designed nor powered to evaluate clinical end-points, the differences favouring automated systems are encouraging. Most of the studies with the closed-loop system have, to date, shown either a reduced weaning time, mechanical ventilation duration and ICU length of stay [63, 64] or equivalent results when compared with protocolised human-driven protocols in highly staffed ICUs [65, 66]. Consequently, this system has the potential to reduce patient morbidity, clinical workload and ICU costs [8]. The SmartCare™ system has one of the highest levels of closed-loop refinement and complexity in mechanical ventilation at the present time [90, 91].

Similarly, ASV™ [45] uses advanced closed-loop technology to deliver controlled and assisted ventilation in pressure preset modes (pressure assist control and PSV) and automates the transition from assisted to controlled ventilation. ASV™ takes into account the patient's respiratory mechanics (resistance and compliance of the respiratory system), using previously described equations [46, 47], in automating the optimal combination of respiratory rate, inspiratory time and inspiratory pressure delivered to obtain a target minute ventilation ($V'E$) to reduce the work of breathing and to minimise the intrinsic PEEP (figs 3 and 4) [93]. This mode was evaluated in patients with ARDS and in the laboratory with simulated ARDS and was considered safe [93, 94]. However, with this mode the target

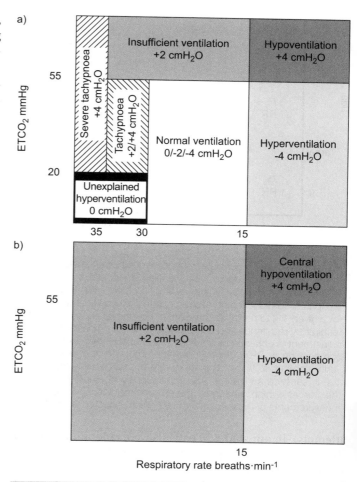

Figure 2. NeoGanseh/SmartCare™ thresholds for the respiratory diagnoses. The respiratory diagnoses are displayed for tidal volumes (VT) a) above minimum VT or b) below VT. For each respiratory diagnosis, the modification of the level of pressure support is indicated. For several respiratory diagnoses, a specific alarm is associated. The minimum VT is 300 mL if the patient's weight is >55 kg and 250 mL if weight is <55 kg. ETCO$_2$: end-tidal CO$_2$.

is the $V'E$ and not VT and, therefore, in some situations VT can increase to 9 mL·kg^{-1} of predicted body weight [94, 95]. ASV™ may be considered a dual mode as it adjusts the pressure level to target a given VT, however, it does not share other known dual mode problems that can be encountered with an increase in ventilator demand [96, 97]. With ASV, $V'E$, PEEP and inspiratory oxygen fraction (F_I,O_2) are manually set by clinicians. Recently, Hamilton Medical AG developed an advanced feature of ASV™, called Intellivent™ that integrates 1) a ventilation controller with the capability of automatically increasing or decreasing the $V'E$ to maintain a stable ETCO$_2$ within a predefined and adjustable range; and 2) an oxygenation controller that automatically adjusts PEEP and F_I,O_2 levels based on the ARDS network tables to maintain an arterial oxygen saturation measured by pulse oximetry (S_p,O_2) within a predefined range. Thus, with Intellivent™ ETCO$_2$ and S_p,O_2 sensors are mandatory. A "heart lung index" based on mechanical ventilation induced plethysmographic variations, reflecting heart lung interactions as previously described [98–100], is used to limit PEEP with unstable haemodynamics. It is also possible for clinicians to manually set the maximal level of PEEP. The only mandatory variables to enter before the start of mechanical ventilation are the patient's sex and height. Initial $V'E$ is calculated from the predicted body weight (obtained from the sex and

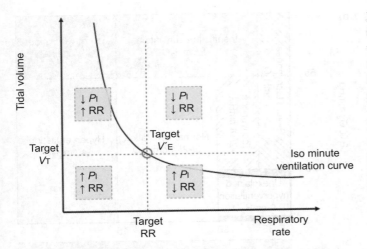

Figure 3. Working principles of adaptive support ventilation (ASV) to maintain the set target minute ventilation (V'_E). The principles of ASV stem from work by OTIS *et al.* [46] and MEAD [47]. They defined an optimal combination of respiratory rate (RR) and tidal volume (V_T) for a given V'_E to minimise the work of breathing, depending on the respiratory resistance and compliance. As it is a pressure mode, V_T adjustment is obtained by varying the inspiratory pressure (P_I). This combination of RR and V_T/P_I defines target V'_E on the iso minute ventilation curve, target respiratory rate and target V_T. After target V'_E is set by the clinician, ASV continuously attempts to maintain the target which changes based on regular and automatic measurements of the respiratory mechanics. Adapted from [38, 92].

height of the patient) and subsequently adjusted to maintain $ETCO_2$ within the selected range. We recently evaluated this new mode in a preliminary safety study in 60 stable patients after cardiac surgery [42]. A fully automated ventilator faces a very dynamic and challenging clinical situation after cardiac surgery. Patients are often hypothermic at ICU arrival and the increased CO_2 production that occurs during rewarming requires ventilator adjustment. Moreover, patients are initially deeply sedated and under the effects of neuromuscular blocking agents and require a controlled mode of ventilation. However, as they progressively awaken, they begin to breathe spontaneously requiring further mechanical ventilation adjustments. Clinicians are usually required (using non-automated ventilators) to continually adjust the respiratory rate or V_T, wean the F_I,O_2 and switch patients from controlled to assisted modes (which often requires several attempts). In our study, 30 patients were randomised to the protocolised ventilation group and 30 to the Intellivent™ group. With Intellivent™, the patients were less frequently in a predefined "non acceptable" zone of ventilation and were in the predefined "optimal" zone of ventilation most of the time. In addition, they all experienced an automatic decrease in V_T, targeted to deliver less than 10 mL·kg^{-1} of predicted body weight [42]. In cardiac surgical patients high V_Ts increase systemic inflammation, promote organ dysfunction and prolong the duration of mechanical ventilation and ICU stay [101–103]. Importantly, the total number of manual interventions was much lower with Intellivent™ compared with the protocolised group (five *versus* 148, p<0.0001). Other preliminary evaluations of this system have been recently conducted by ARNAL *et al.* [104] in medical patients, including some with ARDS, and have shown short-term safety and feasibility with the use of the Intellivent™ software.

In a recent classification of closed-loop ventilation by CHATBURN and MIRELES-CABODEVILA [91], these modes were considered among the most advanced available today. Clinical use of these advanced closed-loop systems will probably become more widely used [70] but rigorous evaluations are still required. Other automated systems have been developed [85, 105], such as mandatory minute ventilation (MMV) [106] or Automode [107]. However, MMV has not been studied adequately in neonates or adults and is infrequently used [105] and Automode like other dual modes has several well-described limitations [96].

Automated ventilation: where do we go from here?

Both systems, SmartCare™ and Intellivent™, have integrated knowledge from physiological studies and from randomised trials. With SmartCare™, it was shown that automated implementation of a weaning protocol was feasible, and at least as efficient as highly staffed centres [63–66]. With Intellivent™, preliminary data showed that fully automated mechanical ventilation can be implemented in stable patients after cardiac surgery including the automated implementation of protective ventilation and automated weaning [42]. Preliminary studies also demonstrated short-term safety in medical patients including those with acute lung injury (ALI)/ARDS [104]. While these studies are encouraging, further evaluation is required to better define both the indications and populations most likely to benefit from the use of these systems. Both systems are modifiable and new rules for ventilator management will need to be incorporated into their software to fit with evolving scientific literature. Therefore it is important that the manufacturers update their software both rapidly and frequently to avoid undue delays in implementing new knowledge into clinical practice.

The systems described here rely on advanced technology, artificial intelligence and controllers. On the contrary, some aspects of automation are much simpler and would only require a spoonful of technology to be implemented. For example, the $Sp,O_2/FI,O_2$ index

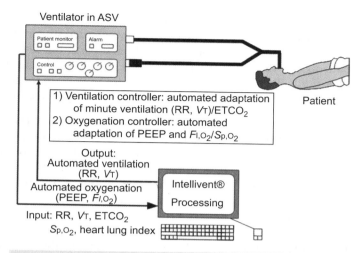

Figure 4. Intellivent™ working principles. This mode is an advanced feature of the adaptive support ventilation (ASV) mode with two additional controllers (closed loops). 1) A ventilator controller adjusts the minute ventilation ($V'E$) to maintain end-tidal CO_2 (ETCO$_2$) within predefined values. Respiratory rate (RR) and tidal volume (VT) are determined by ASV principles. 2) An oxygenation controller adjusts the positive end-expiratory pressure (PEEP) and inspiratory oxygen fraction (FI,O_2) levels to maintain a stable arterial oxygen saturation measured by pulse oximetry (Sp,O_2) within predefined values. PEEP increases can be limited by the user (set the maximum PEEP) or self-limited by the system if pulse oximeter plethysmographic variations induced by the mechanical ventilation suggest hypovolaemia or volume dependence of the cardiac output. At initiation, the height and sex of the patient must be entered to determine the initial $V'E$, which is subsequently adjusted by the ventilation controller.

(which correlates well with arterial oxygen tension (Pa,O_2)/FI,O_2 ratio for Sp,O_2 below 97% [108]), automated plateau pressure (Pplat) or intrinsic PEEP measurement, $VT\cdot kg^{-1}$ of predicted body weight (as opposed to absolute VT) and automated interpretation of ventilator tracings to detect patient ventilator asynchronies or intrinsic PEEP, represent potential targets for monitoring during mechanical ventilation. Monitoring of the $Sp,O_2/FI,O_2$ index could allow for early recognition of patients with potential ARDS. Similarly, $VT\cdot kg^{-1}$ and Pplat monitoring could help reduce the risk of injurious patterns of ventilation in ARDS patients [109] and may reduce the risk of "ICU-acquired ARDS" [110]. Automation of PEEP and FI,O_2 could be easily implemented in ventilators [83] as could automated mechanisms to assess a patients' predicted body weight and appropriate VT [111].

We anticipate that there will be barriers to adopting closed-loop systems into clinical practice. Enhanced acceptance of automated systems may be achieved by organising new consensus conferences or expert meetings to define where, when, how and in whom these new technologies should be used. Updates to these systems will require ongoing collaboration between clinician scientists and industry. Importantly, to improve acceptance of these new systems, adequate clinical evaluation will be required. Currently, among the impressive list of new modes of ventilation, few have been shown to be useful and with clear clinical advantages [112]. Finally, it must be anticipated that novel technology, even closed-loop technology, will require knowledge translation prior to being adopted into clinical practice.

Conclusions

Automation provides one solution to current and forecasted challenges in managing critically ill patients. Automation is a technology that holds promise as a means of facilitating knowledge transfer, reducing healthcare costs and minimising the duration of ventilation. Among the new software developed by manufacturers, several interesting modes of ventilation have emerged in the last decade [38] with a sound physiological basis, but few have been shown to confer benefit to patients and the healthcare system [113, 114]. Considering the forecasted increase in the number of critically ill patients who will be cared for in ICUs in the future and the expanding literature, we expect that automated systems may assume a larger role in the ICU in the future.

Data concerning anticipated ICU demand and difficulties in implementing knowledge transfer should compel us to think about other ways to manage our healthcare system. Anticipated ICU physician shortages in the future and recognising the clinician's desire and obligation to deliver up-to-date care, we will be obliged to rethink the organisation of our ICUs. Automation of several tasks will probably be a cornerstone of this new organisation. Automation of mechanical ventilation is in its infancy and there is a large discrepancy between what can be done and what is currently developed in this field. Currently available systems will probably be refined in the coming years as technology improves and as our understanding of mechanical ventilation and its impact on important patient outcomes evolves. In the meantime, we should continue to develop promising technologies that can deliver safe and effective ventilatory support and formally evaluate their impact on clinically important outcomes and our healthcare system.

Statement of interest

The research laboratory of F. Lellouche received 60,000 Canadian dollars from Hamilton Medical AG (Switzerland) to conduct a clinical evaluation of Intellivent™. F. Lellouche received fees of 1,000 Canadian dollars for speaking at a symposium organised by Hamilton Medical AG. F. Lellouche and K. Burns received a sum of 5,000 Canadian dollars from Dräger Medical (Canada) to cover travel expenses for the WEAN study evaluating the SmartCare™ system in nine Canadian centres.

References
1. Lenfant C. Shattuck lecture – clinical research to clinical practice – lost in translation? N Engl J Med 2003; 349: 868–874.
2. Westfall JM, Mold J, Fagnan L. Practice-based research–"Blue Highways" on the NIH roadmap. JAMA 2007; 297: 403–406.
3. Angus DC, Kelley MA, Schmitz RJ, et al. Caring for the critically ill patient. Current and projected workforce requirements for care of the critically ill and patients with pulmonary disease: can we meet the requirements of an aging population? JAMA 2000; 284: 2762–2770.
4. Needham DM, Bronskill SE, Calinawan JR, et al. Projected incidence of mechanical ventilation in Ontario to 2026: preparing for the aging baby boomers. Crit Care Med 2005; 33: 574–579.
5. Zilberberg MD, de Wit M, Pirone JR, et al. Growth in adult prolonged acute mechanical ventilation: implications for healthcare delivery. Crit Care Med 2008; 36: 1451–1455.
6. Zilberberg MD, Luippold RS, Sulsky S, et al. Prolonged acute mechanical ventilation, hospital resource utilization, and mortality in the United States. Crit Care Med 2008; 36: 724–730.
7. Boles J-M, Bion J, Connors A, et al. Weaning from mechanical ventilation. Eur Respir J. 2007; 29: 1033–1056.
8. Dasta JF, McLaughlin TP, Mody SH, et al. Daily cost of an intensive care unit day: the contribution of mechanical ventilation. Crit Care Med 2005; 33: 1266–1271.
9. Zilberberg MD, Shorr AF. Prolonged acute mechanical ventilation and hospital bed utilization in 2020 in the United States: implications for budgets, plant and personnel planning. BMC Health Serv Res 2008; 8: 242.
10. Moerer O, Plock E, Mgbor U, et al. A German national prevalence study on the cost of intensive care: an evaluation from 51 intensive care units. Crit Care 2007; 11: R69.
11. Cox CE, Carson SS, Govert JA, et al. An economic evaluation of prolonged mechanical ventilation. Crit Care Med 2007; 35: 1918–1927.
12. McGlynn EA, Asch SM, Adams J, et al. The quality of health care delivered to adults in the United States. N Engl J Med 2003; 348: 2635–2645.
13. Pronovost PJ, Rinke ML, Emery K, et al. Interventions to reduce mortality among patients treated in intensive care units. J Crit Care 2004; 19: 158–164.
14. Committee on Quality of Health Care in America, Institute of Medicine. Crossing the quality chasm: a new health system for the 21st century. Washington, National Academy Press, 2001.

15. Cabana MD, Rand CS, Powe NR, *et al*. Why don't physicians follow clinical practice guidelines? A framework for improvement. *JAMA* 1999; 282: 1458–1465.
16. Gravel K, Legare F, Graham ID. Barriers and facilitators to implementing shared decision-making in clinical practice: a systematic review of health professionals' perceptions. *Implement Sci* 2006; 1: 16.
17. Dent EB, Galloway Goldberg S. Challenging resistance to change. *J Appl Behav Sci* 1999; 35: 25–41.
18. Rubenfeld GD, Cooper C, Carter G, *et al*. Barriers to providing lung-protective ventilation to patients with acute lung injury. *Crit Care Med* 2004; 32: 1289–1293.
19. Rubenfeld GD. Implementing effective ventilator practice at the bedside. *Current Opin Crit Care* 2004; 10: 33–39.
20. Sinuff T, Cook D, Giacomini M, *et al*. Facilitating clinician adherence to guidelines in the intensive care unit: a multicenter, qualitative study. *Crit Care Med* 2007; 35: 2083–2089.
21. Scales DC, Adhikari NK. Lost in (knowledge) translation: "All breakthrough, no follow through"? *Crit Care Med* 2008; 36: 1654–165.
22. Villar J, Kacmarek RM, Hedenstierna G. From ventilator-induced lung injury to physician-induced lung injury: why the reluctance to use small tidal volumes? *Acta Anaesthesiol Scand* 2004; 48: 267–271.
23. Ricard JD. Are we really reducing tidal volume – and should we? *Am J Respir Crit Care Med* 2003; 167: 1297–1298.
24. Jones AT. Lost in translation? The pursuit of lung-protective ventilation. *Crit Care* 2008; 12: 122.
25. Rubenfeld GD. Translating clinical research into clinical practice in the intensive care unit: the central role of respiratory care. *Respir Care* 2004; 49: 837–843.
26. Young MP, Manning HL, Wilson DL, *et al*. Ventilation of patients with acute lung injury and acute respiratory distress syndrome: has new evidence changed clinical practice? *Crit Care Med* 2004; 32: 1260–1265.
27. Weinert CR, Gross CR, Marinelli WA. Impact of randomized trial results on acute lung injury ventilator therapy in teaching hospitals. *Am J Respir Crit Care Med* 2003; 167: 1304–1309.
28. Kalhan R, Mikkelsen M, Dedhiya P, *et al*. Underuse of lung protective ventilation: analysis of potential factors to explain physician behavior. *Crit Care Med* 2006; 34: 300–306.
29. Ferguson ND, Frutos-Vivar F, Esteban A, *et al*. Airway pressures, tidal volumes, and mortality in patients with acute respiratory distress syndrome. *Crit Care Med* 2005; 33: 21–30.
30. Wolthuis EK, Korevaar JC, Spronk P, *et al*. Feedback and education improve physician compliance in use of lung-protective mechanical ventilation. *Intensive Care Med* 2005; 31: 540–546.
31. Brun-Buisson C, Minelli C, Bertolini G, *et al*. Epidemiology and outcome of acute lung injury in European intensive care units. Results from the ALIVE study. *Intensive Care Med* 2004; 30: 51–61.
32. Irish Critical Care Trials Group. Acute lung injury and the acute respiratory distress syndrome in Ireland: a prospective audit of epidemiology and management. *Crit Care* 2008; 12: R30.
33. Ely EW. Challenges encountered in changing physicians' practice styles: the ventilator weaning experience. *Intensive Care Med* 1998; 24: 539–541.
34. Ely EW, Bennett PA, Bowton DL, *et al*. Large scale implementation of a respiratory therapist-driven protocol for ventilator weaning. *Am J Respir Crit Care Med* 1999; 159: 439–446.
35. Vitacca M, Clini E, Porta R, *et al*. Preliminary results on nursing workload in a dedicated weaning center. *Intensive Care Med* 2000; 26: 796–799.
36. Checkley W, Brower R, Korpak A, *et al*. Effects of a clinical trial on mechanical ventilation practices in patients with acute lung injury. *Am J Respir Crit Care Med* 2008; 177: 1215–1222.
37. Esteban A, Ferguson ND, Meade MO, *et al*. Evolution of mechanical ventilation in response to clinical research. *Am J Respir Crit Care Med* 2008; 177: 170–177.
38. Lellouche F, Brochard L. Advanced closed loops during mechanical ventilation (PAV, NAVA, ASV, SmartCare). *Best Pract Res Clin Anaesthesiol* 2009; 23: 81–93.
39. Umoh NJ, Fan E, Mendez-Tellez PA, *et al*. Patient and intensive care unit organizational factors associated with low tidal volume ventilation in acute lung injury. *Crit Care Med* 2008; 36: 1463–1468.
40. Dojat M, Brochard L, Lemaire F, *et al*. A knowledge-based system for assisted ventilation of patients in intensive care units. *Int J Clin Monit Comput* 1992; 9: 239–250.
41. Dojat M, Harf A, Touchard D, *et al*. Evaluation of a knowledge-based system providing ventilatory management and decision for extubation. *Am J Respir Crit Care Med* 1996; 153: 997–1004.
42. Lellouche F, Bouchard PA, Wysocki M, *et al*. Prospective randomized controlled study comparing conventional ventilation *versus* a fully closed-loop ventilation (Intellivent) in post cardiac surgery ICU patients. *Am J Respir Crit Care Med* 2010; 181: A6035.
43. Dojat M, Pachet F, Guessoum Z, *et al*. NeoGanesh: a working system for the automated control of assisted ventilation in ICUs. *Artif Intell Med* 1997; 11: 97–117.
44. Dojat M, Sayettat C. A realistic model for temporal reasoning in real-time patient monitoring. *Appl Artif Intell* 1996; 10: 121–143.
45. Laubscher TP, Heinrichs W, Weiler N, *et al*. An adaptive lung ventilation controller. *IEEE Trans Biomed Eng* 1994; 41: 51–59.
46. Otis AB, Fenn WO, Rahn H. Mechanics of breathing in man. *J Appl Physiol* 1950; 2: 592–607.
47. Mead J. Control of respiratory frequency. *J Appl Physiol* 1960; 15: 325–336.
48. Pronovost PJ, Angus DC, Dorman T, *et al*. Physician staffing patterns and clinical outcomes in critically ill patients: a systematic review. *JAMA* 2002; 288: 2151–2162.

49. Tarnow-Mordi WO, Hau C, Warden A, *et al.* Hospital mortality in relation to staff workload: a 4-year study in an adult intensive-care unit. *Lancet* 2000; 356: 185–189.

50. Thorens JB, Kaelin RM, Jolliet P, *et al.* Influence of the quality of nursing on the duration of weaning from mechanical ventilation in patients with chronic obstructive pulmonary disease. *Crit Care Med* 1995; 23: 1807–1815.

51. Amaravadi RK, Dimick JB, Pronovost PJ, *et al.* ICU nurse-to-patient ratio is associated with complications and resource use after esophagectomy. *Intensive Care Med* 2000; 26: 1857–1862.

52. Zilberberg MD, Shorr AF. Projections of growth in adult prolonged acute mechanical ventilation: implications for ICU and hospital bed utilization. *Am J Resp Crit Care Med* 2008; 177: A126.

53. Needham DM, Bronskill SE, Sibbald WJ, *et al.* Mechanical ventilation in Ontario, 1992–2000: incidence, survival, and hospital bed utilization of noncardiac surgery adult patients. *Crit Care Med* 2004; 32: 1504–1509.

54. Boyle D, O'Connell D, Platt FW, *et al.* Disclosing errors and adverse events in the intensive care unit. *Crit Care Med* 2006; 34: 1532–1537.

55. Giraud T, Dhainaut JF, Vaxelaire JF, *et al.* Iatrogenic complications in adult intensive care units: a prospective two-center study. *Crit Care Med* 1993; 21: 40–51.

56. Landrigan CP, Rothschild JM, Cronin JW, *et al.* Effect of reducing interns' work hours on serious medical errors in intensive care units. *N Engl J Med* 2004; 351: 1838–1848.

57. Moyen E, Camire E, Stelfox HT. Clinical review: medication errors in critical care. *Crit Care* 2008; 12: 208.

58. Donchin Y, Seagull FJ. The hostile environment of the intensive care unit. *Current Opin Crit Care* 2002; 8: 316–320.

59. Embriaco N, Papazian L, Kentish-Barnes N, *et al.* Burnout syndrome among critical care healthcare workers. *Current Opin Crit Care* 2007; 13: 482–488.

60. Poncet MC, Toullic P, Papazian L, *et al.* Burnout syndrome in critical care nursing staff. *Am J Respir Crit Care Med* 2007; 175: 698–704.

61. Verdon M, Merlani P, Perneger T, *et al.* Burnout in a surgical ICU team. *Intensive Care Med* 2008; 34: 152–156.

62. Donchin Y, Gopher D, Olin M, *et al.* A look into the nature and causes of human errors in the intensive care unit. *Crit Care Med* 1995; 23: 294–300.

63. Burns KE, Lellouche F, Lessard M, *et al.* Wean earlier and automatically with new technology: preliminary results of the Wean study. *Am J Respir Crit Care Med* 2011; 183: A6248.

64. Lellouche F, Mancebo J, Jolliet P, *et al.* A multicenter randomized trial of computer-driven protocolized weaning from mechanical ventilation. *Am J Respir Crit Care Med* 2006; 174: 894–900.

65. Rose L, Presneill JJ, Johnston L, *et al.* A randomised, controlled trial of conventional *versus* automated weaning from mechanical ventilation using SmartCare/PS. *Intensive Care Med* 2008; 34: 1788–1795.

66. Schädler D, Elke G, Pulletz S, *et al.* The effect of automatic weaning with smartcare/ps on ventilation time in postsurgical patients – a randomized controlled trial. *Am J Respir Crit Care Med* 2009; 179: A3646.

67. Sulzer CF, Chiolero R, Chassot PG, *et al.* Adaptive support ventilation for fast tracheal extubation after cardiac surgery: a randomized controlled study. *Anesthesiology* 2001; 95: 1339–1345.

68. Petter AH, Chiolero RL, Cassina T, *et al.* Automatic "respirator/weaning" with adaptive support ventilation: the effect on duration of endotracheal intubation and patient management. *Anesth Analg* 2003; 97: 1743–1750.

69. Saxton GA Jr, Myers G. A servomechanism for automatic regulation of pulmonary ventilation. *J Appl Physiol* 1957; 11: 326–328.

70. Wysocki M, Brunner JX. Closed-loop ventilation: an emerging standard of care? *Crit Care Clin* 2007; 23: 223–240.

71. East TD, Bohm SH, Wallace CJ, *et al.* A successful computerized protocol for clinical management of pressure control inverse ratio ventilation in ARDS patients. *Chest* 1992; 101: 697–710.

72. East TD, Heermann LK, Bradshaw RL, *et al.* Efficacy of computerized decision support for mechanical ventilation: results of a prospective multi-center randomized trial. *Proc AMIA Symp* 1999; 251–255.

73. Morris AH. Developing and implementing computerized protocols for standardization of clinical decisions. *Ann Intern Med* 2000; 132: 373–383.

74. Tehrani FT. A new decision support system for mechanical ventilation. *Conf Proc IEEE Eng Med Biol Soc* 2007; 2007: 3569–3572.

75. Chopin C, Chambrin MC, Mangalaboyi J, *et al.* Un systeme informaitse de surveillance de la ventilation assistee. Description des premiers resultats [Computerized monitoring system for mechanical ventilation. Description and initial results]. *Agressologie* 1980; 21: 93–100.

76. Samodelov LF, Falke KJ. Total inspiratory work with modern demand valve devices compared to continuous flow CPAP. *Intensive Care Med* 1988; 14: 632–639.

77. Strickland JH, Hasson JH. A computer-controlled ventilator weaning system. *Chest* 1991; 100: 1096–1099.

78. Strickland JH, Hasson JH. A computer-controlled ventilator weaning system. *Chest* 1993; 103: 1220–1226.

79. Nakagawa NK, Macchione M, Petrolino HM, *et al.* Effects of a heat and moisture exchanger and a heated humidifier on respiratory mucus in patients undergoing mechanical ventilation. *Crit Care Med* 2000; 28: 312–317.

80. Nemoto T, Hatzakis GE, Thorpe CW, *et al.* Automatic control of pressure support mechanical ventilation using fuzzy logic. *Am J Respir Crit Care Med* 1999; 160: 550–556.

81. Tehrani F, Rogers M, Lo T, *et al.* A dual closed-loop control system for mechanical ventilation. *J Clin Monit Comput* 2004; 18: 111–129.

82. Tehrani FT, Roum JH. Flex: a new computerized system for mechanical ventilation. *J Clin Monit Comput* 2008; 22: 121–130.

83. Lellouche F, Hernert P, Jouvet P, *et al.* Automatic weaning of PEEP and FiO2 after cardiac surgery. *Intensive Care Med* 2009; 35: S237.

84. Johannigman JA, Muskat P, Barnes S, *et al.* Autonomous control of oxygenation. *Journal Trauma* 2008; 64: S295–S301.

85. Johannigman JA, Muskat P, Barnes S, *et al.* Autonomous control of ventilation. *Journal Trauma* 2008; 64: S302–S320.

86. Dojat M, Harf A, Touchard D, *et al.* Clinical evaluation of a computer-controlled pressure support mode. *Am J Respir Crit Care Med* 2000; 161: 1161–1166.

87. Bouadma L, Lellouche F, Cabello B, *et al.* Computer-driven management of prolonged mechanical ventilation and weaning: a pilot study. *Intensive Care Med* 2005; 31: 1446–1450.

88. Burns KE, Meade MO, Lessard MR, *et al.* Wean earlier and automatically with new technology (the WEAN study): a protocol of a multicentre, pilot randomized controlled trial. *Trials* 2009; 10: 81.

89. Burns KE, Lellouche F, Loisel F, *et al.* Weaning critically ill adults from invasive mechanical ventilation: a national survey. *Can J Anaesth* 2009; 5: 567–576.

90. Chatburn RL. Computer control of mechanical ventilation. *Respir Care* 2004; 49: 507–517.

91. Chatburn RL, Mireles-Cabodevila E. Closed-loop control of mechanical ventilation: description and classification of targeting schemes. *Respir Care* 2011; 56: 85–102.

92. Tassaux D, Dalmas E, Gratadour P, *et al.* Patient-ventilator interactions during partial ventilatory support: a preliminary study comparing the effects of adaptive support ventilation with synchronized intermittent mandatory ventilation plus inspiratory pressure support. *Crit Care Med* 2002; 30: 801–807.

93. Arnal JM, Wysocki M, Nafati C, *et al.* Automatic selection of breathing pattern using adaptive support ventilation. *Intensive Care Med* 2008; 34: 75–81.

94. Sulemanji D, Marchese A, Garbarini P, *et al.* Adaptive support ventilation: an appropriate mechanical ventilation strategy for acute respiratory distress syndrome? *Anesthesiology* 2009; 111: 863–870.

95. Dongelmans DA, Schultz MJ. Adaptive support ventilation: an inappropriate mechanical ventilation strategy for acute respiratory distress syndrome? *Anesthesiology.* 2010; 112: 1295.

96. Jaber S, Delay JM, Matecki S, *et al.* Volume-guaranteed pressure-support ventilation facing acute changes in ventilatory demand. *Intensive Care Med* 2005; 31: 1181–1188.

97. Jaber S, Sebbane M, Verzilli D, *et al.* Adaptive support and pressure support ventilation behavior in response to increased ventilatory demand. *Anesthesiology* 2009; 110: 620–627.

98. Cannesson M, Attof Y, Rosamel P, *et al.* Respiratory variations in pulse oximetry plethysmographic waveform amplitude to predict fluid responsiveness in the operating room. *Anesthesiology* 2007; 106: 1105–1111.

99. Cannesson M, Besnard C, Durand PG, *et al.* Relation between respiratory variations in pulse oximetry plethysmographic waveform amplitude and arterial pulse pressure in ventilated patients. *Crit Care* 2005; 9: R562–R568.

100. Desebbe O, Cannesson M. Using ventilation-induced plethysmographic variations to optimize patient fluid status. *Curr Opin Anaesthesiol* 2008; 21: 772–778.

101. Zupancich E, Paparella D, Turani F, *et al.* Mechanical ventilation affects inflammatory mediators in patients undergoing cardiopulmonary bypass for cardiac surgery: a randomized clinical trial. *J Thorac Cardiovasc Surg* 2005; 130: 378–383.

102. Sundar S, Novack V, Jervis K, *et al.* Influence of low tidal volume ventilation on time to extubation in cardiac surgical patients. *Anesthesiology* 2011; 114: 1102–1110.

103. Lellouche F, Dionne S, Simard S, *et al.* Traditional and high tidal volumes are associated with prolonged mechanical ventilation and organ failure after cardiac surgery. *Am J Respir Crit Care Med* 2010; 181: A6863.

104. Arnal J, Wysocki M, Demory D, *et al.* Prospective randomized cross-over controlled study comparing adaptive support ventilation (ASV) and a fully close loop control solution (Intellivent™) in adult ICU patients with acute respiratory failure. *Am J Respir Crit Care Med* 2010; 181: A3004.

105. Burns KE, Lellouche F, Lessard MR. Automating the weaning process with advanced closed-loop systems. *Intensive Care Med* 2008; 34: 1757–1765.

106. Hewlett AM, Platt AS, Terry VG. Mandatory minute volume. A new concept in weaning from mechanical ventilation. *Anaesthesia* 1977; 32: 163–169.

107. Hendrix H, Kaiser ME, Yusen RD, *et al.* A randomized trial of automated *versus* conventional protocol-driven weaning from mechanical ventilation following coronary artery bypass surgery. *Eur J Cardiothorac Surg* 2006; 29: 957–963.

108. Rice TW, Wheeler AP, Bernard GR, *et al.* Comparison of the SpO_2/FIO_2 ratio and the PaO_2/FIO_2 ratio in patients with acute lung injury or ARDS. *Chest* 2007; 132: 410–417.

109. Ventilation with lower tidal volumes as compared with traditional tidal volumes for acute lung injury and the acute respiratory distress syndrome. The Acute Respiratory Distress Syndrome Network. *N Engl J Med* 2000; 342: 1301–1308.

110. Gajic O, Frutos-Vivar F, Esteban A, *et al.* Ventilator settings as a risk factor for acute respiratory distress syndrome in mechanically ventilated patients. *Intensive Care Med* 2005; 31: 922–926.

111. iAnthropometer ICU 1 and 2. Applestore 2011. http://itunes.apple.com/ca/app/ianthropometer-icu-1/ id428778012?mt=8.

112. Branson RD, Johannigman JA. What is the evidence base for the newer ventilation modes? *Respir Care* 2004; 49: 742–760.

113. Vitacca M. New things are not always better: proportional assist ventilation *vs* pressure support ventilation. *Intensive Care Med* 2003; 29: 1038–1040.

114. Verbrugghe W, Jorens PG. Neurally adjusted ventilatory assist: a ventilation tool or a ventilation toy? *Respir Care* 2011; 56: 327–335.

Chapter 17

Update on sedation and analgesia in mechanical ventilation

T. Strøm and P. Toft

Summary

Routine use of sedation of critically ill patients is not without adverse effects. Evidence shows that the use of protocols and scoring systems for sedatives and daily interruption of sedatives can reduce the duration of mechanical ventilation. A strategy of no sedation is also possible and reduces both time spent on mechanical ventilation and in the intensive care unit, as well as the total length of hospital stay. Less sedation seems not to increase the risk of post-traumatic stress after intensive care. Also evidence shows that less sedation lowers the risk of complications during the intensive care stay. In addition, some evidence shows that organ failure might be less pronounced with the use of no sedation.

Keywords: Analgesics, artificial respiration, critical illness, hypnotics and sedatives, intensive care, length of stay

Dept of Anaesthesia and Intensive Care Medicine, Odense University Hospital, University of Southern Denmark, Odense, Denmark.

Correspondence: T. Strøm, Dept of Anaesthesia and Intensive Care Medicine, Odense University Hospital, Sdr Boulevard 29, 5000 Odense, Denmark.
Email t.s@dadlnet.dk

Eur Respir Mon 2012; 55: 229–238.
Printed in UK – all rights reserved
Copyright ERS 2012
European Respiratory Monograph
ISSN: 1025-448x
DOI: 10.1183/1025448x.10003011

Sedation of critically ill patients is being routinely used to facilitate mechanical ventilation and reduce stress and oxygen consumption [1, 2]. However, no treatment or medication can be administered without side-effects. The patients pay the price for these side-effects with increased length of mechanical ventilation, increased length of stay in the intensive care unit (ICU) and increased total length of hospital stay. Evidence is also emerging that morbidity and mortality is increased with the routine use of sedative drugs. Paracelsus, sometimes called the father of toxicology, wrote: "All things are poison, and nothing is without poison; only the dose permits something not to be poisonous" [3]. In addition, American guidelines for the use of sedative drugs mention sedation as a last resort: "Sedation of agitated critically ill patients should be started only after providing adequate analgesia and treating reversible physiological causes" [4].

Modern intensive care from a historic perspective

A cornerstone in intensive care was the introduction of mechanical ventilation outside of the operating theatre. In Copenhagen in 1952, B. Ibsen, a Danish anaesthetist, was requested to help during the polio epidemic [4]. Standard care was provision of respiratory support by the "iron lung", a whole body ventilator that employed negative pressure to support ventilation. However, these "lungs" were scarce and were outnumbered by the many patients. IBSEN [5] used blood gas analysis to identify that patients were dying of hypoventilation with hypoxaemia and hypercapnia. Initially a well-known procedure from the operating theatre, tracheostomy was performed on a child and she survived. Standard care shifted from negative pressure ventilation to positive pressure ventilation. Medical students were summoned as extra hands were needed to perform manual ventilation. Mortality dropped from 80% to 20% because of this treatment [5–7]. Modern intensive therapy was invented.

Sedative medication and scoring systems

Traditionally, sedation is achieved with a combination of hypnotic and analgesic drugs. These drugs were administered to make the patient comfortable during mechanical ventilation. First-generation ventilators did not have the support modus of modern ventilators and patients almost needed general anaesthesia in order to receive mechanical ventilation. A cornerstone was the introduction of pumps for continuous infusion of medication, such as sedative drugs with a reasonable half-life; however, the half-life of such drugs was far from the half-life of modern medications [8].

Analgesics

The main component of achieving patient comfort is to relieve stress and pain; therefore, analgesics are the cornerstone of such therapy. There is no documentation to say that one analgesic is better than another. The term analgosedation has emerged and it may seem rational to use a drug with a shorter half-life in order to titrate the drug to the patient's need. However, there are no randomised trials to support this choice of drug. A meta-analysis of remifentanil did not show any reduction in the length of ICU stay compared to traditional analgesics [9]. One problem with several of the studies was that both the intervention and control group were too deeply sedated [10]. Again, this highlights the importance of the strategy, rather than the drug itself. A brief overview of common opiod analgesics used in the ICU is shown in table 1.

Sedatives

The most commonly used sedatives in the ICU are benzodiazepines and propofol [1, 2]. Benzodiazepine use has shifted from the long-acting diazepam to lorazepam and towards midazolam. The main problem with benzodiazepines is the long half-life. This problem is especially pronounced with longer periods of continuous sedation. An alternative method would be intermittent bolus sedation [4]. Propofol is a sedative agent with rapid onset and no active

Table 1. Common drugs used as analgesia in the intensive care unit [4]

Agent	Characteristics	Half-life	Adverse effect
Morphine	Reference drug, recommended as a bolus regimen because of the long half-life and active metabolites	3–7 hours	Histamine release can cause hypotension
Fentanyl	Faster onset than morphine	1.5–6 hours	Accumulates with infusion
Sufentanil	Has a better pharmacokinetic profile than fentanyl during infusion with less accumulation	2.7 hours	Dose-dependent
Alfentanil	Short acting compared to morphine, fentanyl and alfentanil	1.5 hours	Risk of muscle rigidity
Remifentanil	Ultra short-acting drug, can only be administered by infusion	3–10 minutes	Risk of muscle rigidity with rapid infusion and a high risk of withdrawal symptoms because of short half-life

metabolites, which are obvious advantages compared to benzodiazepines. However, the risk of propofol infusion syndrome, a syndrome characterised by a rapidly developing lactate acidosis, has limited the use of propofol for long-term sedation [11–14]. Therefore, propofol is only recommended for short-term sedation (<48 hours) and infusion rates <5 mg·kg^{-1}·min^{-1} [14]. Earlier studies have shown that midazolam was the widest used sedative [1]. However, a more recent study by WUNSCH et al. [15] reported that propofol was the most commonly used sedative. The study by WUNSCH et al. [15] was conducted a little differently than former studies. The authors searched the files of 109,671 patients undergoing mechanical ventilation from 2001–2007 and registered the type of drug patients had received for sedation. The author's results probably represent a more accurate picture of the sedatives used. Previous investigations in this area consisted of studies conducted with questionnaires. A brief overview of sedatives used in the ICU is shown in table 2.

Sedative scoring systems

Objective measures for the level of sedation have proved beneficial in terms of minimising over sedation [16]. The oldest and easiest scale is the sedation scale by RAMSAY et al. [17]. The Ramsay Scale ranges from 1–6, with 1 being the awake and alert patient and 6 being the patient with no response to stimulation. The limitation of this scale is its inability to measure the agitated patients. The Richmond Agitation and Sedation Scale (RASS) is one alternative [18]. This scale ranges from +4 to -5 with the highest value being the agitated patient and the lowest the unresponsive patient. Another reason for using the RASS is that it is coupled to delirium scoring using CAM-ICU (Confusion Assessment Method for the ICU). The choice of scale is probably less important; the most important step is using the scale and adjusting the infusion of sedatives to the prescribed level [19].

The last 10 years

An important step towards decreasing the use of sedation was published in 1998 by KOLLEF et al. [20]. This retrospective study reported that patients receiving continuous sedative infusions needed mechanical ventilation for a longer period of time compared to patients only receiving bolus doses of sedatives. In addition, the length of ICU and hospital stay were increased with the use of continuous sedative infusion. This study was limited by its retrospective design. At baseline, patients in the continuous sedation group had a significantly lower arterial oxygen tension (P_{a,O_2})/ inspiratory oxygen fraction (F_{I,O_2}) ratio compared to patients only receiving bolus doses of sedation. The study was accompanied by a very interesting editorial by T.L. Petty from the University of Columbia (New York, NY, USA) who reflected upon the modern use of sedatives: "….But what I see these days are paralyzed, sedated patients, lying without motion, appearing to be dead, except for the monitors that tell me otherwise" [21]. With these words, T.L. Petty had indirectly encouraged the start of an era of less sedation. The study by KOLLEF et al. [20] should probably be viewed as an appetiser for the next study from this group. In 1999, BROOK et al. [22] published a prospective, randomised study reporting that a nurse-driven sedation protocol

Table 2. Common drugs used for sedation in the intensive care unit

Agent	Characteristics	Onset *i.v* minutes	Half-life hour
Diazepam	Oldest sedative drugs with active metabolites	2–5	20–120
Lorazepam	No active metabolites	5–20	8–15
Midazolam	Active metabolites especially with renal failure	2–5	3–11
Propofol	Risk of propofol infusion syndrome, especially with long-term sedation	1–2	3–12 (in practice shorter because of redistribution)
Dexmedetomidine	Cannot be used for deep sedation	30	2

reduced the duration of mechanical ventilation and the length of ICU and hospital stay compared to standard care in which the nurse needed to contact a doctor before adjusting the sedatives. In the intervention group there was also the possibility to only use bolus doses instead of continuous infusion of sedatives. The main message from the study was that patients benefitted from a bedside continuous adjustment of sedative infusions to meet the patient's needs.

Probably the most cited study in this context is the study by KRESS et al. [16]. The authors made two very simple interventions in this prospective, randomised study. They kept patients from the intervention group sedated at a Ramsay level of 3 to 4 and made a daily interruption of the sedative infusions. The control group was treated according to standard care with continuous sedative infusion without any planned interruptions. The authors reported a significant reduction in the duration of mechanical ventilation by almost 2.5 days and a reduction in ICU length of stay of 3.5 days. The authors were not able to show a reduction in total length of hospital stay. Another finding reported by the authors was a reduction in the use of computed tomography (CT) or magnetic resonance scans of the cerebrum by the use of a daily interruption of sedative infusion. The high impact of this single centre study was probably due to the fact it did not dictate a complete cessation of sedative infusion but offered a simple, yet very effective, tool to control the amount of administered sedative medication. Some of the limitations with this study were its single centre nature, the limited number of patients (150 randomised patients) and the inclusion of only medical patients with an APACHE (Acute Physiology, Age and Chronic Health Evaluation) II score of 20 to 22. KRESS et al. [16] also published a follow-up study investigating the psychological consequences of the daily interruption of sedative infusion. They interviewed a total of 32 patients, 18 patients from the original study and 14 patients enrolled after completion of the original study. The authors reported a reduction in post-traumatic stress disorder (PTSD) in the intervention group compared to the control group. This is an important message that daily interruption of sedation does not increase the risk of psychological long-term sequelae. However, the number of patients interviewed was low, only 21% of the original 150 randomised patients; thus, there is a risk that patients suffering from PTSD were overlooked.

GIRARD et al. [23], from Vanderbilt University (Nashville, TN, USA), published a study in 2008. The study was a prospective, randomised multi-centre study and a total of 336 patients were randomised. The study combined a spontaneous breathing trial with a daily interruption of sedation, two interventions that have previously proven beneficial in patients undergoing mechanical ventilation [16, 24]. All patients received spontaneous breathing but only patients in the intervention group received a daily interruption of sedative infusion. The authors reported an increase in the number of ventilator-free days in a 28-day period and a reduction in both the length of stay in the ICU and the hospital. Surprisingly, the authors were also able to report a reduction in the 1-year mortality which further highlighted the impact of sedative infusion, even after patients were discharged from the ICU. In addition, JACKSON et al. [25] performed a psychological follow-up study. Both studies assessed patients at 3 and 12 months after randomisation. 63 patients out of the 336 were interviewed. The authors were able to report a decrease in PTSD after 3 months but no difference after 12 months. 37 patients from the intervention group and 26 from the control group were interviewed after 12 months. It is interesting that daily interruption of sedation has a psychologically beneficial effect after 3 months but not after 12 months. It is unknown if the higher 1-year mortality in the continuously sedated control group might have had any influence on the change in outcome.

A study claiming no effect of a daily interruption of sedation was performed by DE WIT et al. [26]. In this controlled, prospective study the authors randomised patients to either a daily interruption of sedative infusion or a sedation algorithm. DE WIT et al. [26] reported a statistical significant reduction in mechanical ventilation and length of stay in both the ICU and hospital in the group of patients managed by a sedation algorithm compared to the group receiving a daily interruption of sedation. However, there are several problems inherent to this conclusion. Most important is the limited number of patients. The study was designed to randomise a total of 268 patients; however, the study was stopped after inclusion of only 75 patients, 28% of the planned number of patients. The reason for stopping inclusion was an observation of a higher mortality in the group receiving daily interruption of sedatives compared to the group with a sedation algorithm (13 versus seven patients, p=0.04) during an *a priori* planned interim analysis. Since the data at this early point showed a difference in the end-points the study was terminated. The statistical strategy can be questioned since 48% of the randomised patients were censored. Censoring removes patients at any given time and thus loses statistical power. Questionable reasons for censoring were re-intubation and tracheostomy. The design of the study was also problematic because no level of sedation was set for the group of patients randomised to daily interruption of sedation outside of a daily wake-up trial. This carries a risk of over sedation in this group. Because of these limitations with this study the conclusion of no beneficial effect of a daily interruption of sedation needs careful interpretation.

Less is more

The tendency in sedative strategies for critically ill patients undergoing mechanical ventilation from 1998–2010 has been to safely lower the use of sedation and combine other modalities, such as spontaneous breathing trials, to reduce the duration of mechanical ventilation. But can mechanical ventilation patients be managed without the routine use of sedative infusion? Some patients in the ICU require high settings in the ventilator (especially high F_{I,O_2} and positive end-expiratory pressure), for example, those patients with acute respiratory distress syndrome (ARDS) [27]. However, most patients admitted to the ICU do not suffer from severe ARDS and can be managed without the routine use of sedatives (figs 1 and 2). STRØM *et al.* [28] recently conducted and published a study describing this strategy. A total of 140 patients were randomised in two groups, the intervention group receiving only bolus doses of morphine and the control group receiving continuous sedation to a target on the Ramsay Scale of 3 to 4 with daily interruption of sedation. We reported an increase in ventilator-free days of almost 4.5 days, a reduction in ICU length of stay of 10 days and a reduction in the total length of hospital stay of 24 days (figs 3 and 4). We found no change in the need for CT scans of the cerebrum, the number of ventilator-associated pneumonias or the occurrence of accidental extubations. Several limitations need to be highlighted when interpreting the study. First, 10 (18%) patients from the nonsedated intervention group could not be managed with the protocol of no sedation and were sedated in the same manner as the control group. These were mainly patients with severe respiratory distress. However, it is important to note that 82%, the majority of the patients, could be managed according to the no sedation protocol. Secondly, of note is the staffing. The study was conducted at a facility with a 1:1 nurse:patient ratio, which is not common practice outside of Scandinavia. This high nursing ratio provides other opportunities in patient care such as free visiting hours for the patient's family and next of kin. The nurses handle several tasks besides basic care including: ventilator settings according to local algorithms and orders from the doctors; renal replacement therapy; and, very importantly, mobilisation of the patient to a chair several times a day. However, this study gives a very clear picture of the downside of routinely providing continuous sedative infusion and, even in facilities with lower nurse staffing, reduction in sedatives to selected patients would provide the opportunity to improve outcome for these patients. Thirdly, the high frequency of agitated delirium in the nonsedated intervention group was a problem. Delirium was diagnosed using Diagnostic and Statistical Manual of Mental Disorders (DSM)-IV criteria but only diagnosing agitated delirium [29]. A more sensitive method would have been to use the CAM-ICU scoring system which would also have diagnosed silent forms of delirium [30, 31]. The

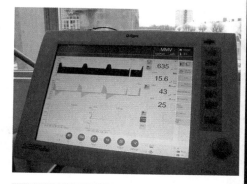

Figure 1. Image of a ventilator with very high settings: peak end-expiratory pressure 26 cmH_2O and inspiratory oxygen fraction 85%.

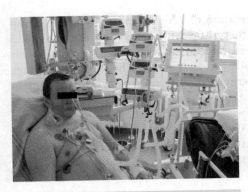

Figure 2. A patient attached to the ventilator shown in figure 1. The patient is orally intubated, awake and mobilised in a chair.

problem with only using DSM-IV criteria is that patients in the sedated control group who had delirium would go undiagnosed. During interruption of sedation, if the patient was agitated, sedative infusion was re-started and the patient was put back to sleep. This probably explains the higher occurrence of delirium in the intervention group which has been noted and has received critique [32]. STRØM *et al.* [33] have also published a follow-up trial, showing no difference in the rate of PTSD with a strategy of no sedation. The psychological follow-up data was necessary because of the fear of an increased rate of psychological sequelae with this no sedation strategy [34, 35].

Using a strategy of no sedation offers a unique opportunity to monitor the cerebral function of the brain. In critically ill patients it is standard care to monitor oxygenation, ventilation, haemodynamics and diuresis. However, no monitoring device exists to monitor the functional status of the brain unless the patient is awake. The underlying disease which resulted in the patient being brought to the ICU can cause ARDS in the lungs, shock in the circulation and acute kidney injury. In addition, the brain can develop acute brain dysfunction which gives an impression of the severity of the underlying disease. Gaining control of the underlying disease is the main treatment of ARDS, shock, acute kidney injury and acute brain dysfunction. When the underlying disease resolves, the affected organs involved in multiple organ failure also resolve and the awakened patient provides an opportunity to monitor this process in the brain.

Under sedation

Much concern has been voiced about not sedating critically ill patients. Alleviating stress and decreasing oxygen consumption has been one of the main reasons for sedating critically ill patients undergoing mechanical ventilation [4, 35, 36]. Are there still ICU patients who need sedation? Can we harm our patients by not giving them sedatives? Obviously, patients admitted to the ICU after cardiac arrest will need sedation while undergoing therapeutic hypothermia [37, 38]. Also, patients with seizures or increased intracranial pressure need sedatives as part of the treatment. Recently, PAPAZIAN *et al.* [39] published a randomised, multi-centre study showing the beneficial effect of neuromuscular blockade in ARDS patients. 340 ARDS patients were randomised to sedation to a Ramsay level of 6. The intervention group also received a 48-hour infusion of a neuromuscular blocking agent (cisatracurium). The authors reported a survival benefit at 28 days and an increase in the number of ventilator-free days with the use of neuromuscular blockade in the intervention group compared to the control group.

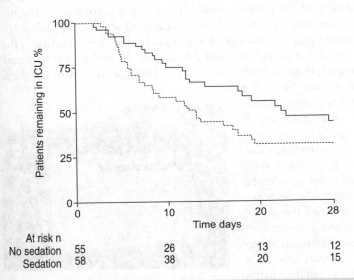

At risk n			
No sedation	55	26	13	12
Sedation	58	38	20	15

Figure 3. Kaplan–Meier plots showing the reduction in the length of stay in the intensive care unit (ICU) with a protocol of no sedation (······). ——: sedation. Reprinted from [28] with permission from the publisher.

However, this benefit was only seen in patients with a $P_{a,O_2}/F_{I,O_2}$ ratio <120. Does this alter the perception that less sedation for the patients undergoing mechanical ventilation is beneficial? Can we harm our patients by not offering them adequate sedation and perhaps neuromuscular blockade? No, as reported in the study by PAPAZIAN et al. [39], only a small fraction of patients admitted to the ICU develops severe ARDS, and only patients with a high oxygen demand profit from neuromuscular blockade. The majority of patients admitted to the ICU will profit from a reduction in the levels of sedatives administered.

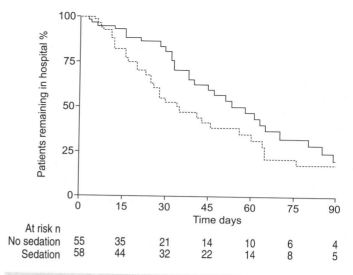

At risk n						
No sedation	55	35	21	14	10	6	4
Sedation	58	44	32	22	14	8	5

Figure 4. Kaplan–Meier plots showing the reduction in the length of stay in hospital with a protocol of no sedation (······). ——: sedation. Reprinted from [28] with permission from the publisher.

Side-effects of sedation

Sedative drugs used in earlier medicine were directly harmful when used for longer periods. LASSEN et al. [40] described the suppression of the bone marrow after prolonged anaesthesia with nitrous oxide. LEDINGHAM and WATT [41] and WATT and LEDINGHAM [42] observed an increased mortality in mechanical ventilation trauma patients sedated with etomidate. It was later described that etomidate resulted in adrenal insufficiency. Drugs commonly used for sedation and analgesia have been shown to have immunmodulatory effects in vitro. However, whether these mechanisms have clinically important in vivo effects has not yet been shown [43, 44]. Only propofol has been shown to have a potentially harmful effect in vivo. Propofol infusion syndrome has been described in patients receiving higher doses (>5 mg·kg^{-1}·hour^{-1}) and for more than 48 hours (refer to the Sedatives section).

Complications because of prolonged exposure to mechanical ventilation have been shown to be clinically important. SCHWEICKERT et al. [45] published a follow-up study reporting the rate of complications in patients from the original study by KRESS et al. [16]. Patient files were searched retrospectively by independent researchers for complications during the patient's ICU stay. When pooling all complications they reported a significantly higher number of complications in the sedated control group compared to the daily awakened intervention group. The study was retrospective and not a priori defined which limits the interpretation of the data. Also, a reduction in ventilator-associated pneumonia had been shown by the introduction of ventilator bundles. These interventions consisted of several factors: daily evaluation of sedation, elevation of the head, deep vein thrombosis prophylaxis and peptic ulcer disease prophylaxis [46, 47].

In the study with a protocol of no sedation it was retrospectively noted that patients from the sedated control group had a lower urine output compared to the awake intervention group [48]. No difference was found with respect to vasopressor use, fluid balance or blood pressure. This retrospective finding could, of course, be by chance but it emphasises the need for further clinical studies on the effects of the routine use of sedative infusions.

Future perspectives

In order to improve the care for critically ill patients we need to improve a lot more than just reducing sedation. Many modalities need to be considered. Traditionally, end-points for sedative studies have been the duration of mechanical ventilation. Many factors affect this parameter. Early and daily mobilisation is a very interesting aspect of care. SCHWEICKERT *et al.* [49] recently published a very interesting study about the beneficial effect of early mobilisation. They performed a randomised controlled study showing that the intervention group receiving early mobilisation had fewer mechanical ventilation dependent days and fewer days with delirium. In addition, more patients from the mobilised intervention group returned to independent functional status after hospital discharge. For critically ill patients to be mobilised and receive active muscle training they need to be either awake or only lightly sedated.

Another aspect is the use of newer drugs with fewer side-effects. A drug that has received much attention is dexmedetomidine; an α_2-adrenergic receptor agonist. Although it is widely used in the USA, it is authorised for use in only a few European countries. Two main advantages of dexmedetomidine are that patients can be sedated and awakened very easily and the rate of delirium seems to be less compared to older drugs. Several studies have shown a reduction in the number of days with delirium [50, 51]. However, a recent meta-analysis did not report any effect on duration of mechanical ventilation, length of hospital stay or duration of delirium [52]. A reduction in length of ICU stay was registered. This conclusion was, however, tempered by the authors because of the great heterogeneity among the pooled studies. Two large studies comparing dexmedetomidine with midazolam (midex/prodex studies) are expected to be published soon showing a reduction in time receiving mechanical ventilation [53]. However, a limitation in the two studies was that sedation could be varied between RASS 0 to -3, which carry a greater risk of over sedation, especially in the midazolam control group. This emphasises that it is not the drug *per se*, but the way each drug is administered that affects outcome [19].

Conclusion

Sedation in the ICU is routinely used for critically ill patients undergoing mechanical ventilation. This is not without adverse effects for the patients. Evidence shows that use of sedatives can cause prolongation in the duration of mechanical ventilation, length of stay in the ICU and total length of hospital stay. In addition, there is evidence of an increased risk of morbidity and mortality. It is possible to use a strategy of no sedation for critically ill patients undergoing mechanical ventilation. This strategy reduces the time patients receive mechanical ventilation, reduces length of stay in the ICU and total length of hospital stay. To date, there is no evidence to support fears that reduced or no sedation increases the risk of post-traumatic stress.

Statement of interest

None declared.

References

1. Mehta S, Burry L, Fischer S, *et al.* Canadian survey of the use of sedatives, analgesics, and neuromuscular blocking agents in critically ill patients. *Crit Care Med* 2006; 34: 374–380.
2. Egerod I, Christensen BV, Johansen L. Trends in sedation practices in Danish intensive care units in 2003: a national survey. *Intensive Care Med* 2006; 32: 60–66.
3. Madea B, Mußhoff F, Berghaus G, eds. Verkehrsmedizin: Fahreignung, Fahrsicherheit, Unfallrekonstruktion. [Traffic medicine: Driving suitability, driving safety, accident reconstruction]. Cologne, Deutscher Ärzte-Verlag, 2007; p. 435.
4. Jacobi J, Fraser GL, Coursin DB, *et al.* Clinical practice guidelines for the sustained use of sedatives and analgesics in the critically ill adult. *Crit Care Med* 2002; 30: 119–141.
5. Ibsen B. The anaesthetist's viewpoint on the treatment of respiratory complications in poliomyelitis during the epidemic in Copenhagen, 1952. *Proc R Soc Med* 1954; 47: 72–74.
6. Ibsen B. Treatment of respiratory complications in poliomyelitis; the anesthetist's viewpoint. *Dan Med Bull* 1954; 1: 9–12.

7. Lassen HC. A preliminary report on the 1952 epidemic of poliomyelitis in Copenhagen with special reference to the treatment of acute respiratory insufficiency. *Lancet* 1953; 1: 37–41.
8. Prien T, Reinhardt C. Die geschichtliche Entwicklung der Intensivmedizin in Deutschland. Zeitgenossische Betrachtungen. Folge 14: Vegetative Blockade und Analgosedierung [History of the development of intensive care medicine in Germany. General considerations. 14. Vegetative blockade and analgesic sedation]. *Anaesthesist* 2000; 49: 130–139.
9. Tan JA, Ho KM. Use of remifentanil as a sedative agent in critically ill adult patients: a meta-analysis. *Anaesthesia* 2009; 64: 1342–1352.
10. Rozendaal FW, Spronk PE, Snellen FF, *et al.* Remifentanil-propofol analgo-sedation shortens duration of ventilation and length of ICU stay compared to a conventional regimen: a centre randomised, cross-over, open-label study in the Netherlands. *Intensive Care Med* 2009; 35: 291–298.
11. Fodale V, La Monaca E. Propofol infusion syndrome: an overview of a perplexing disease. *Drug Saf* 2008; 31: 293–303.
12. Fudickar A, Bein B, Tonner PH. Propofol infusion syndrome in anaesthesia and intensive care medicine. *Curr Opin Anaesthesiol* 2006; 19: 404–410.
13. Kam PC, Cardone D. Propofol infusion syndrome. *Anaesthesia* 2007; 62: 690–701.
14. Vasile B, Rasulo F, Candiani A, *et al.* The pathophysiology of propofol infusion syndrome: a simple name for a complex syndrome. *Intensive Care Med* 2003; 29: 1417–1425.
15. Wunsch H, Kahn JM, Kramer AA, *et al.* Use of intravenous infusion sedation among mechanically ventilated patients in the United States. *Crit Care Med* 2009; 37: 3031–3039.
16. Kress JP, Pohlman AS, O'Connor MF, *et al.* Daily interruption of sedative infusions in critically ill patients undergoing mechanical ventilation. *N Engl J Med* 2000; 342: 1471–1477.
17. Ramsay MA, Savege TM, Simpson BR, *et al.* Controlled sedation with alphaxalone-alphadolone. *Br Med J* 1974; 2: 656–659.
18. Ely EW, Truman B, Shintani A, *et al.* Monitoring sedation status over time in ICU patients: reliability and validity of the Richmond Agitation-Sedation Scale (RASS). *JAMA* 2003; 289: 2983–2991.
19. Skrobik Y, Ahern S, Leblanc M, *et al.* Protocolized intensive care unit management of analgesia, sedation, and delirium improves analgesia and subsyndromal delirium rates. *Anesth Analg* 2010; 111: 451–463.
20. Kollef MH, Levy NT, Ahrens TS, *et al.* The use of continuous *i.v.* sedation is associated with prolongation of mechanical ventilation. *Chest* 1998; 114: 541–548.
21. Petty TL. Suspended life or extending death? *Chest* 1998; 114: 360–361.
22. Brook AD, Ahrens TS, Schaiff R, *et al.* Effect of a nursing-implemented sedation protocol on the duration of mechanical ventilation. *Crit Care Med* 1999; 27: 2609–2615.
23. Girard TD, Kress JP, Fuchs BD, *et al.* Efficacy and safety of a paired sedation and ventilator weaning protocol for mechanically ventilated patients in intensive care (Awakening and Breathing Controlled trial): a randomised controlled trial. *Lancet* 2008; 371: 126–134.
24. Ely EW, Baker AM, Dunagan DP, *et al.* Effect on the duration of mechanical ventilation of identifying patients capable of breathing spontaneously. *N Engl J Med* 1996; 335: 1864–1869.
25. Jackson JC, Girard TD, Gordon SM, *et al.* Long-term cognitive and psychological outcomes in the awakening and breathing controlled trial. *Am J Respir Crit Care Med* 2010; 182: 183–191.
26. de Wit M, Gennings C, Jenvey WI, *et al.* Randomized trial comparing daily interruption of sedation and nursing-implemented sedation algorithm in medical intensive care unit patients. *Crit Care* 2008; 12: R70.
27. Ventilation with lower tidal volumes as compared with traditional tidal volumes for acute lung injury and the acute respiratory distress syndrome. The Acute Respiratory Distress Syndrome Network. *N Engl J Med* 2000; 342: 1301–1308.
28. Strøm T, Martinussen T, Toft P. A protocol of no sedation for critically ill patients receiving mechanical ventilation: a randomised trial. *Lancet* 2010; 375: 475–480.
29. American Psychiatric Association. Task Force on DSM-IV. Diagnostic and Statistical Manual of Mental Disorders. 4th Edn. Washington, American Psychiatric Association, 2000.
30. Ely EW, Inouye SK, Bernard GR, *et al.* Delirium in mechanically ventilated patients: validity and reliability of the confusion assessment method for the intensive care unit (CAM-ICU). *JAMA* 2001; 286: 2703–2710.
31. Ely EW, Margolin R, Francis J, *et al.* Evaluation of delirium in critically ill patients: validation of the Confusion Assessment Method for the Intensive Care Unit (CAM-ICU). *Crit Care Med* 2001; 29: 1370–1379.
32. Spronk PE. Cerebral dysfunction in the intensive care unit: a package deal? *Anesth Analg* 2010; 111: 266–267.
33. Strøm T, Stylsvig M, Toft P. Long-term psychological effects of a no-sedation protocol in critically ill patients. *Crit Care* 2011; 15: R293.
34. Ogundele O, Yende S. Pushing the envelope to reduce sedation in critically ill patients. *Crit Care* 2010; 14: 339.
35. Brochard L. Less sedation in intensive care: the pendulum swings back. *Lancet* 2010; 375: 436–438.
36. Brochard L. Sedation in the intensive-care unit: good and bad? *Lancet* 2008; 371: 95–97.
37. Hypothermia after Cardiac Arrest Study Group. Mild therapeutic hypothermia to improve the neurologic outcome after cardiac arrest. *N Engl J Med* 2002; 346: 549–556.
38. Bernard SA, Gray TW, Buist MD, *et al.* Treatment of comatose survivors of out-of-hospital cardiac arrest with induced hypothermia. *N Engl J Med* 2002; 346: 557–563.

39. Papazian L, Forel JM, Gacouin A, *et al.* Neuromuscular blockers in early acute respiratory distress syndrome. *N Engl J Med* 2010; 363: 1107–1116.
40. Lassen HC, Henriksen E, Neukirch F, *et al.* Treatment of tetanus: severe bone-marrow depression after prolonged nitrous-oxide anaesthesia. *Lancet* 1956; 270: 527–530.
41. Ledingham IM, Watt I. Influence of sedation on mortality in critically ill multiple trauma patients. *Lancet* 1983; 321: 1270.
42. Watt I, Ledingham IM. Mortality amongst multiple trauma patients admitted to an intensive therapy unit. *Anaesthesia* 1984; 39: 973–981.
43. Toft P, Tønnesen E. The systemic inflammatory response to anaesthesia and surgery. *Curr Anaesth Crit Care* 2008; 19: 349–353.
44. Nseir S, Makris D, Mathieu D, *et al.* Intensive care unit-acquired infection as a side effect of sedation. *Crit Care* 2010; 14: R30.
45. Schweickert WD, Gehlbach BK, Pohlman AS, *et al.* Daily interruption of sedative infusions and complications of critical illness in mechanically ventilated patients. *Crit Care Med* 2004; 32: 1272–1276.
46. Blamoun J, Alfakir M, Rella ME, *et al.* Efficacy of an expanded ventilator bundle for the reduction of ventilator-associated pneumonia in the medical intensive care unit. *Am J Infect Control* 2009; 37: 172–175.
47. Papadimos TJ, Hensley SJ, Duggan JM, *et al.* Implementation of the "FASTHUG" concept decreases the incidence of ventilator-associated pneumonia in a surgical intensive care unit. *Patient Saf Surg* 2008; 2: 3.
48. Strøm T, Johansen RR, Prahl JO, *et al.* Sedation and renal impairment in critically ill patients: a *post hoc* analysis of a randomized trial. *Crit Care* 2011; 15: R119.
49. Schweickert WD, Pohlman MC, Pohlman AS, *et al.* Early physical and occupational therapy in mechanically ventilated, critically ill patients: a randomised controlled trial. *Lancet* 2009; 373: 1874–1882.
50. Riker RR, Shehabi Y, Bokesch PM, *et al.* Dexmedetomidine *vs* midazolam for sedation of critically ill patients. *JAMA* 2009; 301: 489–499.
51. Pandharipande PP, Pun BT, Herr DL, *et al.* Effect of sedation with dexmedetomidine *vs* lorazepam on acute brain dysfunction in mechanically ventilated patients. *JAMA* 2007; 298: 2644–2653.
52. Tan J, Ho K. Use of dexmedetomidine as a sedative and analgesic agent in critically ill adult patients: a meta-analysis. *Intensive Care Med* 2010; 36: 926–939.
53. Intensetimes. Issue 12, page 15. April 2011. www.intensetimes.eu/en/archive/Issue-12/

Other titles in the series

ERM 54 – Orphan Lung Diseases
J-F. Cordier

ERM 53 – Nosocomial and Ventilator-Associated Pneumonia
A. Torres and S. Ewig

ERM 52 – Bronchiectasis
R.A. Floto and C.S. Haworth

ERM 51 – Difficult-to-Treat Severe Asthma
K.F. Chung, E.H. Bel and S.E. Wenzel

ERM 50 – Sleep Apnoea
W.T. McNicholas and M.R. Bonsignore

ERM 49 – Exhaled Biomarkers
I. Horvath and J.C. de Jongste

ERM 48 – Interventional Pulmonology
J. Strausz and C.T. Bolliger

ERM 47 – Paediatric Lung Function
U. Frey and P.J.F.M. Merkus

ERM 46 – Interstitial Lung Diseases
R.M. du Bois and L. Richeldi

ERM 45 – Lung Transplantation
A.J. Fisher, G.M. Verleden and G. Massard

ERM 44 – Thoracic Malignancies
S.G. Spiro, R.M. Huber and S.M. Janes

ERM now available on HighWire at: http://erm.ersjournals.com

ORDER INFORMATION

Monographs are priced at £45.00/€53.00/$80.00 each plus postage.
Europe: £7.00/€8.00/$11.00. Non-Europe: £12.00/€13.00/$19.00
For a more detailed postage quote contact
European Respiratory Society publications directly.
**European Respiratory Society Publications Office,
442 Glossop Road, Sheffield, S10 2PX, UK.**
Tel: 44 (0)114 267 2860; Fax: 44 (0)114 2665064; E-mail: info@ersj.org.uk